PAIN MEASUREMENT AND ASSESSMENT

Pain Measurement and Assessment

Editor

Ronald Melzack, Ph.D.
Department of Psychology
McGill University
Montreal, Quebec, Canada

Raven Press ■ New York

Raven Press, 1140 Avenue of the Americas, New York, New York 10036

Library of Congress Cataloging in Publication Data
Main entry under title:

Pain measurement and assessment.

Includes bibliographical references and index.
1. Pain—Psychological aspects.   2. Pain—Measurement.
3. Medical history taking.   4. Questionnaires.
I. Melzack, Ronald.   [DNLM: 1. Pain—Diagnosis.
2. Questionnaires.   WL 704 P1466]
RB127.P33245   1983   616.07′2   82-40296
ISBN 0-89004-893-2

This book is dedicated to
Donald O. Hebb
and
William K. Livingston (1892–1966),
whose concepts of pain inspired many of
the ideas expressed in these pages

Preface

Astonishing advances have been made in recent years in pain research and therapy. In particular, there has been a striking development of techniques for the measurement and assessment of pain. The relevant articles have been published in many different journals, however, and it is increasingly difficult to see all the new approaches in perspective. The time has come, therefore, to bring the important information together so that the new approaches can be evaluated. The purpose of this book is to provide health professionals and students with an overview of the state of the art in the field of pain measurement and assessment.

The contributors to this book are acknowledged experts in the field who have made important contributions to its growth. Their chapters have been organized into six major sections: (i) psychophysical methods of pain measurement, especially in relation to laboratory research; (ii) the use of verbal expression to measure pain in clinical patients; (iii) recent research using verbal measurement methods; (iv) assessment of pain-related behavior; (v) pain assessment in the clinic; and (vi) evaluation of the problems inherent in bridging laboratory and clinical research.

The contributors have written succinct chapters so that the field can be seen as a whole. The emphasis is on an up-to-date review and evaluation of accomplishments rather than on specific details of procedure. The references in each chapter cite the important papers containing these details, where the reader can then pursue any particular technique or field of research in greater detail.

Measurement is an essential ingredient of science, and this century has witnessed the development of increasingly precise measuring tools in the health professions. Pain can be measured and assessed from many points of view, which complement each other and provide a richer, more thorough picture of the patient in pain. The more knowledge we have, the likelier we are to understand the multiple contributing factors in acute and chronic pain and to evaluate the effectiveness of different therapeutic procedures. The beneficiary of this activity will, we hope, be the suffering human being.

Because the field of pain cuts across the traditional boundaries in medicine and other health professions, it is important that all of us who direct our energies to the relief of pain and suffering be able to communicate with each other. An understanding of our basic tools of measurement and assessment is essential for this communication. An attempt has therefore been made to keep jargon at a minimum so that we can communicate more easily and comprehensibly. This is important for those of us already working in this exciting field, and still more important for students who, in the future, will reveal the mechanisms of pain and discover new, more effective forms of therapy. This book, in fact, in addition to providing an up-to-date review of the state of the art, also raises important questions that may serve as a guide for future work in the field.

Ronald Melzack

Acknowledgments

As editor, it is an honor and a pleasure to thank the contributors—all outstanding investigators in the field of pain measurement and assessment—for their excellent, informative chapters. It is also a pleasure to thank Lucy Melzack for her encouragement and suggestions, without which the book would not have been undertaken, and Carol Stokes-Rogolino for her outstanding secretarial assistance.

Contents

I. Psychophysical Methods of Pain Assessment

1. Concepts of Pain Measurement   1
   Ronald Melzack

2. Laboratory Methods of Pain Measurement   7
   B. Berthold Wolff

3. Applications of Sensory Decision Theory to Problems in
   Laboratory and Clinical Pain   15
   W. Crawford Clark and Joseph C. Yang

4. The Tourniquet Pain Test   27
   Richard A. Sternbach

5. Visual Analogue Scales   33
   E. C. Huskisson

II. Verbal Measurement of Pain

6. The McGill Pain Questionnaire   41
   Ronald Melzack

7. The Structure of Pain Descriptors   49
   Warren S. Torgerson and Mohammed BenDebba

8. The McGill Pain Questionnaire: An Appraisal   55
   Anthony E. Reading

9. Factor-Analytic Studies of the McGill Pain Questionnaire   63
   Edward J. Prieto and Kurt F. Geisinger

10. Pain Language and Ideal Pain Assessment   71
    Richard H. Gracely

11. Detecting Psychological Disturbance Using Verbal Pain
    Measurement: The Back Pain Classification Scale   79
    Frank Leavitt

12. Verbal Measurement in Non-English Language: The Finnish Pain
    Questionnaire   85
    P. J. Pöntinen and Heikki Ketovuori

III. Recent Research Using Verbal Measurement Methods

13. Chronic Headache Experience 97
    Clare Philips

14. Laboratory-Induced and Acute Iatrogenic Pain 105
    Robert K. Klepac and Elizabeth Lander

15. Postoperative Pain: Relationships Among Measures of Pain,
    Mood, and Narcotic Requirements 111
    Paul Taenzer

16. Pain Language as a Measure of Affect in Chronic Pain Patients 119
    Edwin F. Kremer and J. Hampton Atkinson, Jr.

17. Relationships between the MMPI and the McGill
    Pain Questionnaire 129
    Laurence A. Bradley

18. Pain Description and Personality Disturbance 137
    Charles McCreary

IV. Assessment of Pain Behavior

19. The Validity of Pain Behavior Measurement 145
    Wilbert E. Fordyce

20. Assessment of Chronic Headache Behavior 155
    Clare Philips

21. Assessment of Pain Behavior: Factors That Distort Self-Report 165
    Edwin F. Kremer, Andrew Block, and J. Hampton Atkinson, Jr.

22. Nonverbal Measures of Pain 173
    Kenneth D. Craig and Kenneth M. Prkachin

V. Pain Assessment in the Clinic

23. The Measurement of Pain in Children 183
    Mary Ellen Jeans

24. Pain Assessment in Rehabilitation Medicine 191
    Etta Rybstein-Blinchik

25. Pain Classification and Vocational Evaluation in
    Chronic Pain States 197
    William Hammonds and Steven F. Brena

26. The Temporal Aspects of Pain: The Pain Chart 205
    Kenneth D. Keele

27. The Pain Chart: Spatial Properties of Pain 215
    Michael S. Margoles

28. Assessment of Body Image in Chronic Pain Patients:
    The Body Parts Problem Assessment Scale 227
    Jon Kabat-Zinn

29. A Comprehensive Pain Questionnaire 233
    Richard Monks and Paul Taenzer

VI. Bridging Laboratory and Clinical Research

30. Interacting Approaches in Pain Research 241
    Ronald Melzack

31. On the Relationship of Human Laboratory and Clinical
    Pain Research 243
    C. Richard Chapman

32. Measurement of Experimental Pain in Chronic Pain Patients:
    Methodological and Individual Factors 251
    Gary B. Rollman

33. Ethical Considerations in Pain Research in Man 259
    Richard A. Sternbach

Appendix 267

    A. McGill Pain Questionnaire 1A

    B. McGill Pain Questionnaire
    Interviewer Guide 10A

Subject Index 283

Contributors

J. Hampton Atkinson, Jr., M.D.
Department of Psychiatry
University of California at San Diego
  Medical School
La Jolla, California 92093
  714-294-5592

Mohammed BenDebba, Ph.D.
Department of Neurosurgery
John Hopkins University
  School of Medicine
601 N. Broadway
Baltimore, Maryland 21205
  301-955-3565/338-7055

Etta Rybstein-Blinchik, Ph.D.
Psychology Service
Department of Rehabilitation Medicine
NYU Medical Center
Goldwater Memorial Hospital
Roosevelt Island, New York 10017
  212-750-6842 or 516-923-1321

Andrew Block, Ph.D.
Department of Psychology
Indiana University–Purdue University
  at Indianapolis
Indianapolis, Indiana 46205
  317-923-1321

Laurence A. Bradley, Ph.D.
Head, Section of Medical Psychology
Bowman Gray School of Medicine of
Wake Forest University
300 South Hawthorne Rd.
Winston-Salem, North Carolina 27103
  919-748-4238

Steven F. Brena, M.D.
Professor and Director
Emory University Pain Control Center
1441 Clifton Road, N.E.
Atlanta, Georgia 30322
  404-329-5492

C. Richard Chapman, Ph.D.
Department of Anesthesiology
University of Washington
  School of Medicine
Seattle, Washington 98195
  206-543-2672

W. Crawford Clark, Ph.D.
Associate Clinical Professor of Psychiatry
College of Physicians and Surgeons of
  Columbia University
New York State Psychiatric Institute
722 West 168th Street
New York, New York 10032
  212-960-2480

Kenneth D. Craig, Ph.D.
Department of Psychology
University of British Columbia
Vancouver, British Columbia
  Canada V6T 1Y5
  604-228-3948

Wilbert E. Fordyce, Ph.D.
Department of Rehabilitative Medicine
University of Washington
  School of Medicine
Seattle, Washington 98195
  206-543-8660

Kurt Geisinger, Ph.D.
Department of Psychology
Fordham University
Bronx, New York 10458
  212-579-2187

Richard H. Gracely, Ph.D.
Research Psychologist
Clinical Pain Section
Neurobiology and Anesthesiology Branch
National Institute of Dental Research
National Institutes of Health
Bethesda, Maryland 20012
  301-496-5237

William Hammonds, M.D.
Department of Anesthesiology
Emory University Clinic
1364 Clifton Road, N.E.
Atlanta, Georgia 30322
404-329-4603

E. C. Huskisson, M.D., F.R.C.P.
Rheumatology Department
St. Bartholomew's Hospital
West Smithfield
London EC1A 7BE, England
01-600-9000 ext. 3304

Mary Ellen Jeans,
B.N., M.Sc.(A), Ph.D.
Director, School of Nursing
McGill University
3506 University St.
Montreal, PQ, Canada H3A 2A7
514-392-5033

Jon Kabat-Zinn, Ph.D.
Director, Stress Reduction and
  Relaxation Program
Department of Medicine
University of Massachusetts
  Medical School
Worcester, Massachusetts 01605
617-856-2656

Kenneth D. Keele, M.D., F.R.C.P.
Leacroft House
Leacroft
Staines, Middlesex TW18 4NN
England
  Staines 52575

Heikki Ketovuori, M.A.
Kipunanpisto 3
71800 Siilinjarvi
Finland

Robert K. Klepac, Ph.D.
Department of Psychology
Florida State University
Tallahassee, Florida 32306

Edwin F. Kremer, Ph.D.
Department of Psychiatry
University of California of San Diego
Medical School
La Jolla, California 92093
714-294-5592

Elizabeth Lander, Ph.D.
Department of Psychology
Florida State University
Tallahassee, Florida 32306

Frank Leavitt, Ph.D.
Rush Medical College
Department of Psychology and
  Social Sciences
1750 West Harrison Street
Chicago, Illinois 60612
312-942-5932

Michael S. Margoles,
B.A. Biochem., M.D.,
F.A.A.N.a.O.S.
Orthopaedic Pain Center of San Jose
Cambrian Park Plaza
14438 Union Ave
San Jose, California 95124
408-371-2137

Charles McCreary, Ph.D.
University of California, Los Angeles
School of Medicine
Department of Psychiatry
760 Westwood Plaza
Los Angeles, California 90024
213-825-0054

Ronald Melzack, Ph.D.
Department of Psychology
1205 Docteur Penfield Avenue
Montreal, PQ, Canada H3A 1B1
514-392-4599

Richard C. Monks, M.D., C.M.,
Dip. Psych., F.R.C.P.(C)
Department of Psychiatry
Montreal General Hospital
1650 Cedar Avenue
Montreal, PQ, Canada H3G 1A4
514-937-6011 ext. 1231

Clare Philips, Ph.D.
Division of Psychology
Department of Psychiatry
Shaughnessy Hospital
4500 Oak Street
Vancouver, British Columbia
* Canada V6H 3N1*
* 604-875-2219 or 875-2222 ext. 8195*

J. Pöntinen, M.D.
Pain Clinic
Palomaentie 34
SF-33230 Tampere 23
Finland
* 358-31-26688*

Edward J. Prieto, M.A.
Bronx Psychiatric Center;
The New York Hospital
Cornell Medical Center; and
Fordham University
* Bronx, New York 10548*
* 914-949-4113*

Kenneth M. Prkachin, Ph.D.
Department of Health Studies
University of Waterloo
Waterloo, Ontario, Canada N2L 3G1
* 519-885-1211 ext. 2839*

Anthony E. Reading, Ph.D.
Visiting Professor
Department of Psychiatry
UCLA School of Medicine
Center for the Health Sciences
760 Westwood Plaza
Los Angeles, California 90024
* 213-825-0565*

Gary B. Rollman, Ph.D.
Psychological Laboratory
University of St. Andrews
St. Andrews, Fife, Scotland KY16 9JU
* St. Andrews 76161*

Richard A. Sternbach, Ph.D.
Head, Section of Psychology and
Director, Pain Treatment Center
Scripps Clinic and Research Foundation
10666 North Torrey Pines Road
La Jolla, California 92037
* 714-455-9100*

Paul Taenzer, Ph.D.
Pain Management Program
Tulsa Rehabilitation Center
Hillcrest Medical Center
Utica on the Park
Tulsa, Oklahoma 74104
* 918-584-1351*

Warren S. Torgerson, Ph.D.
Department of Psychology
The Johns Hopkins University
34th and Charles Streets
Baltimore, Maryland 21218
* 301-338-7080*

B. Berthold Wolff, Ph.D.
Pain Study Group
NYU Medical Center
550 First Avenue
New York, New York 10016
* 212-340-6620*

Joseph C. Yang, M.D.
Department of Anesthesiology
College of Physicians and Surgeons of
Columbia University
722 West 168th Street
New York, New York 10032
* 212-960-2480*

I. PSYCHOPHYSICAL METHODS OF PAIN ASSESSMENT

Pain Measurement and Assessment,
edited by Ronald Melzack,
Raven Press, New York © 1983.

Concepts of Pain Measurement

Ronald Melzack

Department of Psychology, McGill University, Montreal, Quebec, Canada H3A 1B1

The measurement of pain in man is essential for the study of pain mechanisms and for the evaluation of methods to control pain. Historically, there have been two kinds of approach: the use of laboratory techniques to produce and measure pain in people who are normally not in pain (such as healthy university students), and the use of tools to measure or otherwise assess pain in patients who are suffering acute or chronic pain. Both types of methods are essential for the development of pain research and therapy.

Laboratory techniques are often crucial to carry out the precise manipulation of variables in controlled studies—procedures that may not be possible in patients in pain. But it is important to keep in mind that ethical considerations limit the intensity and duration of the pain that can be employed for experimental study. Laboratory pains are usually brief and are stopped when they reach unbearable intensity. Clinical pains, in contrast, are often persistent, unbearable, beyond the patient's control, and accompanied by high levels of anxiety. It is not surprising, therefore, that there are marked differences in drug and placebo effects on clinical and laboratory-produced pains (1).

Clearly, then, it is desirable to study pain in patients who are suffering it for a variety of reasons—acute injury, arthritis, surgical incision, cancer, and so forth. However, there are obvious limitations to the kinds of experiments that are ethically or scientifically feasible in a clinical setting. Such studies often preclude the systematic variation of many psychological, physiological, and pharmacological variables. Healthy students, for example, may be willing subjects for a study of psychological stress on laboratory-produced pain, but it is unlikely that a hospital ethics committee would permit such a study using patients suffering clinical pain. Yet the genuine scientific question regarding the effects of stress on pain remains: Does stress enhance or diminish pain? Research with animals predicts that either effect may occur (12).

THE INTENSITY DIMENSION OF PAIN

Until recently, scientific measuring procedures have treated pain as though it were a specific sensory quality varying only in intensity. Whether pain is measured by a psychophysical "dol" scale (5), words such as "mild," "moderate," and "severe"

1

(6), or numbers or fractions representing pain severity or relief (1), only intensity is specified. It is now evident (10) that the word "pain" refers to an endless variety of qualities that are categorized under a single linguistic label, not to a specific, single sensation that varies only in intensity. Each pain has unique qualities. The pain of a toothache is obviously different from that of a pinprick, just as the pain of a coronary occlusion differs uniquely from that of a broken leg. Describing pain solely in terms of intensity is like specifying the visual world only in terms of light flux without regard to pattern, color, texture, and the many other dimensions of visual experience.

Nevertheless, intensity is, without a doubt, the salient dimension of pain, and a variety of procedures has been developed to measure it. In the laboratory, techniques have been developed to express pain intensity in terms of quantities of stimulus energy, based on the assumption that the intensity of pain experience is proportional to the severity of damage. In the traditional specificity theory of pain, pain is a specific sensation that is determined by a straight-through system from pain receptors in tissue to a pain center in the brain (Fig. 1). Such a concept provides the theoretical foundation for particular approaches to pain research and measurement. This concept of pain as a sensory experience like seeing or hearing led to the search for an invariant pain threshold (the lowest level of potentially injurious energy producing the report of pain) and tolerance level (the lowest level of pain producing the report of pain so intense that the person can no longer tolerate any more of it in either duration or intensity).

Traditional psychophysics, which began with Fechner and Wundt (see Boring, ref. 2), was followed by more complex models of information processing in the nervous system. Input was no longer thought to reach a quiescent brain passively waiting to receive the input, but rather to arrive at an active "noisy" brain in which signals had to be detected in a background of other inputs and ongoing thought (4). The development of the signal detection theory (SDT) represents an important step toward recognizing the complexity of neural processes in pajin. Whether signal detection theory is the right approach for the study of pain remains controversial (see Rollman, ref. 14). However, Clark (3), a leading exponent of this approach, makes a strong case for its use.

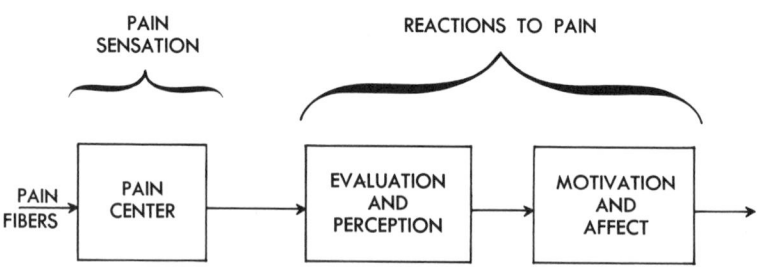

FIG. 1. Conceptual model of pain sensation and reactions to pain.

THE MOTIVATIONAL–AFFECTIVE DIMENSION OF PAIN

The rapid development of sensory physiology and psychophysics since the beginning of this century has given momentum to the concept of pain as a sensation and has long overshadowed the role of affective and motivational processes. The sensory approach to pain, however, valuable as it has been, fails to provide a complete picture of pain processes. Even the concept of pain as a perception, with full recognition of past experience, attention, and other cognitive determinants of sensory quality and intensity (7,8), still neglects the crucial motivational dimension. Pain has a unique, distinctly unpleasant, affective quality that differentiates it from sensory experiences such as sight, hearing, and touch. It becomes overwhelming, demands immediate attention, and disrupts ongoing behavior and thought. It motivates or drives the organism into activity aimed at stopping the pain as quickly as possible. To consider only the sensory features of pain and ignore its motivational and affective properties is to look at only part of the problem, and not even the most important part at that (9).

The assumption that pain is a primary sensation has relegated motivational and cognitive processes to the role of "reactions to pain" (see Fig. 1), making them only secondary considerations in the whole pain process (5,15). But the notion that motivational and cognitive processes occur only after the primary pain sensation fails to account for even relatively simple data. For example, Beecher's observation that most American soldiers wounded at the Anzio beachhead "entirely denied pain from their extensive wounds or had so little that they did not want any medication to relieve it (1)" is interpreted by specificity theorists (1,15) to mean that their joy at having escaped alive from the battlefield blocked only their reaction to pain, but not the pain sensation itself. If this is the case, then pain sensation is not painful, even after extensive bodily damage. Rather than face the paradox of nonpainful pain (13), it seems more reasonable to say simply that these men felt no pain after their extensive injuries, that the input was blocked or modulated by cognitive activities before it could evoke the motivational–affective processes that are an integral part of the total pain experience. The gate control theory of pain proposed by Melzack and Wall (11) provides the basis for precisely this kind of modulation.

Melzack and Casey (9) specifically examined the role of motivation in pain processes and proposed a model, shown in Fig. 2, to account for the multidimensional properties of pain experience and behavior. They propose that: (a) the sensory–discriminative dimension of pain is determined primarily by activity in the rapidly conducting spinal systems; (b) the powerful motivational drive and unpleasant affective characteristic of pain are subserved by activities in reticular and limbic structures that are influenced predominantly by the slowly conducting spinal systems; and (c) neocortical or higher central nervous system processes, such as evaluation of the input in terms of past experience, exert control over activity in both the discriminative and motivational systems. They assume that these three categories of activity interact with one another to provide perceptual information regarding the location, magnitude, and spatiotemporal properties of the noxious stimulus,

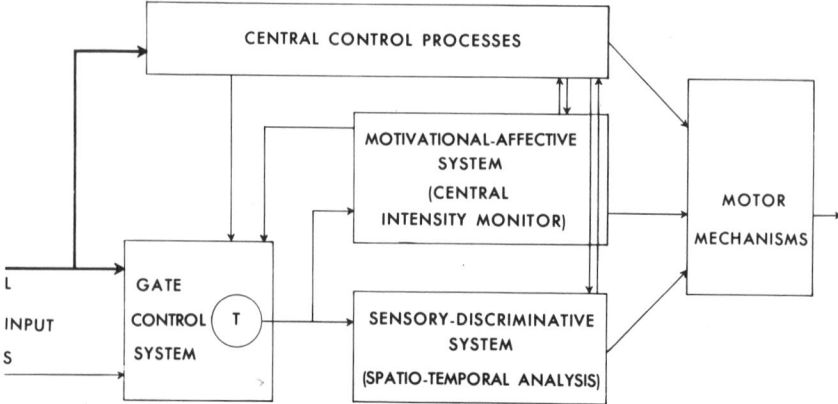

FIG. 2. Conceptual model of the sensory, motivational, and central control determinants of pain. The output of the transmission (T) cells of the gate control system projects to the sensory–discriminative and the motivational–affective systems. The central control trigger is represented by a line running from the large (L) fiber system to central control processes; these, in turn, project back to the gate control system and to the sensory–discriminative and motivational–affective systems. All three systems interact with one another, and project to the motor system. (From Melzack and Casey, ref. 9.)

motivational tendency toward escape or attack, and cognitive information based on analysis of multimodal information, past experience, and probability of outcome of different response strategies. All three forms of activity may then influence motor mechanisms responsible for the complex pattern of the overt responses that characterize pain.

THE LANGUAGE OF PAIN

Melzack and Casey's model provided a conceptual framework for the study of the language of pain (9). Verbal descriptions have always played a crucial role in diagnosis and therapy related to pain. Melzack and Torgerson (10) carried out a systematic study of these descriptors that formed the basis of the McGill Pain Questionnaire (MPQ). The status of this method of pain measurement will be discussed in a later chapter. Here it need only be noted that although the MPQ permits measurement of the sensory, affective, and evaluative dimensions of pain, it also provides information on the relative intensity of each, as well as several measures of the patient's evaluation of the overall intensity of the pain.

This first section of the book deals primarily with the intensity dimension of pain. The emphasis is on laboratory-produced pain and laboratory studies, but the approaches clearly deal with the full range of problems that confronts the researcher and clinician concerned with pain. Huskisson's chapter on the visual analogue scale is based largely on clinical considerations and observations, but is presented in this section because it is predominantly a measure of overall intensity.

REFERENCES

1. Beecher, H. K. (1959): *Measurement of Subjective Responses*. Oxford University Press, New York.
2. Boring, E. G. (1942): *Sensation and Perception in the History of Experimental Psychology*. Appleton-Century-Crofts, New York.
3. Clark, W. C. (1978): Measurement of pain in humans: Signal detection theory and pain. *Neurosci. Res. Prog. Bull.*, 16:14–27.
4. Green, D. M., and Swets, J. A. (1966): *Signal Detection Theory and Psychophysics*. John Wiley, New York.
5. Hardy, J. D., Wolff, H. G., and Goodell, H. (1952): *Pain Sensations and Reactions*. Williams & Wilkins, Baltimore.
6. Keele, K. D. (1948): The pain chart. *Lancet*, 2:6–8.
7. Livingston, W. K. (1953): What is Pain? *Sci. Am.*, 196:59–66.
8. Melzack, R. (1961): The perception of pain. *Sci. Am.*, 204:41–49.
9. Melzack, R., and Casey, K. L. (1968): Sensory, motivational, and central control determinants of pain: A new conceptual model. In: *The Skin Senses*, edited by D. Kenshalo, pp. 423–439. Charles C Thomas, Springfield.
10. Melzack, R., and Torgerson, W. S. (1971): On the language of pain. *Anesthesiology*, 34:50–59.
11. Melzack, R., and Wall, P. D. (1965): Pain mechanisms: A new theory. *Science*, 150:971–979.
12. Melzack, R., and Wall, P. D. (1982): *The Challenge of Pain*. Basic Books, New York.
13. Nafe, J. P. (1934): The pressure, pain, and temperature senses. In: *Handbook of General Experimental Psychology*, edited by C. A. Murchison, pp. 1037–1087. Clark University Press, Worcester.
14. Rollman, G. B. (1977): Signal detection theory measurement of pain: A review and critique. *Pain*, 3:187–211.
15. Sweet, W. H. (1959): Pain. In: *Handbook of Physiology. Section I: Neurophysiology*, edited by J. Field, pp. 459–506. American Physiological Society, Washington, D.C.

Pain Measurement and Assessment,
edited by Ronald Melzack,
Raven Press, New York © 1983.

Laboratory Methods of Pain Measurement

B. Berthold Wolff

Pain Study Group, New York University Medical Center, New York, New York 10016

The application of laboratory methods to the study of human pain began a century ago with the psychophysical studies of von Frey (13) in which he used tactile and pressure stimulation to evoke pain. However, Hardy et al. (4,5) are usually credited with laying the foundations for the systematic investigation and measurement of human pain in the laboratory. These investigators (5) listed the following eight requirements for the laboratory measurement of the threshold sensation of pain: (a) the measurable aspect of the stimulus should be closely associated with changes causing pain, that is, with noxious stimulation; (b) the stimulus should be one for which, under the same conditions, reproducible quantitative measurements of the pain threshold are obtained; (c) the intensity of the stimulus should be controllable and measurable to a degree higher than the difference between two stimuli that evoke a just noticeable difference in pain sensation; (d) the stimulus should be one for which the ability of the subject to discriminate differences in pain intensity can be ascertained throughout the effective range of the stimulus, that is, from threshold to "ceiling" pain; (e) the stimulus should cause minimal tissue damage at pain threshold and should be a minor hazard to the subject even at highest intensities; (f) the stimulus should be capable of evoking separately one of the qualities of pain—burning, pricking, aching; (g) the stimulus should be one that can be conveniently applied; (h) the stimulus should be one for which the perception and identification of pain are clear-cut, whether or not other sensations are evoked before, during, or after the pain.

These requirements, published 30 years ago, are generally still relevant to modern investigations, except for (e) and (f). It is no longer accepted that tissue damage or injury is a *sine qua non* for pain. In fact, ethical guidelines now prohibit any but the most minimal tissue damage. Furthermore, although at least two major types of pain exist (7), there may be many more, and we prefer a larger number of pain descriptors than three.

Pain is a response and consists in humans, at least, of two major groups of components, often labeled sensory and psychological. The former refers to anatomical, physiological, and chemical factors, whereas the latter designates psychosocial and affective variables—the "suffering." In the laboratory, pain measurement usually involves more of the sensory components, whereas in clinical practice pain assessment generally involves a significant proportion of the affective components.

Modern laboratory methods tend to compensate for the emphasis on sensory variables by the use of several pain response parameters, ranging from pain threshold to pain tolerance. As the experimentally induced pain increases from threshold—the point at which pain is first experienced—to tolerance—the point at which the subject withdraws and refuses to accept more pain—the "suffering" components also tend to increase. Therefore, laboratory-induced pain has some advantage over clinical pain in permitting comparison of minimal with maximal pain within the same experimental session—a manipulation that is not that easy in the clinical situation. However, to reiterate, pain is a very complex response modulated by a multitude of factors; its division into sensory and psychological components is simplistic, but originally of practical value to the investigator (18). The complexity of the response is underscored by the neurochemical substratum of pain and the presence of endogenous opioid peptides in analgesia. The interaction and integration of these various factors make the separation of sensory and psychological components somewhat of a scientific anachronism. Nevertheless, in some behavioral pain-relieving therapies, the distinction between sensory and the affective or "suffering" components is of major significance in the treatment.

It should be noted that the eight requirements for laboratory pain measurement listed by Hardy et al. (5) refer continuously to the stimulus but rarely to the response. This reflects the "indirect" approach to pain measurement as used in classic psychophysics. The stimulus is controlled and varied systematically, and the resultant response is measured in terms of such stimulus changes. Several classic psychophysical techniques for such measurement exist and they have previously been described (16). The great advantage of this indirect psychophysical approach is that a stimulus is chosen that is known, easily controllable and changeable, and easily measured. Therefore, in the laboratory such pain induction methods are preferred. In contrast, clinical pain usually lacks a definitely known and manipulable stimulus, and thus direct measurement techniques are preferred.

An important issue for laboratory pain induction methods is whether or not the resultant experimental pain bears any relationship to clinical pain. There are three common approaches to deal with this issue: correlational studies with clinical pain; mimicry techniques; and manipulation of psychosocial variables, especially those related to anxiety, under controlled experimental conditions during laboratory noxious stimulation. These three procedures are not exclusive, and it is even possible to use all three in the same study.

In the first approach, laboratory-induced pain is compared with clinical pain. Perhaps the simplest technique consists of matching the intensity of an existing clinical pain with that of an experimentally induced pain, such as comparing clinical pain in one knee with pressure-induced pain in the other (8). Thus, changes in the clinical pain over time can be measured by proportional changes in the experimentally induced pain. However, although this matching procedure can be of value for clinical pain localized in one area in which the healthy contralateral side is used for comparison, it tends to present problems for many clinical states with diffuse or multiple pains. A more sophisticated and valid but also much more complex method is to record various pain-response parameters induced by laboratory stimuli in a group of patients and then measure intensity or intensity change of clinical pain in the same group of patients and subject the data to some kind of correlational analysis.

Some time ago we conducted a study of patients with chronic arthritis who were undergoing corrective or reconstructive joint surgery (14). Each patient was given a battery of physical and psychological tests before surgery, which included five different laboratory pain induction methods, three cutaneous (electrical, cold pressor, and radiant heat) and two deep somatic (electrical and hypertonic saline). Pain thresholds, pain tolerance levels, and pain sensitivity ranges (PSRs) were measured. Pre- and postoperative self-ratings of the clinical pain were made by the patients, and, in addition, three experienced physicians rated the patients' clinical pain behavior. The patients were required to exercise the operated joint within 24 hr postoperatively in order to maximize range of motion, and such physical therapy tended to be very painful initially. Postoperative success or failure was largely dependent on the patient's active participation. Potent analgesic drugs were contraindicated as they interfered with the patient's physical exercise program. Each patient was evaluated 6 months postoperatively, and the outcome, largely dependent on the patient's ability to tolerate clinical pain, was used as the criterion with which the laboratory-induced pain parameters were compared. The many clinical and laboratory measures were correlated with each other and the resultant correlation matrix subjected to factor analysis. A pain-specific factor that was significantly correlated with the clinical criterion was isolated, and was subsequently labeled "pain endurance" (14). More recently, Timmermans and Sternbach (12), using patients with low back pain, also isolated a pain-specific factor, resembling the pain endurance factor previously isolated. It would appear that this pain-specific factor is relatively stable for a given individual and might even be considered to be a personality trait.

The techniques just described can be termed "direct" correlational methods, because the laboratory-induced pain is directly correlated with clinical pain. A different procedure utilizing an indirect approach, which can also be classified as correlational, consists of comparing laboratory-induced pain with an independent standard, such as an analgesic drug; the latter in turn is compared with its effect on clinical pain. Specifically, the effect of an analgesic agent, such as codeine, can be measured in the laboratory with healthy volunteers. If the produced changes resemble those known to be produced by that drug on clinical pain, then it can be used as a control. This is important for human analgesic assays with laboratory-induced pain because a new drug can be compared with a standard drug and placebo. There are many advantages to using healthy volunteers instead of patients with clinical pain for such assays with laboratory-induced pain. The noxious stimulus is known and can be manipulated at will, which is not generally the case with clinical pain. Furthermore, cross-over studies with statistical power much greater than that with single-dose studies are easier to do in the laboratory than in the clinic, as base-line (no pain) measures can be obtained in each session (19). The U.S.

Federal Drug Agency has left the door open for such laboratory investigational studies of new drugs.

Mimicry techniques refer to methods in which an attempt is made to let the induced pain resemble or mimic clinical pain in quality. Ischemic methods, such as the cold pressor test (6,15) in which a hand is immersed in ice water and the tourniquet method (10) in which pain is induced after occluding the blood flow to an arm with an inflated blood pressure cuff, are probably the best known. The tooth pulp stimulation method (3) is another in which the induced pain, usually by electrical stimulation of the tooth pulp, is said to be very similar to clinical pain. Some investigators believe that this mimicry establishes a link between clinical and laboratory-induced pain. It should be noted that in our experience most individuals, be they patients or healthy volunteers, find it much easier to use pain descriptors for laboratory-induced pain that mimics clinical pain than for induced pain that is not similar to frequently experienced clinical pain. Electrical stimulation, at least in our hands, is most often described as "discomfort" rather than "pain," as it has a unique quality rarely encountered in clinical pain states.

The third approach employs manipulation of psychosocial variables, most frequently associated with anxiety, during noxious stimulation (9). In an experimental study in our laboratory, a healthy volunteer was placed in a sound-attenuated and electrically shielded isolation chamber for 4 hr. The subject was hooked up to and prepared to receive several types of noxious or aversive stimuli, including electricity, cold pressor, radiant heat, white noise, and brightness. Previously, the subject's pain-response parameters had been determined in a standard fashion. During the experimental sessions in the isolation chamber, the subject never received noxious stimuli greater than two-thirds of the previously established pain sensitivity range. In one session, termed the pain-response session, the subject's pain response parameters to either electrical or radiant heat stimulation were measured at irregular intervals while other types of noxious or aversive stimuli were presented (a) immediately after a signal, a tone, (b) after a 15-sec latency following the tone, and (c) after a 30-sec latency following the tone. The subject did not know which of five possible aversive or noxious stimuli or which of three possible intensity levels would be presented with or following the tone. As was predicted, an aversive or noxious stimulus immediately following the signal had only minor distracting effects on pain measurements with the dependent technique. In contrast, latencies of both 15 and 30 sec after which the independent stimulus was presented had highly significant ($p < 0.001$) distorting effects on both the dependent pain threshold and pain tolerance levels, decreasing both (17). The longer latency evoked greater distortion than the 15-sec latency. We interpret these results to indicate that anxiety is rapidly generated on presentation of the tone without immediate association with the independent stimulus by production of uncertainty, yielding significant sensory distortion. In other words, the dependent noxious stimuli were perceived as more painful during anxiety than under standard conditions. Anxiety plays a major role in a patient's suffering while in clinical pain. Therefore, a link between clinical and experimental pain can be claimed with this approach. Incidentally, our investigation also demonstrated the difference between aversion and pain—the aversion threshold was always greater than the pain threshold.

Four pain response parameters can usually be measured with laboratory-induced pain utilizing classic psychophysical methodology. Pain threshold is that point at which pain is first felt on ascending stimulus trials or at which pain just disappears on descending trials. With numerous trials, it is that point at which pain is felt 50% of the time. The pain threshold is a fairly stable parameter in healthy and cooperative subjects under the same experimental conditions. However, different pain induction methods differ in their repeat reliability. In our hands, cutaneous electrical stimulation has the highest repeat reliability for pain threshold with a reliability coefficient ≤ 0.95 for immediate test–retest and ≥ 0.85 for between-sessions retest. The pain threshold, however, is readily modulated by changes in the experimental conditions, although it is less sensitive to many analgesic drugs than some other parameters. Pain tolerance is that point at which the subject terminates or withdraws from the noxious stimulation. It is thus an upper threshold. Pain tolerance is somewhat less stable than pain threshold and easily manipulated by experimental changes. It is a very useful parameter for evaluating pain relief treatment modalities, especially narcotic analgesics. Drug request point is that point at which the subject would prefer to take a mild painkiller were he to experience a similar pain intensity level in a real life situation. It is a rather useful parameter for analgesic assays as it has the widest spectrum of sensitivity to mild, moderate, and potent analgesic drugs. Pain sensitivity range (PSR) is the arithmetical difference between pain tolerance and pain threshold. It is more stable than pain tolerance and the response parameter most closely related to the pain endurance factor. A more detailed discussion of these pain-response parameters has previously been published (16).

There are probably as many pain induction methods as there are investigators. On a practical basis, it is useful to classify them into cutaneous, deep somatic, and visceral pain techniques in terms of the locus of the stimulus application. One may also categorize these methods in terms of the nature of their stimuli, such as chemical (e.g., cantharidin blister), mechanical (e.g., pressure algometer), thermal (e.g., radiant heat), electrical (e.g., tooth pulp), etc. Detailed descriptions of these methods have been published (15).

Clinical pain should be separated into acute and chronic pain states. Acute pain refers to pain usually associated with tissue damage, in which the pain decreases as the tissue heals—the traditional medical concept. Chronic pain, on the other hand, is pain that persists usually for 6 months or more and no longer signals real or impending tissue damage. Bonica (2) termed chronic pain a malefic force and was one of the first to recognize that it must be differentiated from acute pain. Many pain clinicians now consider that an independent syndrome exists—the chronic pain syndrome—associated with certain psychological changes and requiring a multidisciplinary treatment approach. Very generally, it is chronic pain and the chronic pain syndrome that predominate in pain clinics. Unfortunately, a serious criticism of laboratory-induced pain is that it serves as a model for acute and not for chronic pain. Theoretically, it is probably quite feasible to develop chronic pain models in the laboratory, but certainly for human subjects such models would be unethical and probably illegal and thus totally unacceptable.

We have been interested in developing broader applications of laboratory-induced pain to clinical problems in spite of its apparent limitation as an acute pain model. Several years ago we started to administer three standardized pain induction methods, namely, cutaneous electrical stimulation, radiant heat, and cold pressor, to nearly every patient of the New York University Comprehensive Pain Center. Previously we had collected similar data from large numbers of healthy volunteers as well as from certain diagnostic groups, especially arthritis and cancer. Different pain states appeared to yield different types of pain-response patterns when compared to the healthy norms if corrected for sex, age, and ethnocultural subgroup. These differences were found to be related to both deviations from mean values and within-test scatter. It now appears that the total pattern of pain responses to these three laboratory methods can differentiate four diagnostic groups from the healthy norms: acute pain, chronic pain, pain secondary to psychological problems, and malingerers. This is very exciting because it suggests that laboratory pain can in fact play an important practical role in differential pain diagnosis.

This chapter, so far, has discussed indirect pain measurement methods using a classic psychophysical approach, with the focus on the stimulus rather than on the response, as the resultant response parameters are described in terms of stimulus values. In essence this is the domain of laboratory-induced pain. However, direct measurement of pain is also possible utilizing direct scaling (magnitude estimation) of the pain intensity. This approach is used primarily with clinical pain. Beecher (1) introduced direct measurement of "subjective" pain responses as a valid procedure for clinical pharmacology, whereas Stevens (11) demonstrated that sensory modalities, including pain, obeyed a power rather than a linear function. The U.S. Federal Drug Administration now requires such magnitude estimation for human analgesic assays with clinical pain. Certain pain groups are selected, such as postoperative pain, postpartum pain, and molar extraction pain, and a trained nurse-observer requests the patient to rate his intensity along a 4- or 5-point scale from no pain to excruciating pain. Provided that the pain is at least moderate or greater, the patient is accepted into the study and given the drug under double-blind conditions. The nurse-observer returns to the patient on an hourly basis and has him rate his pain each time along the same scale. Changes in pain intensity are then used as a measure of the efficacy of the drug—a simple technique, but very valid.

Finally, this chapter has discussed the relation of laboratory-induced pain to clinical pain, demonstrating that these methods do play a useful role in our understanding of pain mechanisms. These techniques also can serve as valid and practical tools for clinical pain evaluations.

ACKNOWLEDGMENTS

Some of the studies reported in this chapter were in part supported by Grant No. CA-20652 from the National Cancer Institute.

REFERENCES

1. Beecher, H. K. (1959): *Measurement of Subjective Responses*. Oxford University Press, New York.
2. Bonica, J. J., editor (1974): *Advances in Neurology, Vol. 4: International Symposium on Pain*. Raven Press, New York.
3. Goetzl, F. R., Burrill, D. Y., and Ivy, A. C. (1943): A critical analysis of algesimetric methods with suggestion for a useful procedure. *Q. Bull. Northwest. Univ. Med. School*, 17:280–291.
4. Hardy, J. D., Wolff, H. G., and Goodell, H. (1940): Studies on pain: A new method for measuring pain threshold observations on the spatial summation of pain. *J. Clin. Invest.*, 19:649–657.
5. Hardy, J. D., Wolff, H. G., and Goodell, H. (1952): *Pain Sensations and Reactions*. Williams & Wilkins, Baltimore.
6. Hilgard, E. R., Ruch, J. C., Lance, A. F., Lenox, J. R., Morgan, A. H., and Sachs, L. B. (1974): The psychophysics of cold pressor pain and its modification through hypnotic suggestion. *Am. J. Psychol.*, 87:17–31.
7. Jarvik, M. E., and Wolff, B. B. (1962): Differences between deep pain responses to hypertonic and hypotonic saline solutions. *J. Appl. Physiol.*, 17:841–843.
8. Kast, E. C. (1962): The measurement of pain: A new approach to an old problem. *J. New Drugs*, 2:344–351.
9. Kornetsky, C. (1954): Effects of anxiety and morphine on the anticipation and perception of painful radiant thermal stimuli. *J. Comp. Physiol. Psychol.*, 47:130–132.
10. Smith, G. M., Egbert, L. D., Markowitz, R. A., Mosteller, F., and Beecher, H. K. (1966): An experimental pain method sensitive to morphine in man. The submaximum effort tourniquet technique. *J. Pharmacol. Exp. Ther.*, 154:324–332.
11. Stevens, S. S. (1959): Cross-modality validation of subjective scales for loudness, vibration and electric shock. *J. Exp. Psychol.*, 57:201–209.
12. Timmermans, G., and Sternbach, R. A. (1974): Factors of human chronic pain: An analysis of personality and pain reaction variables. *Science*, 184:806–808.
13. von Frey, M. (1894): Beiträge zur Physiologie des Schmerzsinnes. *Ber.ü.d.Verhandl.d.k. sächs.Ges.d.Wiss.z.Leipzig*, 46:185–196; 288–296.
14. Wolff, B. B. (1971): Factor analysis of human pain responses: Pain endurance as a specific pain factor. *J. Abnorm. Psychol.*, 78:292–298.
15. Wolff, B. B. (1977): The role of laboratory pain induction methods in the systematic study of human pain. *Acupunct. Electro-Ther. Res. Int. J.*, 2:271–305.
16. Wolff, B. B. (1978): Behavioral measurement of human pain. In: *The Psychology of Pain*, edited by R. A. Sternbach, pp. 129–168. Raven Press, New York.
17. Wolff, B. B., Cohen, P., and Greene, C. T. (1976): Behavioral mechanisms of human pain: Effects of expectancy, magnitude and type of cross-modal stimulation. In: *Advances in Pain Research and Therapy, Vol. 1*, edited by J. J. Bonica and D. Albe-Fessard, pp. 327–333. Raven Press, New York.
18. Wolff, B. B., and Horland, A. A. (1967): Effect of suggestion upon experimental pain: A validation study. *J. Abnorm. Psychol.*, 72:402–407.
19. Wolff, B. B., Kantor, T. G., Jarvik, M. E., and Laska, E. (1969): Response of experimental pain to analgesic drugs. III: Codeine, aspirin, secobarbital and placebo. *Clin. Pharmacol. Ther.*, 10:217–228.

Pain Measurement and Assessment,
edited by Ronald Melzack,
Raven Press, New York © 1983.

Applications of Sensory Decision Theory to Problems in Laboratory and Clinical Pain

*W. Crawford Clark and **Joseph C. Yang

*New York State Psychiatric Institute and Department of Psychiatry, and **Department of Anesthesiology, College of Physicians and Surgeons, Columbia University, New York, New York 10032*

In the behavioral sciences, as in the physical sciences, progress is often paced by new mathematical models that specify novel ways of making observations and interpreting data. Signal detection theory, or more descriptively, sensory decision theory (SDT), is one such model. The SDT pain literature is too vast to review here; instead, critical studies that have increased our understanding of pain, or promise to point the way, have been selected. Recent work will be emphasized since reviews and discussion by Lloyd and Appel (26), Hall (23), Clark (7), Rollman (30), Chapman (3), and Jones (25) have appeared. Procedures for parametric (6,7,9,14) and nonparametric (12,28,29) data analyses have been described.

At a simple level, pain may be viewed as possessing both sensory and emotional components. The latter is closely related to Beecher's concept of the "reaction to pain" (1a), that is, the significance of the pain to the patient and its arousal of psychological distress. The strength of the SDT approach resides in the fact that it quantifies both a sensory and an attitudinal parameter. The index of discriminability [d' or $P(A)$] measures the accuracy with which an individual distinguishes among stimuli of various intensities; it is related to the functioning of the neurosensory system. High values suggest that the neurosensory input is adequate for decision making, low values that sensory processes have been interfered with. This index of perceptual performance is little influenced by attitudinal variables. The other measure of perceptual performance is the report criterion (L_x or B), which measures the willingness or reluctance of a subject to use a particular response; it is related to the subject's attitude toward the sensory experience. A high criterion reflects stoicism, a low criterion that the subject readily reports pain. A brief and simple introduction to these concepts is available (12). There are other quantitative models for viewing pain behavior—for example, traditional threshold, magnitude estimation, and multidimensional scaling—but none of these yields measures that can be readily identified with the sensory and the emotional components of pain.

It is well known that a person's report of pain can be altered by psychological means such as suggestion, placebo, hypnosis, attention, biofeedback, and psychotherapy. However, there is little agreement concerning the mechanism. One view holds that these manipulations alter the neurosensory activity underlying the pain percept in much the same way as an analgesic. The mistaken belief that the pain threshold depends only on neurosensory and not psychological variables is partly responsible for this view. The contrary view is that manipulations of these nonsensory variables merely produce a more conservative or stoic attitude toward reporting pain; the underlying neurosensory activity and pain experience remain unchanged. Any attempt to resolve this dispute requires a methodology that can (a) provide estimates of an individual's pain report criterion, and (b) independently yield a measure—of necessity indirect—related to the underlying neurosensory activity.

INTRODUCTION TO THE SDT MODEL

An example of the stimulus-response matrix of sensory decision theory appears in Table 1. In the simple binary decision case, high- (stimulus) and low- (blanks) intensity stimuli are presented randomly, and the subject responds "high" or "low," or "painful" or "not painful." The report of "high" or "pain" to high-intensity stimulus is a hit; the same report to a low-intensity stimulus is a false alarm. A plot of hit rate against false alarm rate yields the receiver-operating characteristic curve of the SDT. In pain research, more than two intensities of stimulation are typically presented, and the binary choice is extended to a rating scale of 8 to 16 categories. The analysis of the data, however, is essentially the same as for the binary task described in this example.

The two parameters of decision theory—discriminability and response bias—may be understood by viewing the response matrices of 4 subjects who differ in their ability to discriminate between high- and low-intensity stimuli, and who differ in where they locate their subjective criterion for reporting pain (see Table 2). Subject 1 (S-1) was presented 10 high- and 10 low-intensity stimuli in random order. When the high stimulus was presented, he reported "pain" or "high" nine times and "hot" or "low" once, a hit rate of 0.90. When the low-intensity stimulus was presented, he reported "pain" or "high" four times, a false alarm rate of 0.40. The difference of 5 reflects discriminability, which yields a $P(A)$ of 0.85; thus S-1 and S-2 show superior discriminability to S-3 and S-4. The discriminability

TABLE 1. *Stimulus-response matrix for the binary decision task*

Stimulus	Response	
	"Pain" or "high"	"No pain" or "low"
Higher intensity	Hit	Miss
Lower intensity	False alarm	Correct rejection

TABLE 2. *Relationships between hit and false-affirmative rates and values of discriminability [P(A)] and report criterion (B)*

		Low criterion response $B = 0.57$				High criterion response $B = 1.23$	
		S-1				**S-2**	
		"Pain"	"Hot"			"Pain"	"Hot"
High discriminability $P\ (A) = 0.85$	10 high-intensity stimuli	9	1	10 high-intensity stimuli		6	4
		——(5)——				——(5)——	
	10 low-intensity stimuli	4	6	10 low-intensity stimuli		1	9
	Total	13	7	Total		7	13
		S-3				**S-4**	
		"Pain"	"Hot"			"Pain"	"Hot"
Low discriminability $P(A) = 0.60$	10 high-intensity stimuli	7	3	10 high-intensity stimuli		4	6
		——(1)——				——(1)——	
	10 low-intensity stimuli	6	4	10 low-intensity stimuli		3	7
	Total	13	7	Total		7	13

measure reflects the functional state of the pain system without any dependence on the total frequency of the subject's report of pain. A low $P(A)$ could be caused by a small physical difference between the high- and low-intensity stimuli, by a sensory defect, or by any treatment, such as an analgesic (32) that decreases sensory information arriving centrally. The other index of perceptual performance is the subject's report criterion *(B)*. S-1 and S-3 emitted 13 pain reports; they were much less stoic than S-2 and S-4. A suggestion that less pain will be felt has been demonstrated (10) to move a subject toward a high *B*, whereas the suggestion that more pain will be felt will shift a subject toward a low *B* without changing the subject's discriminability.

EMPIRICAL FINDINGS: RESPONSES TO CALIBRATED NOXIOUS STIMULI

Effect of Suggestion

Clark (5) found that a placebo described and accepted as a powerful analgesic markedly raised the pain threshold, that is, decreased the sensitivity to noxious thermal stimulation. However, application of SDT to the same data demonstrated that this decrease in the report of pain was caused by a raised pain report criterion and not by a decrease in thermal discriminability. It was concluded that the analgesia typically believed to be produced by placebos was entirely a psychological response to the social demand characteristics of the experimental situation, and was not due to altered neurosensory activity that would be expected to reduce discriminability. In a related study, Clark and Goodman (10) demonstrated that suggestion alone could produce the same effect.

Although reports of hypnoanalgesia in clinical pain are very dramatic, most studies of the effects of hypnosis on experimental pain thresholds are not very convincing. Clark and Goodman (10) demonstrated that although instructions can raise the thermal pain threshold by 50 mCal, the change is entirely due to a criterion shift. Thus, those hypnosis studies that achieve a threshold change of this amount or less reflect only a criterion shift, not hypnoanalgesia. Interestingly, Hall (23) has reported that individuals who are highly hypnotizable do show a decrease in discriminability, suggestive of analgesia.

Effect of Attitude and Anxiety

The demonstration that pain thresholds reflect decision processes in addition to sensory input has forced a reevaluation of studies in which experimental pain thresholds have been reported to differ with age, sex, ethnocultural differences, personality, and anxiety. People bring their own attitudes into a study. Even with no, or with neutral instructions, every participant covertly instructs himself.

Pain thresholds do differ in different groups, but are these differences neurosensory or attitudinal? Clark and Mehl (13) found that older subjects possessed a much higher thermal pain threshold. SDT treatment of the data revealed that the higher threshold of the older subjects was almost entirely due to their high response criterion. This finding supports the adaptation level concept, according to which internal standards of stimulus characteristics provide a context that influences perceptual judgments. In comparison to the endogenous aches and pains of old age, experimentally induced pain probably seems quite inconsequential. Harkins and Chapman (24) studied the response of young and elderly women to electrical dental stimulation. No difference in the pain threshold was found; however, the finer analysis permitted with SDT revealed both a higher pain report criterion and a reduced ability to discriminate among the noxious intensities in the elderly. This study illustrates an important methodological point. The fact that two pain thresholds are the same does not mean that discriminability and criteria are the same for each. Discriminability and criteria may differ, yet interact in such a way as to mask this difference when they are blended into the traditional threshold measure.

Various investigators have found women to have higher, the same, or lower pain thresholds than men. Who is right? And does the difference have an attitudinal or a physiological basis? Clark and Goodman (10) studied a college-age population and found men to have a higher threshold and a higher criterion. However, the two sexes were identical with respect to thermal discriminability, indicating the absence of neurosensory differences. Furthermore, considerable differences were found in the way the sexes changed their criterion in response to various suggestions. The unmeasured presence of these attitudinal variables undoubtedly caused the considerable confusion found in the earlier pain threshold literature.

People from non-Western cultures are often thought to be more tolerant of pain, perhaps because of genetically based physiological differences. Clark and Clark (8) studied a group of Sherpas in Nepal and found that their ability to discriminate electrical stimuli was the same as that of Western controls. However, the Sherpas had a much higher pain threshold, probably owing to a culturally and perhaps climatically determined stoical pain report criterion. This study suggests that many, if not all, of the differences in pain thresholds reported to exist among various ethnic, religious, and "racial" groups are due to differences in the criterion for reporting pain, and not to the sensory experience itself.

Personality also influences pain report. Yang et al. (32) have found that those chronic pain patients who score high on hostility and paranoid ideation scales report moderate thermal stimuli to be painful, that is, they set a relatively low pain report criterion. The effect of trait anxiety on SDT parameters was examined by Dougher (20), who found that anxious students had a much lower threshold for reporting focal pressure pain. SDT analysis revealed that this effect was due solely to a lowered pain report criterion since discriminability remained unchanged. Malow (27) compared responses to intervals signaled as threat of shock (high anxiety) to intervals signaled as no shock (low anxiety). He found that induced state anxiety decreased discriminability and raised the pain report criterion, changes suggestive of analgesia, perhaps owing to attentional effects. These studies show that different types of anxiety can have quite different effects on the pain criterion, and that in general the increased reports of pain in anxious individuals do not necessarily mean that they are experiencing more pain. Malow's results, however, suggest that further studies should be undertaken.

Effect of Analgesics and Anxiolytics

Analgesics would be expected to decrease discriminability by attenuating the amount of neurosensory information reaching higher centers. In addition, the pain report criterion probably would be raised. These effects on discriminability and criterion have been found with nitrous oxide, morphine, and codeine using thermal and electrical stimulation to skin and tooth pulp. At low-dose levels, codeine has yielded mixed results (20). Demonstration of the effectiveness of weaker analgesics on experimentally induced pain using traditional procedures has proven difficult. However, Buchsbaum et al. (1) have demonstrated that aspirin, as well as morphine, reduces discriminability. Their success with the weak analgesic may be due to the use of a new nonparametric technique based on SDT principles. This method integrates the information provided by responses to a large number of intensities instead of only a pair of intensities as in the standard procedure.

The ultimate standard by which analgesic effectiveness is judged, of course, must be the amelioration of clinical pain. However, studies of experimental pain within the context of SDT provide a deeper insight into the mechanisms involved. Analgesia is not the only cause for a decrease in pain report. Analgesics possess mood-altering properties, and it is possible that improved mood, rather than an analgesic effect *per se*, is responsible for some of the analgesic effects reported clinically. For example, cannabinoids and their synthesized analogs have been reported to ameliorate cancer pain. However, studies by Clark and co-workers (12), using calibrated thermal stimuli, demonstrated that smoking an average of 12 marijuana cigarettes a day for 4 weeks failed to produce any analgesia. Indeed, there was some evidence of hyperalgesia, namely, an increase in discriminability and a lower pain report criterion. These results conflict with reports that cannabinoids and certain analogs are effective in the treatment of cancer-related pain. However, the reputed analgesic effect of marijuana in these double-blind studies could be due to a feeling of increased well-being resulting from its antiemetic properties, or to a placebo effect. The use of the double-blind control does not necessarily eliminate the placebo effect; often the subjective effects produced by most analgesics permit the subject to "peek through the double-blind." The discrimination measure of SDT obtained in an experimental pain study is not influenced by placebo responses or mood changes. Thus experimental pain offers a useful supplement to clinical trials by elucidating the mechanisms behind the decreased pain report.

The separate neurosensory and attitudinal parameters of SDT have proved useful in the examination of the effect of mood-altering drugs on the pain threshold. Yang et al. (31) found that intravenous diazepam raised the pain threshold almost as much as morphine did, suggesting a surprisingly strong analgesic effect for the anxiolytic. However, dissection of the threshold into its sensory and attitudinal components revealed that whereas the raised morphine threshold was due equally to reduced discriminability and a raised pain report criterion, the increased diazepam threshold was due mostly to an increase in the pain report criterion. Diazepam also produced a slight but significant decrease in discriminability, suggesting the presence of a slight analgesic effect as well. This study illustrates the point that SDT, because it possesses both an emotional and a neurosensory parameter, represents the only possible approach to the study of those drugs that influence both the subject's mood and perception of pain (17). Although it would be wrong to equate decreased discriminability with analgesia in every instance, there is mounting evidence that discriminability will prove to be a useful correlate of analgesia.

Variables Reputed to Influence Discriminability

Between those procedures that manipulate attitudinal variables and alter only the criterion and those procedures involving strong analgesics that alter discriminability as well, lies a group of controversial approaches to the alleviation of pain. These maneuvers clearly influence pain report, but whether this change is due to altered sensitivity, to changed pain report criterion, or to both is unclear. Psychological and physiological variables could act either separately or jointly to influence pain report after transcutaneous electrical nerve stimulation (TENS), acupuncture, stress, and cyclic hormonal changes.

Callaghan et al. (2) used SDT to study the effect of TENS in patients with chronic pain in one limb. Without TENS the painful limb showed impaired thermal discriminability compared with the patient's normal limb, indicating impaired neurosensory input, perhaps in the large fibers. TENS increased thermal discriminability in the painful limb of the chronic patient, but tended to decrease discriminability in the nonpainful limb, as well as in normal control subjects. Poor thermal discriminability and pain in the injured limb suggest that inadequate large fiber input had opened the Melzack-Wall pain gate. In the painful limb, TENS improved the functioning of the large fiber system, which caused both increased discriminability and closed the pain gate. For the uninjured limb and for the normal control subjects possessing intact large fiber systems, TENS closed the gate, decreasing discriminability and decreasing pain. Since TENS influenced discriminability, the SDT analysis demonstrated that more than a placebo-mediated criterion shift in pain report had occurred in this group of patients.

The question of acupunctural analgesia has generated considerable controversy. In normal volunteers, Clark and Yang (16) found that electroacupuncture at traditional sites raised the pain criterion without influencing discriminability. They concluded that acupunctural analgesia was a placebo effect. In a recent cross-cultural study using tooth pulp stimulation, Chapman et al. (4) found a small but statistically significant reduction in discriminability as well as a raised criterion after bilateral facial acupuncture stimulation. Clark et al. (11) proved in normals that TENS stimulation of the median nerve lowered discriminability and raised the pain report criterion to thermal stimuli applied to the region of the hand subserved by the median nerve. The effect appeared in the TENS-treated hand, not in the control hand, and furthermore only briefly outlasted cessation of TENS. It was concluded that the decrease in discriminability was not an acupunctural effect, but rather a result of direct synaptic inhibition. Thus, these studies do not necessarily confirm or disprove the claims of classic acupuncture regarding clinical pain.

Possible Endocrine and Neurotransmitter Effects

Pain thresholds have been reported to vary with the ovulatory cycle, to vary diurnally, to be raised after exercise stress, and to be altered in psychiatrically depressed patients and in patients suffering intractable pain. Because pain threshold changes during the menstrual cycle are poorly understood, Goolkasian (22) used SDT to demonstrate that discriminability for radiant heat stimuli markedly increased during the ovulation phase, and that no such phase effect could be found in women using oral contraceptives. Response bias did not vary in any of the groups. This study has done much to clarify a hitherto confused literature. Using SDT to study diurnal variation, Davis et al. (18) found that normal subjects tested in the morning were poorer discriminators of electrical stimulation and set a higher pain report criterion than when they were tested in the afternoon. Their response to naloxone suggested that the naturally occurring morning analgesia was related to raised endorphin levels. Stress-induced analgesia has been difficult to prove in man, since criterion shifts related to changes in mood could explain the decreased pain report. Recently, Janal et al. *(in preparation)*, using SDT, found that a 6-mile run by long-distance runners improved their mood and decreased their discriminability to thermal stimulation. This analgesic effect was blocked only partially by naloxone, suggesting that substances other than endogenous opioids participate in stress-induced analgesia.

It has been demonstrated by SDT that compared with normal volunteers, chronic pain patients are far less able to discriminate among thermal stimuli and set a much more stoic pain report criterion (32). Both of these changes could be due to mobilization of endogenous opioids. It was also found that within the patient group, those patients who were high on self-report measures of psychological distress tended to set a low criterion and, interestingly, had previously been prescribed stronger (narcotic) medication. The SDT has permitted a penetrating look into the relationships among personality, pain response bias, and the medication given to chronic pain patients.

Using the SDT approach, psychiatrically depressed patients have been found to be more stoic and generally less able to discriminate among the various noxious intensities (15,19). The high pain report criterion could be due to a context or adaptation level effect. However, the inability of the patients to discriminate among the noxious stimuli demonstrated that some hypoanalgesia was present in addition to a stoic attitude. The physiological basis of this effect is unknown. The depressed patients, in contrast with the chronic pain patients, suffered no loss in ability to detect minimal warmth stimulation, suggesting that different physiological mechanisms are involved.

EMPIRICAL FINDINGS: PATIENTS' RESPONSES TO SDT PAIN QUESTIONNAIRES

In an attempt to extend the analytic power of SDT to the solution of problems encountered with clinical pain, four questionnaires based on SDT principles have been developed recently (21,33).

The Situational Pain Questionnaire (SPQ) was developed to measure discriminability and attitude toward imaginary painful situations. Its entries portray situations that are painful (signals) and that are relatively nonpainful (blanks). Signals are represented by 12 situations such as getting a tooth drilled without a painkiller, whereas blanks are represented by minor pain situations such as pulling out a strand of hair. In a recent study (32,33), outpatients suffering chronic pain rated the degree of pain they thought they would feel in each situation on a visual analogue scale anchored at "no pain at all" and at "pain as bad as it could be." A relatively painful response on the scale to a severe pain situation is interpreted as a hit, whereas a relatively painful response to a minor pain situation is scored as a false alarm.

Decision theory analysis yielded measures for discriminability (how well the patient distinguished between the two types of situations) and for response criterion (the patient's general tendency to see both kinds of situations as painful or not). These scores were then related to measures of personality obtained from the Derogatis Brief Symptom Inventory (BSI), to SDT measures of responses to calibrated thermal stimuli, and to the strength and type of medication prescribed.

Chronic pain patients who were high on the hostility and paranoid ideation scales of the BSI tended to perceive a lot of pain (low criterion) in both painless and painful situations. These symptoms may reflect the frustration and suspiciousness that accompany the chronic patient's search for a cure. This low pain report criterion appears to carry over into their behavior concerning the reporting of their chronic pain, since these patients were found to be more likely to receive medications with a stronger effect on the central nervous system. A generally low criterion for reporting all types of pain could reflect an unconscious attempt by the patient to convince the treating physician of the reality of his pain in order to obtain more powerful treatment. Obviously the patients succeeded! The discriminability measure on the SPQ revealed that chronic pain patients who obtained high scores on measures of psychological distress and phobic anxiety on the BSI were less able to discriminate between painful and relatively painless situations on the SPQ. This suggests the possibility that these patients may also be less able to discriminate the quality and intensity of their own chronic pain. These psychologically disturbed chronic pain patients also set a low criterion for reporting pain to thermal stimulation.

Of special interest is the striking parallel between the low pain report criteria obtained from both thermal stimulation and the SPQ and the two independently obtained estimates of personal distress and strength of medication prescribed. The fact that two such different SDT tests yield similar correlations strongly suggests that SDT successfully measures the patient's covert attitude toward pain.

CONCLUSIONS

The failure to quantify pain has seriously handicapped our ability to relieve it, for without measurement, it is almost impossible to compare the efficacy of the various treatments available for the relief of pain. This lack of progress has been due to the widely held belief that the report of pain is a relatively objective and exact description of a purely sensory experience. The concept of pain threshold best exemplifies this trap. Nevertheless, at a descriptive, or qualitative, level, the sensory and emotional components of pain have long been recognized. SDT now permits the quantification of these two components into indices of discriminability and pain report criterion.

Although SDT cannot be applied to the direct measurement of clinical pain, experimental pain studies using calibrated stimuli have provided a number of insights into general pain behavior that have direct clinical implications. SDT questionnaires may prove to be useful in understanding clinical pain, since they appear to be sensitive to otherwise hidden influences on pain behavior. It is too early to determine if this approach will prove fruitful, but the initial results are encouraging.

ACKNOWLEDGMENT

This report was supported in part by NIH Grant GM-26461-03.

REFERENCES

1a. Beecher, H. K. (1959): *Measurement of Subjective Responses*, p. 157. Oxford University Press, New York.

1. Buchsbaum, M., Davis, G. C., Coppola, R., and Naber, D. (1981): Opiate pharmacology and individual differences. 1. Psychophysical pain measurements. *Pain*, 10:357–366.

2. Callaghan, M., Sternbach, R. A., Nyquist, J. K., and Timmerman, G. (1978): Changes in somatic sensitivity during transcutaneous electrical analgesia. *Pain*, 5:115–127.

3. Chapman, C. R. (1977): Sensory decision theory methods in research: A reply to Rollman. *Pain*, 3:295–305.

4. Chapman, C. R., Sato, T., Martin, R. W., Tanaka, A., Okazaki, N., Colpitts, Y. M., Mayens, J. K., and Gagliardi, G. J. (1982): Comparative effects of acupuncture in Japan and the United States on dental pain perception. *Pain*, 12:319–328.

5. Clark, W. C. (1969): Sensory-decision theory analysis of the placebo effect on the criterion for pain and thermal sensitivity *(d')*. *J. Abnorm. Psychol.*, 74:363–371.

6. Clark, W. C. (1974): Pain sensitivity and the report of pain: An introduction to sensory decision theory. *Anesthesiology*, 40:272–287.

7. Clark, W. C. (1978): Measurement of pain in humans: Signal detection theory and pain. *Neurosci. Res. Prog. Bull.*, 16:14–27.

8. Clark, W. C., and Clark, S. B. (1980): Pain responses in Nepalese porters. *Science*, 209:440–442.

9. Clark, W. C., and Dillon, D. J. (1973): Signal detection theory analysis of binary decisions and sensory intensity ratings to noxious thermal stimuli. *Percep. Psychophys.*, 13:491–493.

10. Clark, W. C., and Goodman, J. S. (1973): The effect of suggestion on d' and C for pain detection and pain tolerance. *J. Abnorm. Psychol.*, 83:364–372.

11. Clark, W. C., Hall, W., and Yang, J. (1976): Changes in thermal discriminability and pain report criterion after acupunctural or transcutaneous electrical stimulation. In: *Advances in Pain Research and Therapy, Vol. 1*, edited by J. J. Bonica and D. Albe-Fessard, pp. 769–773. Raven Press, New York.

12. Clark, W. C., Janal, M. N., Zeidenberg, P., and Nahas, G. G. (1981): Effects of moderate doses of marihuana on thermal pain: A sensory decision theory analysis. *J. Clin. Pharmacol.*, 21:299s–310s.

13. Clark, W. C., and Mehl, L. (1971): Thermal pain: A sensory decision theory analysis of the effect of age and sex on d', various response criteria, and 50% threshold. *J. Abnorm. Psychol.*, 78:202–212.

14. Clark, W. C., and Mehl, L. (1973): Signal detection theory procedures are not equivalent when thermal stimuli are judged. *J. Exp. Psychol.*, 97:148–153.

15. Clark, W. C., and Mehl, L. (1976): Thermal pain: Sensory (d') and criterion (L_x) differences between psychiatric patients and normals. 21st International Congress of Psychology, Paris, France.

16. Clark, W. C., and Yang, J. C. (1974): A signal detection theory evaluation of acupunctural analgesia. *Science*, 184:1096–1098.

17. Clark, W. C., and Yang, J. C. (1980): The consequences of not applying sensory decision theory to studies of analgesics with psychotropic properties. *Anesthesiology*, 53:265–266.

18. Davis, G. C., Buchsbaum, M. S., and Bunney, W. E. (1978): Naloxone decreases diurnal variation in pain sensitivity and somatosensory evoked potentials. *Life Sci.*, 23:1449–1459.

19. Davis, G. C., Buchsbaum, M. S., and Bunney, W. E. (1979): Analgesia to painful stimuli in affective illness. *Am. J. Psychiatry*, 136:1148–1151.

20. Dougher, M. J. (1979): Sensory decision theory analysis of the effects of anxiety and experimental instructions on pain. *J. Abnorm. Psychol.*, 88:134–144.

21. Ferrer-Brechner, T., Clark, W. C., Wagner, J., and Yang, J. C. (1982): Side-effects of analgesics in cancer patients: A sensory decision theory approach. American Society for Clinical Pharmacology and Therapeutics, Florida.

22. Goolkasian, P. (1980): Cyclic changes in pain perception: An ROC analysis. *Percept. Psychophys.*, 27:499–504.

23. Hall, W. (1977): Psychological processes in pain perception: The prospects of a signal detection theory analysis. Unpublished doctoral dissertation. The University of New South Wales, Kensington, N.S.W., Australia.
24. Harkins, S. W., and Chapman, C. R. (1977): The perception of induced dental pain in young and elderly women. *J. Gerontol.*, 32:428–435.
25. Jones, B. (1979): Signal detection theory and pain research. *Pain*, 7:305–312.
26. Lloyd, M. A., and Appel. J. B. (1976): Signal detection theory and psychophysics of pain: Introduction and review. *Psychosomatic Medicine*, 38:79–94.
27. Malow, R. M. (1981): The effects of induced anxiety on pain perception: A signal detection analysis. *Pain*, 11:397–405.
28. McNicol, D. (1972): *A Primer of Signal Detection Theory*, pp. 18–49. Allen & Unwin, London.
29. Myers, S. J., Janal, M. N., and Clark, W. C. (1982): A model of clinical pain: Technique for evaluation of analgesic agents. *Am. Phys. Med.*, 61:1–10.
30. Rollman, G. B. (1977): Signal detection theory measurement of pain: A review and critique. *Pain*, 3:187–211.
31. Yang, J. C., Clark, W. C., Ngai, S. H., Berkowitz, B. A., and Spector, S. (1979): Analgesic action and pharmacokinetics of morphine and diazepam in man: An evaluation by sensory decision theory. *Anesthesiology*, 51:495–502.
32. Yang. J. C., Clark, W. C., and Wagner, J. M. (1982): Relationship of thermal sensory decision indices and psychological distress in chronic pain patients. American Pain Society, Florida.
33. Yang, J. C., Wagner, J. M., and Clark, W. C. (1983): Psychological distress and mood in chronic pain and surgical patients: A decision theory analysis. In: *Advances in Pain Research and Therapy, Vol. 5*, edited by J. J. Bonica et al., pp. 901–906. Raven Press, New York.

Pain Measurement and Assessment, edited by
Ronald Melzack, Raven Press, New York ©
1983.

The Tourniquet Pain Test

Richard A. Sternbach

*Pain Treatment Center, Scripps Clinic and Research Foundation,
La Jolla, California 92037*

It is important to obtain an accurate assessment of how much pain a patient is experiencing. The intensity of the pain, as well as its other qualities, has a bearing on the diagnosis in some cases, and frequently determines the extent to which major intervention is considered.

If one were to rely solely on the patient's description of the intensity of the pain, one would expect considerable influence from personality variables and other sociocultural factors (11). A result of such influences may be the needless suffering of overly stoic patients, whereas overly expressive ones may undergo unnecessary procedures.

Beecher (3) has shown that the results of studies that use experimental pain are often not comparable with those obtained in the clinic when the effects of analgesic drugs are examined. This, he argued, is because experimental pain is usually less intense, less threatening, and of shorter duration than pathological pain, and can be discontinued deliberately.

DEVELOPMENT OF THE TOURNIQUET PAIN TECHNIQUE

To overcome some of the shortcomings of experimental pain, Beecher's group (7–10) adapted Lewis' ischemic pain test into a standardized "submaximum effort tourniquet technique." Briefly, a pressure cuff is applied to and inflated on the upper arm of a subject who then closes and opens the hand at a fixed rate. This procedure produces a deep, slowly increasing intensity of pain similar to that of many pathological pains. Even in experienced subjects it produces the marked sympathetic responses (sweating, pupillary dilatation, tachycardia) that frequently accompany pain of pathological origin. The reports of Beecher et al. suggested that normal subjects' responses (pain ratings at specified times after induction of ischemia) were sensitive to even mild analgesics such as 600 mg of aspirin.

There was some suggestion by other investigators, however, that the technique was not in fact sensitive to mild analgesics unless experimental or statistical manipulations of anxiety were performed (1,2,5,18). Without such manipulations there were no differences among subjects' responses to mild analgesics and placebo. Similarly, real versus placebo acupuncture could not be differentiated (8).

The technique nonetheless seemed to have promise as a measure of clinical pain levels in patients. We proposed that the induced ischemic pain could provide: (a) a clinical pain level—the time (in sec) to match the intensity of the patient's clinical pain; (b) a maximum pain tolerance—the duration (in sec) of the ischemic pain the patient can endure; and (c) a tourniquet pain score, [(a)/(b)] × 100—the ratio of the patient's clinical pain to his own pain tolerance.

Our preliminary report on the technique (15) described excellent reliability and good validity as the score varied appropriately with pain intervention techniques and seemed to correlate well with numerical pain estimates. Subsequently, using factor analysis and a canonical correlation analysis of pain scores and psychological test scores, we were able to show that numerical pain estimates by patients were associated with the impact of pain on daily activities, whereas the tourniquet pain ratio score was associated with the patient's level of depression; and the two scores seemed clearly to reflect different factors (16,17).

The tourniquet pain test also seemed useful in inferring mechanisms of pain-relieving techniques. For example, the clinical pain level, but not the maximum pain tolerance, was affected by the analgesia provided by transcutaneous electrical neurostimulation (13). However, the maximum pain tolerance, but not the clinical pain level, was increased with the administration of chlorimipramine (14). Thus, the clinical pain level component of the tourniquet pain test seems to reflect peripheral phenomena, and the maximum pain tolerance component seems to reflect central phenomena.

FURTHER STUDIES

The question remained, however, whether the tourniquet pain test, as a measure of clinical pain, is adequately sensitive. Doubts were raised by the failure of the submaximum effort tourniquet technique to differentiate between mild analgesics and placebo in normals (1,2,5). Accordingly, a study was designed to address this issue specifically (12).

Following 12 hr of abstention from any chemical or electrical analgesia, each of 24 chronic pain patients was given, on each of 4 successive days, oral doses of 60 mg of morphine, 60 mg of codeine, 600 mg of aspirin, and placebo. Each of the subjects received the drugs in a different 1 of the 24 possible orders, in a double-blind counterbalanced design. Two hours after ingestion, numerical pain estimates on a 0 to 100 scale and tourniquet pain scores were obtained.

The variability of results in all scores was so great as to preclude achieving statistical significance. This was true for both the clinical pain level and the maximum pain tolerance scores, as well as the indirect tourniquet pain (ratio) scores. This last score failed as well to show any differences among the means for each of the analgesics. Interestingly, the patients' numerical pain estimates showed some trend of scores in the expected direction, but the variability here too was sufficiently great as to preclude significance of differences among the scores. It was concluded that the tourniquet technique was an insensitive measure—perhaps because of the chronicity of the pain, perhaps because the "washout" period between analgesics was inadequate; but in this study the method was clearly unable to discriminate among analgesics of differing strengths (12).

Moore et al. (6) performed a methodological evaluation of the submaximum effort tourniquet technique. They were interested to see if differences in exercise effort and duration would affect the rate of pain induction, and to examine the relationship between pain intensity and elapsed time. Using 5 normal subjects who underwent the ischemic test (12 trials each), the investigators studied the effect of two levels of grip strength and two levels of exercise (grip squeeze) duration. The subjects rated pain on a visual analogue scale. The results showed clearly that the amount of exercise used during the test (both duration of squeeze and force of contraction required) significantly affected the levels of reported pain intensity as time elapsed. Also it was clear that the pain ratings were not a linear function of time but followed a sigmoid form. This could explain some of the variability in data from patients, especially if the clinical pain level component of the ratio score occurred at low or high intensities.

Moore et al. suggested that if the tourniquet pain test is to be used in the clinical situation, then (a) measurement of elapsed time should begin with inflation of the cuff; (b) grip strength should be assessed first, and a fixed percentage (e.g., 50%) should be used to reduce variability among patients; and (c) the duration of each grip squeeze should also be made constant. Extreme scores should be interpreted in light of the sigmoid response curve and not as a function of individual communicative style (6).

Fox et al. (4) studied the submaximum effort tourniquet technique on 19 normal subjects and 12 chronic pain patients, standardizing the squeeze force to 50% of grip strength. Pain estimates were made on a 0 to 100 scale. These investigators also showed that individual linear functions of pain by elapsed time were quite exceptional, although the group average of the pain patients seemed linear when compared with normals who showed more negative acceleration in their scores. The difference in slopes between patients and normals was very significant (patients were also significantly more neurotic), although pain tolerance levels were similar between the groups. From their results, Fox et al. drew similar conclusions about the need for caution in interpreting tourniquet pain scores in ways that assume, implicitly, linearity of functions (e.g., percentage change). Interestingly, they also concluded that with appropriate precautions the technique may yet be useful in pain evaluations (4).

INDICATIONS FOR FUTURE RESEARCH

There may yet be promise in adapting the submaximum effort tourniquet technique into a tourniquet pain test of clinical significance. Several of the aforementioned papers commented on the similarity of pain descriptors used by subjects when describing the ischemic pain to those used by patients. The test clearly has some face validity to it. More work must be done to specify the standardization of the necessary parameters, such as shown by Moore et al. (6) with normal subjects but applied to patient populations.

There seems to be a practice effect in the tourniquet pain test (18), which must be accounted for in repeated measures by means of statistical analyses or by means of counterbalanced or crossover designs. This practice effect, however, is variable depending on whether subjects are initially relatively pain tolerant or intolerant. This in turn seems to be a function of neuroticism (4) or, more specifically, anxiety levels (18). The need for the use of homogeneous matched groups in comparing treatment techniques or the use of covariance analysis to account for pretreatment group differences in anxiety or similar variables is indicated.

From the studies performed thus far, it is clear that the linearity assumed in the ratio (percentage) score of the tourniquet pain test may not be supportable. At least on the basis of studies with the submaximum effort tourniquet technique on normals, ischemic pain appears to have a sigmoid curve when plotted against time, and the scores at the extremes have a flatter slope than those in the middle of the distribution (4,6). However, it is not clear whether this makes a difference in any "typical" sample of pain patients. It is quite likely that the matching clinical pain level scores will be in the middle of the distribution, especially if the recommendation of Moore et al. (6) that timing begin with the inflation of the cuff rather than with the completion of the exercise is followed. If the other recommendations are also adopted, i.e., standardization of percentage of grip strength required and duration of squeeze, much more linear functions might very possibly be obtained, justifying the use of the pain score concept. In this regard, it is interesting that the simple standardization of percentage of grip strength by Fox et al. (4) seemed to be associated with a rather linear function for the patient group. However, this is really an empirical question that has not yet been addressed systematically, and suggests the need for additional studies in this area.

If the tourniquet pain test could be standardized in the ways mentioned and thus prove to be not merely reliable but more sensitive than shown thus far, we may have a clinically useful measure for assessing the severity of patients' pains. We have already shown that it reflects a different dimension than simple numerical estimates (16,17), and patients themselves often volunteer that the test is a truer measure of their pain than paper-and-pencil estimates.

REFERENCES

1. Adler, R., Gervasi, A., Holzer, B., and Hemmeler, W. (1974): Mild analgesics evaluated with the "submaximum effort tourniquet technique." II. The influence of a tranquilizer on their effect. *Psychopharmacologia*, 38:357–362.
2. Adler, R., and Lomazzi, F. (1974): Mild analgesics evaluated with the "submaximum effort tourniquet technique." I. The influence of psychological factors on their effect. *Psychopharmacologia*, 38:351–356.
3. Beecher, H. K. (1959): *Measurement of Subjective Responses: Quantitative Effect of Drugs*, pp. 12–64. Oxford University Press, New York.
4. Fox, C. D., Steger, H. G., and Jennison, J. H. (1979): Ratio scaling of pain perception with the submaximum effort tourniquet technique. *Pain*, 7:21–29.

5. Moore, J. D., Weissman, L., Thomas, G., and Whitman, E. N. (1971): Response of experimental ischemic pain to analgesics in prisoner volunteers. *J. Clin. Pharmacol.*, 11:433–439.
6. Moore, P. A., Duncan, G. H., Scott, D. S., Gregg, J. M., and Ghia, J. N. (1979): The submaximal effort tourniquet test: Its use in evaluating experimental and chronic pain. *Pain*, 6:375–382.
7. Smith, G. M., and Beecher, H. K. (1969): Experimental production of pain in man: Sensitivity of a new method to 600 mg of aspirin. *Clin. Pharmacol. Ther.*, 10:213–216.
8. Smith, G. M., Chiang, H. T., Kitz, R. J., and Antoon, A. (1974): Acupuncture and experimentally induced ischemic pain. In: *Advances in Neurology, Vol. 4*, edited by J. J. Bonica, pp. 827–832. Raven Press, New York.
9. Smith, G. M., Egbert, L. D., Markowitz, R. A., Mosteller, F., and Beecher, H. K. (1966): An experimental pain method sensitive to morphine in man: The submaximum effort tourniquet technique. *J. Pharmacol. Exp. Ther.*, 154:324–332.
10. Smith, G. M., Lowenstein, E., Hubbard, J. H., and Beecher, H. K. (1968): Experimental pain produced by the submaximum effort tourniquet technique: Further evidence of validity. *J. Pharmacol. Exp. Ther.*, 163:468–474.
11. Sternbach, R. A. (1974): *Pain Patients: Traits and Treatment*, pp. 20–78. Academic Press, New York.
12. Sternbach, R. A., Deems, L. M., Timmermans, G., and Huey, L. Y. (1977): On the sensitivity of the tourniquet pain test. *Pain*, 3:105–110.
13. Sternbach, R. A., Ignelzi, R. J., Deems, L. M., and Timmermans, G. (1976): Transcutaneous electrical analgesia: A follow-up analysis. *Pain*, 2:35–41.
14. Sternbach, R. A., Janowsky, D. S., Huey, L. Y., and Segal, D. S. (1976): Effects of altering brain serotonin activity on human chronic pain. In: *Advances in Pain Research and Therapy, Vol. 1*, edited by J. J. Bonica and D. Albe-Fessard, pp. 601–606. Raven Press, New York.
15. Sternbach, R. A., Murphy, R. W., Timmermans, G., Greenhoot, J. H., and Akeson, W. H. (1974): Measuring the severity of clinical pain. In: *Advances in Neurology, Vol. 4*, edited by J. J. Bonica, pp. 281–288. Raven Press, New York.
16. Timmermans, G., and Sternbach, R. A. (1974): Factors of human chronic pain: An analysis of personality and pain reaction variables. *Science*, 184:806–808.
17. Timmermans, G., and Sternbach, R. A. (1976): Human chronic pain and personality: A canonical correlation analysis. In: *Advances in Pain Research and Therapy, Vol. 1*, edited by J. J. Bonica and D. Albe-Fessard, pp. 307–310. Raven Press, New York.
18. Von Graffenried, B., Adler, R., Abt, K., Nuesch, E., and Spiegel, R. (1978): The influence of anxiety and pain sensitivity on experimental pain in man. *Pain*, 4:253–263.

Pain Measurement and Assessment,
edited by Ronald Melzack,
Raven Press, New York © 1983.

Visual Analogue Scales

E. C. Huskisson

St. Bartholomew's Hospital, London EC1A 7BE, England

The visual analogue scale is a line, the length of which is taken to represent the continuum of some experience like pain. It is a simple, robust, sensitive, and reproducible instrument that enables a patient to express the severity of his pain in such a way that it can be given a numerical value. It has been useful for studies of pain severity in different groups of patients and particularly in clinical trials. Visual analogue scales can be used to compare pain severity in the same patient at different times or in groups of patients receiving different treatments. The design of a scale may profoundly affect its performance. Problems with visual analogue scales include failure to understand the concept, variation in reproducibility along the length of the line, and doubts about the relationship of the measurement to the true pain experience. Nevertheless, visual analogue scales are widely used and very useful.

CONCEPT AND BEHAVIOR OF THE VISUAL ANALOGUE SCALE

A visual analogue scale is a line, usually 10 cm in length, the extremes of which are taken to represent the limits of the pain experience; one end is therefore defined as "no pain" and the other as "severe pain" (Fig. 1). The patient is asked to mark the line at a point corresponding to the severity of his pain. The distance of the mark from the end of the scale is then taken to represent his pain severity. Most patients with pain understand the concept and can quickly make the measurement (4). Children aged 5 and over can usually manage it (10). The distribution of results in an unselected population of patients is uniform (4); there are equal numbers of measurements at all points on the line. This uniformity is crucial for the sensitivity of the scale, one of its greatest advantages. It is difficult to measure the sensitivity of pain measurements especially since there is no absolute standard. But the visual analogue scale has a greater capacity to change in response to a stimulus such as treatment than the simple verbal descriptive scale. There are not enough descriptions that can reliably be placed in ascending order of severity for pain (9). There is a very high correlation between successive measurements of pain severity on a visual analogue scale, confirming the reproducibility of the method (12). Good correlation also exists between measurement of pain severity by visual analogue scale and other methods (3).

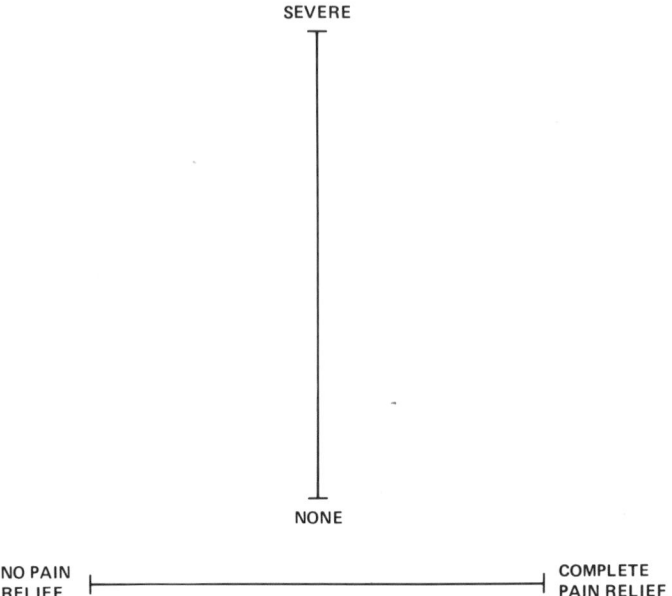

FIG. 1. Visual analogue scales for pain **(top)** and pain relief **(bottom)**. These scales may be oriented either vertically or horizontally.

DESIGN OF VISUAL ANALOGUE SCALES

A 10-cm line is the basis of the visual analogue scale. It should have "stops" at each end, at right angles to the line, to limit the distribution of results (8), and descriptions at each end beyond the stops. Such a simple scale may be vertical or horizontal (13).

The addition of descriptions along the length of the line may affect the distribution of results (11); along a vertical scale they will cause the majority of the results to be grouped around the descriptions. For those results, the scale behaves like a simple descriptive scale, and the sensitivity of the visual analogue will be reduced. This grouping of results does not occur when the line is horizontal, provided that the descriptions are spread out from one end of the line to the other. Numbers should not be placed on visual analogue scales, since preferred numbers like 5 and 10 will attract an unfair share of the results. Scales running from left to right behave similarly to those running from right to left, and it therefore does not matter which is the severe end of the scale (11).

USES OF VISUAL ANALOGUE SCALES

Visual analogue scales are now widely used in clinical trials designed to establish the value of some sort of treatment. Comparisons can be made among groups of patients, although it cannot be assumed that different patients would use the scale in the same way. The same is true of any other method of pain measurement, and the term "moderate" is as open to interpretation as the middle part of a visual analogue scale. The scale is ideal for crossover experiments, enabling one patient to express an opinion about the relative value of different treatments. It can also be used to compare pain scores in different groups of patients, having been used to show, for example, that children with arthritis have little pain by comparison with adults (10).

Visual analogue scales provide a satisfactory method for documenting diurnal variation in disease and differences between diseases (6). They can be used to study the effects of treatment on diurnal variation (5) and to show the time course of the action of a treatment (7).

CONDUCT OF THE EXPERIMENT

Careful explanation is clearly necessary for the patient who is required to use a visual analogue scale. Measurement must also be set within the context of a satisfactory experimental design, and carried out under carefully defined conditions. For example, the person who presents the scale and the form of words used may influence the result. When possible, it is better to measure pain relief directly rather than to measure absolute pain on two occasions and subtract the second from the first (4). The latter technique introduces a mathematical artifact: the change in pain will always be related to the initial score so that differences between groups of patients may explain apparent differences in response. It has been a traditional rule of clinical trials that patients not be allowed to see previous measurements. This introduces an error, especially after long periods of time, in which patients tend to overestimate pain severity (12). It is better that patients be reminded of their previous assessments; many think in terms of change rather than in absolute terms.

SOURCES OF ERROR IN VISUAL ANALOGUE SCALES

The particular advantages of the visual analogue scale are its sensitivity, simplicity, reproducibility, and universality. Although the explanation must be translated, the scale itself is independent of language. All measurements have potential sources of error, and the visual analogue scale is no exception. Some are equally applicable to other methods such as the effects of depression. Others arise in the production or administration of the scale; e.g., photocopying makes the line longer, and an inadequate explanation may lead to failure.

More serious is the suggestion that the scale is not a good reflection of the condition to be measured. In a study of grip strength (2), the correlation between measured grip and a subjective assessment of it using a visual analogue scale was not as good as might have been expected—not even as good as a physician's assessment of grip. It is interesting but perhaps not surprising that patients' views of their impairment do not necessarily reflect the objective phenomenon. But if a patient says he feels weak, he feels weak even if he is not weak; if he says he has pain, he has pain. Another source of error is variation in reproducibility in different parts of the line (1). Normal volunteers asked to reproduce the position of a mark on a scale show their least reproducibility in the region of the golden section (defined as that point on a line that divides it into two segments such that the smaller is to the larger as the larger is to the whole line). This point lies about 6.2 cm along a 10-cm visual analogue scale. Again, it is perhaps not surprising that reproducibility is greatest at the extremes of the line and at its midpoint. But expressing pain severity on a visual analogue scale may not be the same as remembering a point on a line and trying to reproduce it. The correlation coefficients between successive measurements of pain on a visual analogue scale have been as high as 0.99, suggesting that reproducibility is not a big problem in patients (13).

Another problem common to all scales is the limitation imposed by the extremes. If a patient rates his pain at the top of the scale and then gets worse, his measurement can only remain unchanged. This is another argument for the use of pain relief scales whenever possible. The ends are defined as "no relief" and "complete relief." It is impossible to be more than completely relieved. Although it is possible to become worse, the term "no relief" is still appropriate. Deterioration could be measured separately if it were a source of interest—usually it is not.

Very occasional patients are unable to understand the concept of the scale. Intelligent people may have the greatest difficulty, thinking it must be more complicated than it is. They see the top of the vertical scale as the head and the bottom as the feet; the left end of a horizontal scale may be perceived as the morning and the right end as the evening. But failures are very rare with careful explanation and perhaps a little practice. These latter tasks are the responsibility of a physician or clinical metrologist. The actual measurement is the sole responsibility of the patient. No one else knows.

COMPARISON WITH OLDER METHODS

The traditional method for assessing pain or pain relief is the simple descriptive scale devised by Keele (9a). Pain is defined as severe, moderate, mild, and absent; pain relief can similarly be defined as none, slight, moderate, and good. This type of scale is simple and robust but insensitive. Patients with mild pain must be free of pain to show a difference, and it would be nice to measure smaller changes. Nevertheless, this type of methodology forms the basis of most trials of simple analgesics. A pain relief scale is used hourly for 6 hr after drug administration. Differences between drug and placebo are used to calculate the area under the analgesia curve known as the sum of pain intensity difference. Alternatives to the use of words include numbers for absolute pain and fractions or percentages for relief. It is certainly possible to measure the number of patients achieving a particular amount of pain relief, such as 50%, but this is another insensitive method. It will fail to detect a drug with slight but probably worthwhile analgesic properties and will underestimate the value of a curve. It is wise to avoid the temptation of devising new scales. Simple descriptive scales provide a well-tried method, with visual analogue scales preferred because of their additional sensitivity.

REFERENCES

1. Dixon, S., and Bird, H. A. (1981): Reproducibility along a 10cm visual analogue scale. *Ann. Rheum. Dis.*, 40:87–89.
2. Downie, W. W., Leatham, P. A., Rhind, V. M., Pickup, M. E., and Wright, V. (1978): The visual analogue scale in the assessment of grip strength. *Ann. Rheum. Dis.*, 37:382–384.
3. Downie, W. W., Leatham, P. A., Rhind, V. M., Wright, V., Brancho, J. A., and Anderson, J. A. (1978): Studies with pain rating scales. *Ann. Rheum. Dis.*, 37:378–381.
4. Huskisson, E. C. (1974): Measurement of pain. *Lancet*, 2:1,127–1,131.
5. Huskisson, E. C. (1976): Chronopharmacology of anti-rheumatic drugs with special reference to indomethacin. In: *Inflammatory Arthropathies*, edited by E. C. Huskisson and G. P. Velo, pp. 99–105. Excerpta Medica, Amsterdam.
6. Huskisson, E. C., Dieppe, P. A., Tucker, A. K., and Cannell, L. B. (1979): Another look at osteoarthritis. *Ann. Rheum. Dis.*, 38:423–428.
7. Huskisson, E. C., Jaffe, I. A., Scott, J., and Dieppe, P. A. (1980): 5-Thiopyridoxine in rheumatoid arthritis: Clinical and experimental studies. *Arthritis Rheum.*, 23:106–110.
8. Huskisson, E. C., and Scott, P. J. (1977): Floctafenine: A new analgesic for use in rheumatic diseases. *Rheumatol. Rehabil.*, 16:54–57.
9a. Keele, K. D. (1948): *Lancet*, 2:6.
9. Melzack, R., and Torgerson, W. S. (1971): On the language of pain. *Anesthesiology*, 34:50–59.
10. Scott, J., Ansell, B. M., and Huskisson, E. C. (1977): The measurement of pain in juvenile chronic polyarthritis. *Ann. Rheum. Dis.*, 36:186–187.
11. Scott, J., and Huskisson, E. C. (1976): Graphic representation of pain. *Pain*, 2:175–184.
12. Scott, J., and Huskisson, E. C. (1979): Accuracy of subjective measurements made with or without previous scores: An important source of error in serial measurements of subjective states. *Ann. Rheum. Dis.*, 38:558–559.
13. Scott, J., and Huskisson, E. C. (1979): Vertical or horizontal visual analogue scales. *Ann. Rheum. Dis.*, 38:560.

II.
VERBAL MEASUREMENT
OF PAIN

Pain Measurement and Assessment,
edited by Ronald Melzack,
Raven Press, New York © 1983.

The McGill Pain Questionnaire

Ronald Melzack

Department of Psychology, McGill University, Montreal, Quebec, Canada H3A 1B1

Clinical investigators have long recognized the varieties of pain. Descriptions of the burning qualities of causalgic pain (9) and the stabbing, cramping qualities of visceral pains (8) frequently provide the key to diagnosis and may even suggest the course of therapy (8,9). The layman is equally aware of the many qualities and dimensions of pain. An evening of radio, television, or newspaper commercials makes us aware of the splitting, pounding qualities of headaches, the gnawing, nagging pain of rheumatism and arthritis, and the cramping heavy qualities of menstrual pain. The word "pain," then, refers to an endless variety of qualities that are categorized under a single linguistic label (4,9).

In 1971, Melzack and Torgerson (13) began the specification of the qualities of pain. Words used to describe pain were brought together and categorized, and an attempt was made to scale them on a common intensity dimension. Their aim was to develop new approaches to the problem of describing and measuring pain.

CLASSIFICATION OF PAIN DESCRIPTORS

Dallenbach (1), in 1939, compiled a list of 44 words describing pain qualities, and classified some of the words into five groups characterizing (a) the temporal course of the experience, e.g., palpitating, throbbing; (b) its spatial distribution, e.g., penetrating, radiating; (c) its fusion or integration with pressure, e.g., heavy, pressing; (d) its affective coloring, e.g., savage, ugly; and (e) purely qualitative attributes, e.g., achey, bright, clear, dull, itchy, prickling, and quick.

Starting with Dallenbach's words, Melzack and Torgerson obtained additional words relating to pain from the clinical literature and from descriptions given by patients at hospital clinics. The final list contained 102 words. In the course of compiling the words, it was immediately apparent that the list, arranged in alphabetical order, was a meaningless jumble. They therefore attempted to put the words into classes and subclasses describing different aspects of the experience of pain.

In the first part of the study, physicians and other university graduates were asked to classify the words into small groups describing distinctly different qualities of pain. On the basis of the data, the words were categorized into 3 major classes

41

and 16 subclasses. The distribution of a portion of the words is shown in Fig. 1. The classes are: words that describe the sensory qualities of the experience in terms of temporal, spatial, pressure, thermal, and other properties; words that describe affective qualities in terms of tension, fear, and autonomic properties that are part of the pain experience; and evaluative words describing the subjective overall intensity of the total pain experience. Each subclass, given a descriptive label, consisted of a group of words that were considered by most subjects to be qualitatively similar. Some of these words were undoubtedly synonyms, others seemed to be synonymous but varied in intensity, whereas many had subtle differences or nuances (despite their similarities) that may be of importance to a patient who is trying desperately to communicate to a physician.

The second part of the study was an attempt to determine the pain intensities implied by the words within each subclass. Groups of doctors, patients, and students were asked to assign an intensity value to each word, using a numerical scale ranging from least (or mild) to worst (or excruciating) pain. When this was done, it was apparent that several words within each subclass had the same relative intensity relationships in all three sets. For example, in the spatial subclass, "shooting" was found to represent more pain than "flashing," which in turn implied more pain than "jumping." Although the precise intensity scale values differed for the three groups, all three agreed on the positions of the words relative to each other. The scale values of the words for patients, based on the precise numerical values listed by Melzack and Torgerson (13), are indicated in Fig. 1.

Because of the high degree of agreement on the intensity relationships among pain descriptors by subjects who had different cultural, socioeconomic, and educational backgrounds, a pain questionnaire (Fig. 2) was developed as an experimental tool for studies of the effects of various methods of pain management. In addition to the list of pain descriptors, the questionnaire contained line drawings of the body to show the spatial distribution of the pain, words that describe temporal properties of pain, and the overall present pain intensity (PPI). The PPI was recorded as a number from 1 to 5, in which each number was associated with the following words: 1, mild; 2, discomforting; 3, distressing; 4, horrible; 5, excruciating. The mean scale values of these words, which were chosen from the evaluative category, were approximately equally far apart (13), so that they represented equal scale intervals, thereby providing "anchors" for the specification of overall pain intensity.

In a preliminary study, the pain questionnaire consisted of the 16 subclasses of descriptors shown in Fig. 1, as well as the additional information deemed necessary for the evaluation of pain. It soon became clear, however, that many of the patients found certain key words to be absent. These words were then selected from the original word lists used (13), categorized appropriately, and ranked according to their mean scale values. A further set of words—cool, cold, freezing—was used by patients on rare occasions but was indicated to be essential for an adequate description of some types of pain. Thus, four supplementary, or "miscellaneous," subclasses were added to the word lists of the questionnaire (Fig. 2). The final classification, then, appeared to represent the most parsimonious and meaningful

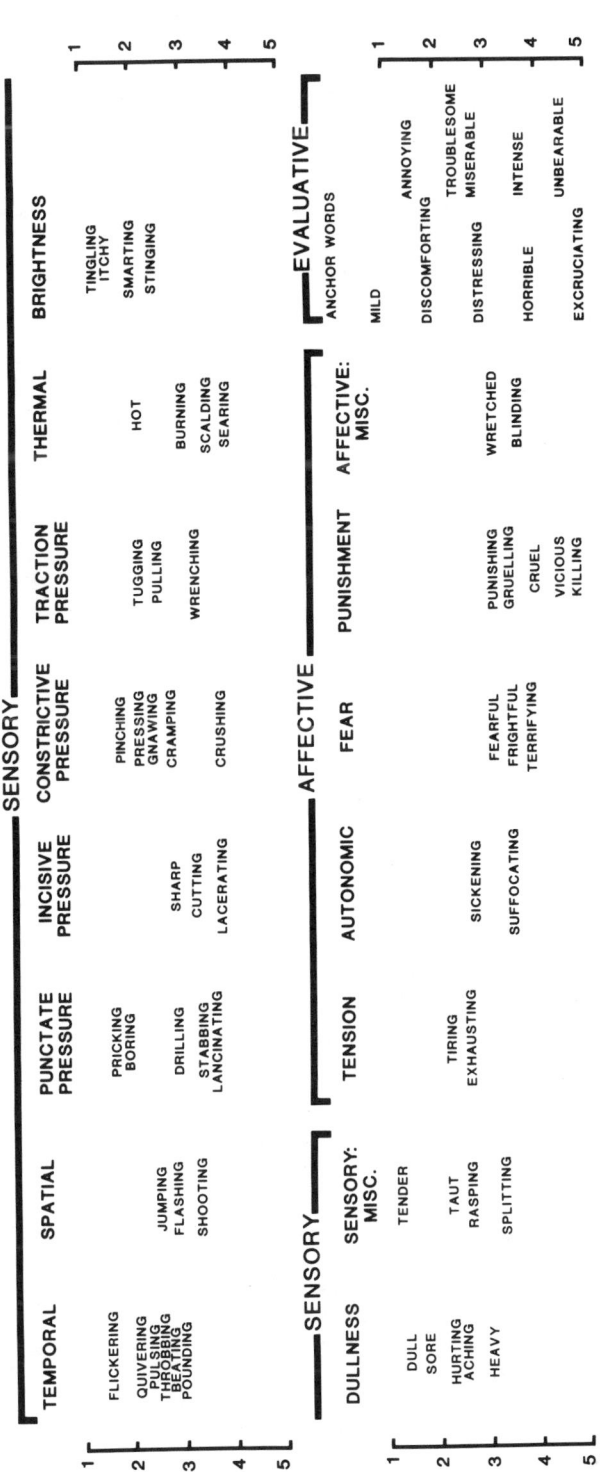

FIG. 1. Spatial display of pain descriptors based on intensity ratings by patients. The intensity scale values range from 1 (mild) to 5 (excruciating). (From Melzack and Torgerson, ref. 13.)

McGill Pain Questionnaire

Patient's Name ————————————— Date ——————————— Time————am/pm

PRI: S————— A ————— E———— M————— PRI(T)———— PPI ——
      (1–10)   (11–15)   (16)   (17–20)   (1–20)

1 FLICKERING	11 TIRING
QUIVERING	EXHAUSTING
PULSING	
THROBBING	12 SICKENING
BEATING	SUFFOCATING
POUNDING	13 FEARFUL
2 JUMPING	FRIGHTFUL
FLASHING	TERRIFYING
SHOOTING	14 PUNISHING
3 PRICKING	GRUELLING
BORING	CRUEL
DRILLING	VICIOUS
STABBING	KILLING
LANCINATING	15 WRETCHED
4 SHARP	BLINDING
CUTTING	16 ANNOYING
LACERATING	TROUBLESOME
5 PINCHING	MISERABLE
PRESSING	INTENSE
GNAWING	UNBEARABLE
CRAMPING	17 SPREADING
CRUSHING	RADIATING
6 TUGGING	PENETRATING
PULLING	PIERCING
WRENCHING	18 TIGHT
7 HOT	NUMB
BURNING	DRAWING
SCALDING	SQUEEZING
SEARING	TEARING
8 TINGLING	19 COOL
ITCHY	COLD
SMARTING	FREEZING
STINGING	20 NAGGING
9 DULL	NAUSEATING
SORE	AGONIZING
HURTING	DREADFUL
ACHING	TORTURING
HEAVY	PPI
10 TENDER	0 NO PAIN
TAUT	1 MILD
RASPING	2 DISCOMFORTING
SPLITTING	3 DISTRESSING
	4 HORRIBLE
	5 EXCRUCIATING

BRIEF	RHYTHMIC	CONTINUOUS
MOMENTARY	PERIODIC	STEADY
TRANSIENT	INTERMITTENT	CONSTANT

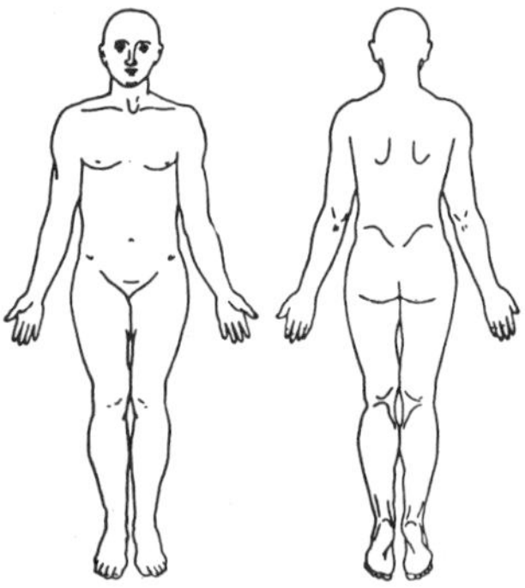

E = EXTERNAL
I = INTERNAL

COMMENTS:

FIG. 2. McGill Pain Questionnaire. The descriptors fall into four major groups: sensory, 1 to 10; affective, 11 to 15; evaluative, 16; and miscellaneous, 17 to 20. The rank value for each descriptor is based on its position in the word set. The sum of the rank values is the pain rating index (PRI). The present pain intensity (PPI) is based on a scale of 0 to 5. Copyright 1970 Ronald Melzack.

set of subclasses without at the same time losing subclasses that represented important qualitative properties.

The questionnaire, during this stage of preliminary investigation, did not have a name but was occasionally referred to as the Melzack-Torgerson questionnaire, or simply as the Pain Questionnaire. As more people became familiar with it, particularly with its use in research at McGill University, it came to be referred to in correspondence among investigators as the McGill Pain Questionnaire (MPQ). A paper describing the properties and scoring methods of the questionnaire (10) was published in 1975. It demonstrated that the questionnaire provides reliable, valid indices of pain, and that it is sufficiently sensitive to detect differences among different methods to relieve pain.

MEASURES OF PAIN EXPERIENCE

Direct Measures

Three types of measures are commonly obtained from the MPQ (10). (a) The pain rating index (PRI) based on the rank values of the words is a scoring system in which the word in each subclass implying the least pain is given a value of 1, the next word is given a value of 2, etc., and the values of the words chosen by a patient are then added up to obtain a score for each category, and a total score for all categories; (b) the number of words chosen; and (c) the PPI, the number–word combination chosen as the indicator of overall pain intensity at the time of administration of the questionnaire. In initial studies, a fourth measure was obtained: a PRI based on the scale values obtained by Melzack and Torgerson (13). However, the PRI scores obtained from rank values and from scale values were found to correlate so highly that the rank value procedure has been used almost exclusively.

Recently, an additional scoring procedure has been used. Kremer et al. (6) calculate a score for each dimension "by summing the rank order intensity value for each dimension and dividing that summated value by the total possible score on that dimension. This procedure yields values ranging from 0 to 1.0, with 0 indicating that the patient selected no words from a particular dimension to describe his pain and 1.0 indicating that the patient selected all of the highest ranked descriptors in a particular dimension to describe his pain."

Measures of Change

Each type of data represents a quantitative index of pain and can also be used to indicate the extent of change in pain quality and intensity as a result of some manipulative procedure. The questionnaire is administered before and after the procedure, and the difference can be expressed as a percentage change from the initial value. If different groups take part in a study of, for example, hypnotic training compared with a control base-line session (11), it is essential that the initial (pretreatment or precontrol) values are not significantly different for the two groups. Several problems are encountered in these computations, such as the great variability in the subjects' initial pain scores. For example, some patients may have low PRI scores, whereas others have high scores. Are changes from the initial values comparable, for example, if 1 patient's score is reduced from 4 to 2 and another's from 30 to 15? Or, if initial scores of 4 or 30 are reduced to 0, both are counted as a 100% change, but does this provide an adequate way to compare procedures since the latter change is relatively more dramatic? Problems such as these are discussed (though not necessarily solved) by Melzack (10). In order to reduce the intersubject variability and to overcome some of the problems raised above, Hartman and Ainsworth (3) have proposed transformation of the data into a pain ratio or fraction: the "pain ratio was calculated for each session by dividing the post-session rating by the sum of the pre- and post-session ratings." They found this procedure effective in the analysis of their data.

A final form of computation may be useful, although work with it is preliminary (R. Melzack and J. D. Katz, *in preparation*). Figure 1 shows that the affective descriptors generally have higher scale values than the sensory words. Yet this information is lost by using only the rank values. Consequently, Melzack and Katz *(in preparation)* have multiplied each subclass by a constant value derived from the mean scale values for doctors and patients (13). The constants for each subclass are the following: 1 (0.69); 2 (1.38); 3 (0.93); 4 (1.59); 5 (0.81); 6 (1.19); 7 (1.28); 8 (0.70); 9 (0.72); 10 (0.94); 11 (1.74); 12 (2.22); 13 (1.87); 14 (1.32); 15 (2.33); 16 (1.01); 17 (1.22); 18 (0.81); 19 (1.0); 20 (1.15). Future research will determine if this procedure allows greater discriminability and sensitivity of the measures.

USEFULNESS OF THE MPQ

The most important requirement of a measure is that it be valid, reliable, consistent, and above all useful. The MPQ appears to meet all of these requirements (see the following chapters in sections II and III), providing a relatively rapid way of measuring subjective pain experience. When administered to a patient by reading each subclass, it can be completed in approximately 5 min. It can also be filled out by the patient in a more leisurely way as a paper-and-pencil test, although the scores are somewhat different (5).

The MPQ has now been used in many studies by investigators at McGill University (2,11,14). Recently, a study of labor pain was undertaken (12) in which it was found that (a) pain levels in labor are generally extremely high, (b) there is great variability among women, and (c) prepared childbirth training diminishes pain by statistically significant amounts, but the pain still remains at a high level, so that the title of a major book in the field—*Painless Childbirth* (7)—is obviously misleading. Although the sensitivity and usefulness of the MPQ is no longer in doubt, there is still much work to be done, and undoubtedly, changes to be made. Melzack and Torgerson pioneered in the measurement of subjective pain experience. New studies, described in the following chapters by many scientists working in several countries, indicate the scope, the problems, and the future of verbal approaches to the measurement of pain.

REFERENCES

1. Dallenbach, K. M. (1939): Somesthesis. In: *Introduction to Psychology*, edited by E. G. Boring, H. S. Langfeld, and H. P. Weld, pp. 608–625. John Wiley, New York.
2. Dubuisson, D., and Melzack, R. (1976): Classification of clinical pain descriptions by multiple group discriminant analysis. *Exp. Neurol.*, 51:480–487.
3. Hartman, L. M., and Ainsworth, K. D. (1980): Self-regulation of chronic pain. *Can. J. Psychiatry*, 25:38–43.
4. Hebb, D. O. (1949): *The Organization of Behavior*. John Wiley, New York.
5. Klepac, R. K., Dowling, J., Rokke, P., Dodge, L., and Schafer, L. (1981): Interview vs. paper-and-pencil administration of the McGill Pain Questionnaire. *Pain*, 11:241–246.
6. Kremer, E. F., Atkinson, J. H., and Ignelzi, R. J. (1982): Pain measurement: The affective dimensional measure of the McGill Pain Questionnaire with a cancer pain population. *Pain*, 12:153–163.
7. Lamaze, F. (1970): *Painless Childbirth: Psychoprophylactic Method*. H. Regnery, Chicago.
8. Livingston, W. K. (1935): *The Clinical Aspects of Visceral Pain*. Charles C Thomas, Springfield.
9. Livingston, W. K. (1943): *Pain Mechanisms*. Macmillan, New York.
10. Melzack, R. (1975): The McGill Pain Questionnaire: Major properties and scoring methods. *Pain*, 1:277–299.
11. Melzack, R., and Perry, C. (1975): Self-regulation of pain: The use of alpha-biofeedback and hypnotic training for the control of chronic pain. *Exp. Neurol.*, 46:452–469.
12. Melzack, R., Taenzer, P., Feldman, P., and Kinch, R. A. (1981): Labour is still painful after prepared childbirth training. *Can. Med. Assoc. J.*, 125:357–363.
13. Melzack, R., and Torgerson, W. S. (1971): On the language of pain. *Anesthesiology*, 34:50–59.
14. Veilleux, S., and Melzack, R. (1976): Pain in psychotic patients. *Exp. Neurol.*, 52:535–543.

Pain Measurement and Assessment,
edited by Ronald Melzack,
Raven Press, New York © 1983.

The Structure of Pain Descriptors

*Warren S. Torgerson and **Mohammed BenDebba

*Department of Psychology, The Johns Hopkins University,
and **Department of Neurosurgery, The Johns Hopkins University School of Medicine,
Baltimore, Maryland 21218

Subjective pain experiences vary not only in intensity but in quality or kind as well. The verbal descriptors people use to describe their pain experiences reflect both types of differences. In 1971, Melzack and Torgerson (6) compiled a list of 102 words that patients use to describe pain. They grouped the words into three broad classes, based on whether they seemed to be primarily descriptive of sensory, affective, or evaluative aspects of experienced pain. Within each of these classes, the words were further categorized into a number of more specific subclasses. Their initial assignments were based in part on their own subjective judgments. The validity of these assignments was then checked by subjects who were asked to agree or disagree with each descriptor's class membership, and some were subsequently reassigned to reflect the subjects' judgments. In addition, several psychophysical scaling experiments, using Thurstone's law of categorical judgments, were carried out on all descriptors, regardless of their class membership. These resulted in numerical scale values of intensity on a single scale for all descriptors.

Melzack (5) used the results of these studies to construct the McGill Pain Questionnaire for the specification of both qualitative and quantitative properties of experienced clinical pain. Despite its rough nature and the simple indices used, the questionnaire has repeatedly proven to be clinically useful (2,4,5).

Melzack and Torgerson (6) realized that the procedures they used to assign descriptors to classes were based largely on *a priori* considerations that were verified using rather primitive techniques. Hence, the resulting classification structure of pain quality was considered to be suggestive rather than definitive. Their aim was "to present an approach which, hopefully, will provide some guidelines for future studies using one or another of the newer, more elaborate multidimensional scaling or classification models."

The general class of multidimensional scaling procedures begins with observations of the relative degree of similarity of pairs of elements from a domain, relates the elements to points in an abstract space and their dissimilarities to distances in the space, and solves for the configuration of points in terms of their projections on an arbitrary set of orthogonal axes that span the space.

It should be noted that the representation of the configuration in terms of projections of elements on axes or dimensions of the space is merely a convenience. The important result is the configuration. Virtually any type of underlying similarity structure can be imbedded in a multidimensional space, with the configuration described by projections on coordinate axes. Hence. additional steps are required to determine whether the structure is in fact dimensional in nature or whether some other structure is more appropriate (10). The key to the solution of this problem lies in the fact that all underlying structures, other than the purely dimensional, place restrictions on the "shape" of the spatial configuration of points. For a pure, nominal class structure, all of the points must lie on the vertices of a multidimensional tetrahedron, with each vertex corresponding to a class (with erroneous data, points within a class would cluster about the vertex rather than lying exactly on it). If the similarity structure is determined both by class membership and by variation on a quantitative dimension, then all stimulus points must lie along the edges of a multidimensional triangular prism (the clusters defining the classes are now clusters about lines rather than clusters about points). This is the geometric representation of the tentative classification model for pain descriptors developed by Melzack and Torgerson (6).

An analytical procedure that can rotate an observed configuration to reveal any nominal class structure or structure resulting from a mixture of class and dimensional variables is now available (3). Research by Bradshaw (1) has shown, however, that the perceived relationships among the pain descriptors are not well represented by a mixed-class dimensional structure. Others have shown that a totally dimensional representation is also inappropriate (7).

Preliminary studies carried out in our laboratory have indicated that the domain of pain descriptors requires a structural model in which, in addition to quantitative variation owing to intensity, each word varies relative to a number of ideal types. Here, instead of each descriptor being a member of one and only one class, it can be similar in different degrees to several different ideal types.

THE IDEAL-TYPE MODEL

In the geometric representation of the ideal-type model, degree of dissimilarity is interpreted as a geodesic distance in hyperspherical space rather than as a Euclidean distance. All stimulus points lie on or within the boundaries of a hyperspherical triangle; pure ideals are represented by points at the vertices of the triangle; stimuli that are completely dissimilar are represented by points separated by a distance of 90°. An efficient iterative solution for this model has been obtained and applied successfully to empirical data in the domain of visual forms (11). The generalization of the ideal-type model to allow for variation in one or more quantitative dimensions leads to a geometric representation in hypercylindrical space. The general model represents stimuli as points in a hypercylindrical space, with distances between points in this space corresponding to dissimilarities between stimuli. The hypercylindrical space can be partitioned into two orthogonal subspaces: a hyperspherical subspace and a dimensional Euclidean subspace. When stimulus points are projected into the hyperspherical subspace, the spherical distances among them reflect stimulus variations due to the underlying ideal type structure. When stimulus points are projected into the dimensional Euclidean subspace, the distances reflect stimulus variations in continuous quantitative dimensions. Computer algorithms for the model have been developed by Satalich, and an operational program is now available (8).

The domain of pain descriptors appears to call for this type of geometric representation. The dimensional portion is Euclidean, and is needed because the descriptors vary in the intensity of the pain they imply. The hyperspherical portion specifies quality in terms of the great circle distance of a descriptor from each of a number of ideal types.

RECENT RESEARCH

A large-scale study is now underway to determine the structure of meaning for the entire set of 102 terms considered in the original Melzack and Torgerson paper (6). Ideally, similarity judgments for all pairs of descriptors would be obtained from each subject. But this would require over 5,000 evaluations of similarity—a task much too formidable for even the most dedicated subject We have found that 20 to 25 stimuli are about all a subject can deal with in a stable, nonsuperficial manner. The research thus requires an extensive series of interlocking studies, involving overlapping sets of approximately 20 descriptors each. The final stage will involve merging the results obtained in the separate studies into a single overall structure.

Empirical data have been obtained and preliminary analyses carried out for several overlapping sets of descriptors. Since the experimental methods, population, and analytical procedures have been, and will be, essentially the same for all separate studies, only one will be described here to illustrate the technique and the results obtained through its use.

The subjects were 16 student volunteers from the Johns Hopkins University. They either received course credit or were paid for their participation. The stimuli for this study are listed in Table 1. They were chosen to represent the brightness, temporal, and thermal subclasses of the original Melzack-Torgerson subclasses (6), plus the descriptor "jumping," which we thought might be close to stimuli in the temporal subclass.

The subject's task was to rate all possible pairs of descriptors on a numerical scale of similarity from 0 (identical) to 9 (very dissimilar). The subjects were asked to use the following context for their judgments: "If the single word ———— best describes a particular pain, how close would each of the words listed below be in describing the same pain?" The blank was filled with a "key" stimulus, and the list was composed of all remaining words. Each word served in turn as the key word.

Each pair of stimuli was presented twice for each of the 16 subjects, once when one word of the pair served as the key term and a second time when the other word served as the key. Judgments with respect to different keys, however, were ex-

TABLE 1. *Projections of descriptors on the quantitative dimension and on four orthogonal ideal-type axes*

Stimuli	Intensity	Ideal-type axes			
		1	2	3	4
Flickering	−0.445	0.388	0.618	0.589	0.352
Quivering	−0.313	0.215	0.577	0.573	0.539
Pulsing	0.003	0.214	0.939	0.260	0.075
Throbbing	0.114	0.175	0.972	0.150	0.014
Thumping	0.012	−0.128	0.939	0.138	0.049
Beating	0.152	0.078	0.970	0.216	−0.064
Pounding	0.133	0.073	0.996	0.039	0.014
Jumping	0.013	−0.098	0.886	0.212	0.395
Tickling	−0.672	0.242	0.259	0.863	0.357
Tingling	−0.424	0.327	0.249	0.871	0.267
Itching	−0.545	0.319	0.125	0.939	−0.038
Smarting	−0.090	0.457	0.299	0.810	−0.209
Stinging	0.098	0.334	0.105	0.937	−0.015
Hot	0.379	0.973	0.055	0.223	0.002
Burning	0.419	0.920	0.064	0.378	−0.068
Scalding	0.588	0.945	0.044	0.289	0.143
Searing	0.579	0.845	0.190	0.489	0.106

pressed in different units of measurement. The first step, therefore, was to convert all judgments to a common scale. The least-square solution developed by Satalich et al. (9) was used.

Once the judgments were standardized, individual subject reliabilities were determined by computing for each subject the correlation between the two scaled ratings of the 136 pairs of stimuli. These correlations (centering around 0.70) indicated that reasonably reliable judgments were obtained from most subjects. For each subject, the two scaled ratings obtained for each pair of stimuli were then averaged and the average ratings then subjected to inverse principle component analyses to determine if systematic individual differences existed. None were found. The ratings for each pair of stimuli were then averaged across subjects. These average ratings, with reliabilities well over 0.90, were used to construct the matrix of dissimilarities. The dissimilarity matrix thus obtained served as input to the hypercylindrical scaling program developed by Satalich (8).

The general program transforms the observed measures of similarity into distances in a K-dimensional hypercylindrical space embedded in a $K + 1$-dimensional Euclidean space. The program then rotates the configuration of points so that the first r axes span the Euclidean portion of the space, and the remaining $K + 1 - r$ dimensions the hyperspherical portion. Two procedures exist to orient the configuration in the correct direction for the precise identification of the ideal types and quantitative dimensions: one is exploratory, the other confirmatory. The exploratory procedure uses the special properties of the model to orient the configuration correctly. The confirmatory procedure relies on information supplied by the investigator about the quantitative subspace to find the proper orientation. The procedure uses this information to rotate the configuration so that its quantitative dimensions correspond best to those provided by the investigator. Varimax rotation procedures are then used on the hyperspherical portion to rotate to ideal types. Because Varimax is an orthogonal simple structure technique and the ideal types need not be orthogonal to one another, an option is available that will allow for temporary adjustments to be made to the radius of the hypersphere as a device for increasing the accuracy of the Varimax rotation procedure.

In the present application, the confirmatory procedure was used. A single quantitative dimension was hypothesized and the intensity scale values of the stimuli, as reported in the original Melzack-Torgerson study (6), served as the target vector for the single dimension of the quantitative subspace.

The results of the analysis showed a very close fit in a one-quantitative dimension, four ideal-type hypercylindrical space. Stress, the usual overall index of a bad fit, had a value of only 0.04. The projections of the stimuli on the quantitative dimension correlated 0.93 with the original Melzack-Torgerson intensity values of the stimuli. Their values are shown in the first data column of Table 1. The configuration of the projections of the descriptors in the four ideal-type hyperspherical subspace is easily interpretable. The projections of the stimuli onto each ideal-type axis are given in the last four columns of Table 1. The first ideal-type axis can be interpreted as brightness, the second is a slow, rhythmic, temporal type of pain, the third is thermal, and the fourth describes a rapid, almost vibratory and perhaps arrhythmic pain sensation. It is interesting to note that no single descriptor closely approximates this type. Flickering and especially quivering are similar to the type, but shade off in the directions of both the temporal and brightness types. Jumping is also related, but is closer to the temporal. In like manner, tickling and tingling are somewhat related although they are both closer to brightness.

The results of the study reported here, along with initial results from five other sets of descriptors, show that the hypercylindrical model describes the structure of meaning of the pain descriptors very well. It appears to be the appropriate structural model for representing both the quantitative and the qualitative variations in pain as revealed by the subjective meaning of the verbal descriptors used by patients when describing the nature of their pain. The quantitative dimension obtained corresponds closely to independent measures of intensity of pain implied by the descriptors, and the ideal types revealed by this completely objective procedure make very good subjective sense. Projections of the descriptors in the hyperspherical subspace do not in general form the tight clusters that would exist if the original Melzack-Torgerson classification (6) structure were correct. Many of the words are descriptive of pains that are intermediate in various degrees between two or more of the ideal types.

A substantial amount of work remains to be done before a complete ideal-type structure of pain descriptors is realized. However, the theory appears sound, and the experimental methodology used appears to yield reliable and consistent results, both within and across data sets. The only theoretical problem remaining is the development of an efficient algorithm for merging the structures obtained in the separate experiments into a single overall structure. This remaining mathematical problem is challenging but does not appear to be intractable.

ACKNOWLEDGMENT

This work is supported in part by National Institutes of Health Grant # GM-29772.

REFERENCES

1. Bradshaw, M. H. (1979): *The effect of context on the structure of pain.* Doctoral dissertation. The Johns Hopkins University, Baltimore, Maryland.
2. Crockett, D. J., Prkachin, K. M., and Craig, K. D. (1977): Factors of the language of pain in patient and volunteer groups. *Pain*, 4:175–182.
3. Degerman, R. (1970): Multidimensional analysis of complex structure: Mixture of class and quantitative variation. *Psychometrika*, 35:475–491.
4. Kremer, E., and Atkinson, T. H. (1981): Pain measurement: Construct validity of the affective dimension of the McGill Pain Questionnaire with chronic benign pain patients. *Pain*, 11:93–100.
5. Melzack, R. (1975): The McGill Pain Questionnaire: Major properties and scoring methods. *Pain*, 1:277–299.
6. Melzack, R., and Torgerson, W. S. (1971): On the language of pain. *Anesthesiology*, 34:50–59.
7. Reading, A. E., Everitt, B. S., and Sledmere, G. M. (1981): The McGill Pain Questionnaire: A replication of its construction. Paper presented at the Third World Congress on Pain, Edinburgh, Scotland.
8. Satalich, T. A. (1981): Hypercylindrical multidimensional scaling: The ideal type model. Doctoral dissertation. The Johns Hopkins University, Baltimore, Maryland.
9. Satalich, T. A., Torgerson, W. S., and Green, B. F. (1982): An analytic solution for the scaling constants in the method of multidimensional category rating. Unpublished.
10. Torgerson, W. S. (1965): Multidimensional scaling of similarity. *Psychometrika*, 30:379–393.
11. Torgerson, W. S., and Satalich, T. A. (1980): Hyperspherical and hypercylindrical multidimensional scaling: The ideal type model. Paper presented at the spring meeting of the Psychometric Society, Iowa City, Iowa.

Pain Measurement and Assessment,
edited by Ronald Melzack,
Raven Press, New York © 1983.

The McGill Pain Questionnaire: An Appraisal

Anthony E. Reading

Department of Psychiatry and Biobehavioral Sciences, Neuropsychiatric Institute, UCLA School of Medicine, Center for the Health Sciences, University of California Los Angeles, Los Angeles, California 90024

The McGill Pain Questionnaire (MPQ) (27) emerged from research demonstrating the feasibility of achieving a meaningful grouping of pain descriptors (29). Since its introduction, it has become a frequently reported dependent measure in both clinical evaluations (16,35) and treatment trials (11,38). It has been also used in laboratory studies in which noxious stimulation is applied to normal volunteers (5,20). It is noteworthy that in describing the questionnaire, Melzack (27) remarked, "The questionnaire presented here, it is hoped, will eventually be refined by investigators in other laboratories and clinics" and "lead to universal tools for the measurement and assessment... of clinical pain phenomena...." The MPQ marked an initial, important step in this direction, by providing patients with an opportunity to describe their pain on a number of dimensions of experience. This explicit recognition of the primacy of verbal report was based on an early collection of words by Dallenbach (6) and the use of patients' pain language in clinical interview. Attempts to relate verbal descriptions to the location of the pain (19) and to psychiatric origin (1,7) had already been documented. The MPQ represented an attempt to systematize verbal description by imposing an organization on the pain adjectives, thereby achieving the quantification of the language of pain.

In the present evaluation, commonly accepted psychometric standards will be utilized in order to judge the degree to which the MPQ satisfies these criteria. The issues to be addressed include: reliability, because pain measures must demonstrate their ability to yield reproducible data; issues relating to validity, in terms of face, construct, concurrent and discriminant validity; and a reappraisal of its internal composition.

RELIABILITY

Considerations of reliability are relevant to all assessment instruments and become particularly problematic where the variable under study is subject to variation across time, as is the case with pain. Assessing the reliability of pain scales is confounded by memory capacity, because the patient may recall the pattern of responses of an earlier occasion, and by the inherent fluctuating quality of the pain experience. In cases in which the pain has changed, what appears to be low reliability may be a reflection of a scale's sensitivity to change. If it is accepted that the generic term "pain" subsumes a number of dimensions of experience, a problem with rating scales may be that they ensure that only one aspect of the experience is responded to consistently. Certain properties of scales are likely to augment their reliability. This issue becomes most salient in the context of the administration of a single rating scale. In a scale that requires a number of judgments for each dimension under study, the reliability of the scores obtained is likely to be increased. Similarly, the complexity of the task will influence reliability; when this is simple, as in the case of paired comparisons involving a choice between only two alternatives, reliability will be enhanced.

Repeated administrations of the questionnaire to cancer patients have yielded a consistency index of 75% (range 35 to 90%) between the first two administrations, which decreased to 66% and then increased to 80% over the course of weekly assessments (14). These figures are comparable with those reported by Melzack (27), in which the consistency of word choices by 10 cancer patients over 3 days ranged from 50 to 100%, with a mean of 70.3%. The profiles obtained in a response to laboratory pain have been examined according to administration format (interview or self-administration), with a broadly similar pattern emerging, even though the mean levels were consistently higher on the interview (21). The words selected on the MPQ have been compared with those chosen from a checklist format, and a broadly similar profile was obtained (A. E. Reading, D. Hand, C. M. Sledmere, *unpublished data*, 1982).

A study by Hunter et al. (18) is also relevant to this issue. They studied the ability of patients to remember their pain and to report it consistently. The MPQ was administered to 16 patients experiencing pain resulting from a neurosurgical procedure (such as lumbar puncture, myelogram). None had organic disorders that would have impaired their recall ability. Pain recall was assessed after an interval of 1 or 5 days. The results indicated high consistency in score profiles among the three occasions. These results lend support to the reliability of patients' retrospective pain reports.

VALIDITY

Face Validity

The increase in the number of studies from a variety of clinical settings that include the MPQ as a dependent measure testifies to its acceptability in this setting. Supplying the patient with pain adjectives may overcome the language barriers that exist in the free-report situation. Moreover, the inclusion of emotional–affective words sanctions their use if they are indicated. It is noteworthy that a preference for verbal scales emerged from a comparison of verbal, visual analogue, and numerical rating scales (23).

Construct Validity

Melzack (27) originally postulated that the MPQ reflected three main dimensions: sensory, affective, and evaluative (29). A number of studies have attempted to replicate these dimensions by subjecting responses to principal-component analysis. Crockett et al. (5) derived a five-factor solution with combined sensory and affective subgroup content, although the degree to which the heterogeneity of the sample (volunteers and patients) and the pain described (clinical, threshold, tolerance) confounded the results is unclear. A survey of back-pain patients (24) yielded seven factors, with the main dimension reflecting emotional adjectives and the remainder specific sensations. However, in this study a checklist format was used, which failed to provide a straightforward test of the MPQ structure. The problems of subjecting binary data, of the form derived from a checklist, to principal-component analysis also deserve consideration.

In a study of dysmenorrheic patients, four factors were derived, comprising two specific sensory dimensions, an affective dimension (descriptor groups 13 and 15), and a principal component accounting for 38% of the variance with loadings on Melzack's evaluative group (group 16), as well as groups 14 and 20 (31). Prieto et al. (31) reported the results of oblique and orthogonal rotation of factors for a mixed-sex sample of back-pain patients. Employing oblique rotation, a discrete evaluative factor emerged (group 16), although this was less pronounced when the data were subjected to orthogonal rotation, with groups 17 and 20 also loading on this factor. Distinctive sensory, sensory–affective, and evaluative factors also emerged from an analysis of 102 back-pain patients (26). Finally, Reading (33) examined the comparability of dimensions to emerge from chronic and acute (benign) pain groups. The factors derived reflected specific sensory qualities and combined emotional–sensory dimensions. The results were interpreted as suggesting that acute pain may involve less differentiation of the sensory, affective, and evaluative components than chronic pain. The results of these studies confirm the distinction between sensory and affective subgroups and lend support to the practice of deriving representative scale scores. An evaluative component has also been distinguished, albeit less consistently.

Construct validity has been also addressed by investigating the relationship between MPQ scores and concomitant assessments of psychological state. Elevations on the affective scale in oncology patients have been related to increased scores on depression inventories (22). Similarly, McCreary et al. (26) attempted to study Minnesota Multiphasic Personality Inventory (MMPI) profiles in relation to MPQ scores. Utilizing multiple regression analysis, with the MMPI results as criterion variables and the MPQ scales as predictors, it was found that affective scores contributed to the prediction of MMPI profiles, with intensity emerging as the best predictor.

Concurrent Validity

The MPQ has been utilized in a number of clinical trials, and information is available on both its concurrent and predictive validity. MPQ scores have been reported to be associated with analgesia requirements (31) and recovery from oral surgery (3). In an experimental setting, MPQ scores for tolerance of noxious stimulation exceeded those for threshold (20). Correlations between MPQ-derived scores and verbal rating and visual analogue rating scales have also been examined. Correlations of 0.39 and 0.10 between the total rank score for the MPQ and verbal and visual analogue rating scales have been reported (33). Similarly, Hunter and Philips (16) found significant correlations between MPQ scores and diary card ratings of headache intensity and duration but not frequency. The magnitude of the correlations that were obtained compared favorably with those obtained from comparisons of linear rating scales (32).

Discriminant Validity

A further approach is to examine the efficiency of the questionnaire in distinguishing among patient groups. This reflects the diagnostic potential of the MPQ and is consistent with clinical observations that patients display distinctive score profiles according to the nature of the pain. A comparison of MPQ profiles of women experiencing pelvic pain showed that acute pain patients displayed greater use of sensory word groups, testifying to the pronounced sensory input from the damaged perineum; in contrast, chronic pain patients used affective and evaluative groups with greater frequency (33).

An extension of this approach has been to subject the MPQ responses of a number of discrete patient groups to discriminant function analysis. Dubuisson and Melzack (8) reported the results of this approach in a survey of 95 patients covering eight clinical pain syndromes. The analysis yielded a correct classification rate of 77% on the basis of the MPQ scores, although this figure may be overly optimistic in the absence of a validation sample (15).

INTERNAL STRUCTURE

In parallel with investigations of the clinical and experimental utility of MPQ scores, research has also concerned its internal composition. The adjective groupings have been investigated, employing maximally different methodological and statistical techniques from those used originally (34). In this study a direct grouping or classification technique was used (39), and the resulting similarity matrix (4) was subjected to cluster analysis (9). The resulting 20-group solution was examined. Considerable similarity emerged between this and the MPQ, although several interesting differences were evident, particularly with respect to sensory groups. It was encouraging that the subjects completed the task without difficulty and that the mean number of groups used was 19, with a range from 7 to 31, indicating this to be a meaningful and manageable task. As in the original study, a clear distinction was observed between groups representing sensory and affective–evaluative words.

A further question concerned the extent to which words within each group lend themselves to ordering along an intensity dimension. A derived 16-group solution was subjected to intensity scaling procedures and multidimensional scaling. The results indicated that although a unidimensional intensity dimension might not be an unreasonable assumption, for a number of groups two or more dimensions were necessary. Moreover, where a one-dimensional solution was appropriate, the scale values assigned to each word indicated that they were not necessarily equally spaced along the intensity dimension (34).

CONCLUSIONS AND IMPLICATIONS

Information is accumulating on the clinical and experimental utility of the MPQ. The questionnaire has performed favorably, displaying acceptable reliability and face, construct, discriminant, and concurrent validity. Greater attention has to be paid to its prognostic precision and questions of incremental validity relative to alternative measures. The attempts to relate MPQ profiles to concomitant state and trait measures have produced encouraging results, and further research of this kind is indicated. Melzack's (27) original objective of developing a universal language of pain is being implemented, as indicated by a comparable form in Finnish (18). Although the authors suggest their methodology is applicable to other cultures, considerable variation in pain vocabulary has been documented (10).

Efforts have been made to tailor abbreviated formats of the MPQ to particular groups (16,25). Unless such formats enhance reliability, a case can be made for using the MPQ unchanged in order to ensure comparability across studies. However, there are indications that the structure and scoring practices of the MPQ may require modification. In particular, the practice of deriving scale score values may be inadvisable until further work has been conducted to determine realistic intensity values for descriptor groups (34). In addition, the degree to which groups uniformly display a unidimensional structure warrants further study. Bailey and Davidson (2) suggest that intensity may be more appropriate for evaluative–affective descriptors than for sensory descriptors. The latter may have greater utility in understanding the nature of the complaint and reaching a diagnosis. This introduces the possibility of imposing different instructions for the different sections of the questionnaire. Sensory words may lend themselves to descriptive interpretation, with greater attention given to the intensity relationships within the affective–evaluative groups. As such a modification would attenuate the questionnaire's ability to quantify the descriptors used, further attempts to define the feasibility of retaining this feature are required.

This leads to a consideration of ways of deriving an index of reliability on each testing occasion rather than relying on normative properties—an important objective with many clinical advantages. Establishing confidence limits would be useful where it is believed that patients have an incentive to project a more severe presentation, or where narcotic analgesia may be distorting perceptual processes (37). Reliability has been assessed by examining the internal consistency of response patterns (36). If it is assumed that words can be ordered along a dimension such as intensity, balanced and repeated presentations of permutations of these permit an empirical test of consistency. Gracely (*personal communication*, 1981) has developed this notion by requiring respondents to complete a number of rating scales, thereby permitting the consistency of responses to be examined.

In conclusion, since its introduction in 1975, the MPQ has proved to be a valuable addition to the range of assessment measures available. No test can be relied on in isolation, and the MPQ is part of a broader assessment battery. Future work is needed to explore the covariation between MPQ responses and other indices, particularly behavioral and physiological. Whatever its future, by introducing this questionnaire, Melzack (27) has accomplished his objectives of focusing attention on verbal report (12,14) and stimulating research on innovative and multidimensional assessment methods.

ACKNOWLEDGMENT

I am grateful to the Nuffield Foundation of the U.K. for a grant to investigate the McGill Pain Questionnaire.

REFERENCES

1. Agnew, D. C., and Merskey, H. (1976): Words of chronic pain. *Pain*, 2:73–81.
2. Bailey, C. A., and Davidson, P. O. (1976): The language of pain: Intensity. *Pain*, 2:319–324.
3. Buren, J. V., and Kleinknecht, R. A. (1979): An evaluation of the McGill Pain Questionnaire for use in dental pain assessment. *Pain*, 6:23–33.
4. Burton, M. (1972): Semantic dimensions of occupation names. In: *Multidimensional Scaling, Vol. 2*, pp. 55–71. Seminar Press, New York.
5. Crockett, D. J., Prkachin, K. M., and Craig, K. D. (1977): Factors of the language of pain in patient and normal volunteer groups. *Pain*, 4:175–182.
6. Dallenbach, K. M. (1939): Somesthesis. In: *Introduction to Psychology*, edited by E. E. Boring, H. S. Langfield, and H. P. Wald, pp. 608–625. John Wiley, New York.
7. Devine, L., and Merskey, H. (1965): The description of pain in psychiatric and general medical patients. *J. Psychosom. Res.*, 9:311–316.
8. Dubuisson, D., and Melzack, R. (1976): Classification of clinical pain descriptions by multiple group discriminant analysis. *Exp. Neurol.*, 51:480–487.
9. Everitt, B. S. (1980): *Cluster Analysis*. Heinemann Educational Books, London.
10. Fabrega, H., and Tyma, S. (1976): Culture, language and shaping of illness: An illustration based on pain. *J. Psychosom. Res.*, 20:323–337.
11. Fox, E. J., and Melzack, R. (1976): Transcutaneous electrical stimulation and acupuncture: Comparison of treatment for low back pain. *Pain*, 2:141–148.
12. Gracely, R. H. (1980): Pain measurement in man. In: *Pain, Discomfort and Humanitarian Care*, edited by J. J. Bonica, pp. 111–137. Elsevier, Amsterdam.
13. Gracely, R. H., and Dubner, R. (1981): Pain assessment in humans—A reply to Hall. *Pain*, 11:109–120.
14. Graham, C., Bond, S. S., Gerkousch, M. M., and Cook, M. R. (1980): Use of the McGill Pain Questionnaire in the assessment of cancer pain: Replicability and consistency. *Pain*, 8:377–387.
15. Hand, D. (1981): *Discriminant Function Analysis*. John Wiley, London.
16. Hunter, M., and Philips, C. (1981): The experience of headache—An assessment of the qualities of tension headache pain. *Pain*, 10:209–220.
17. Hunter, M., Philips, C., and Rachman, S. (1979): Memory for pain. *Pain*, 6:35–46.
18. Ketovuori, H., and Pontinen, P. J. (1981): A pain vocabulary in Finnish: The Finnish Pain Questionnaire. *Pain*, 11:247–253.
19. Klein, R. F., and Brown, W. A. (1967): Pain descriptions in the medical setting. *J. Psychosom. Res.*, 10:367–372.
20. Klepac, R. K., Dowling, J., and Hauge, E. (1981): Sensitivity of the McGill Pain Questionnaire to intensity and quality of laboratory pain. *Pain*, 10:199–207.

21. Klepac, R. K., Dowling, J., Rokke, P., Dodge, L., and Schafer, L. (1981): Interview vs. paper and pencil administration of the McGill Pain Questionnaire. *Pain*, 11:241–246.
22. Kremer, E., and Atkinson, J. H. (1981): Pain measurement: Construct validity of the affective dimension of the McGill Pain Questionnaire with chronic benign pain patients. *Pain*, 11:93–100.
23. Kremer, E., Atkinson, J. H., and Ignelzi, R. J. (1981): Measurement of pain: Patient preference does not confound pain measurement. *Pain*, 10:241–248.
24. Leavitt, F., Garron, D. C., Whisler, W. W., and Sheinkop, M. B. (1978): Affective and sensory dimensions of pain. *Pain*, 4:273–281.
25. McCreary, C. P., Turner, J., and Dawson, E. (1979): The MMPI as a predictor of response to conservative treatment for low back pain. *J. Clin. Psychol.*, 35:278–284.
26. McCreary, C., Turner, J., and Dawson, E. (1981): Principal dimensions of the pain experience and psychological disturbance in chronic low back pain patients. *Pain*, 11:85–92.
27. Melzack, R. (1975): The McGill Pain Questionnaire: Major properties and scoring methods. *Pain*, 1:275–299.
28. Melzack, R., and Casey, K. L. (1968): Sensory, motivational and central control determinants of pain. In: *The Skin Senses*, edited by D. R. Kenshalo, pp. 423–443. Charles C Thomas, Springfield.
29. Melzack, R., and Torgerson, W. S. (1971): On the language of pain. *Anesthesiology*, 34:50–59.
30. Prieto, E. J., Hopson, L., Bradley, L. A., Byrne, M., Geisinger, K. F., Midax, D., and Marchisello, P. J. (1980): The language of low back pain: Factor structure of the McGill Pain Questionnaire. *Pain*, 8:11–20.
31. Reading, A. E. (1979): The internal structure of the McGill Pain Questionnaire in dysmenorrhea patients. *Pain*, 7:353–358.
32. Reading, A. E. (1980): A comparison of pain rating scales. *J. Psychosom. Res.*, 24:119–126.
33. Reading, A. E. (1982): An analysis of the language of pain in chronic and acute patient groups. *Pain*, 13:185–192.
34. Reading, A. E., Everitt, B. S., and Sledmere, C. M. (1982): The McGill Pain Questionnaire: A replication of its construction. *Br. J. Clin. Psychol., (in press)*.
35. Reading, A. E., and Newton, J. R. (1977): On a comparison of dysmenorrhea and intra-uterine device related pain. *Pain*, 3:265–276.
36. Reading, A. E., and Newton, J. R. (1978): A card sort method of pain assessment. *J. Psychosom. Res.*, 22:503–512.
37. Revill, S. I., Robinson, J. O., Rosen, M., and Hogg, M. I. J. (1976): The reliability of a linear analogue for evaluating pain. *Anaesthesia*, 31:1191–1198.
38. Rybstein-Blinchik, E. (1979): Effects of different cognitive strategies on chronic pain experience. *J. Behav. Med.*, 2:93–101.
39. Wexler, K. N., and Romney, A. K. (1972): Individual variations in cognitive structures. In: *Multidimensional Scaling, Vol. 2*, pp. 73–92. Seminar Press, New York.

Pain Measurement and Assessment,
edited by Ronald Melzack,
Raven Press, New York © 1983.

Factor-Analytic Studies of the McGill Pain Questionnaire

*Edward J. Prieto and **Kurt F. Geisinger

*Bronx Psychiatric Center, *The New York Hospital-Cornell Medical Center, and
*Fordham University; **Department of Psychology, Fordham University,
Bronx, New York 10458

Early efforts to measure pain concentrated on global evaluations of intensity by using numerical or verbal scales (4). Although the overall intensity of pain is an important consideration in understanding pain experience, measures that reflect only intensity are insensitive to variations in qualitatively different aspects of pain. Pain is a subjective, multidimensional experience that encompasses sensory and affective components. Verbal descriptions of pain provide terms that reflect the subjectively felt experience and, hence, allow investigators and clinicians to understand the pain experience more fully. The McGill Pain Questionnaire (MPQ) (15,17), which comprises 78 descriptors arranged in 20 subclasses (Table 1), is increasingly being used to measure pain experience.

Several investigators have provided positive evidence regarding the reliability (15), validity (8,16,21), and objectivity (7) of the MPQ. Nonetheless, some of the assumptions underlying the development and structure of the MPQ have been questioned. Factor-analytic studies have been introduced to attempt to determine empirically the dimensions of pain (intensity) and question Melzack's *a priori* conceptualization of the three major pain dimensions.

FACTOR ANALYSIS

Factor analysis is a quantitative technique with which researchers may attempt to analyze the relationships among variables in a set into a smaller set of explanatory super-order dimensions. If a factor-analytic solution is a good one, the relationships among the original variables in the set will be well represented using a reduced set of dimensions. Thus, the most useful factor-analytic solution is one that maximally reproduces the information presented in the original set of variables while employing the smallest possible number of new, super-order-level variables—or factors. Factors are weighted combinations of the original variables that may be used in a predictive and explanatory manner.

Factor analysis may be used to explore new ideas as well as to confirm old ones. In addition, statements may be made regarding what is essentially convergent and

TABLE 1. *Scale names and anchor words of the McGill Pain Questionnaire*

Word group	Scale name	Anchor words
Sensory		
1	Temporal	Flickering/pounding
2	Spatial	Jumping/shooting
3	Punctate pressure	Pricking/lancinating
4	Incisive pressure	Sharp/lacerating
5	Constrictive pressure	Pinching/crushing
6	Traction pressure	Tugging/wrenching
7	Thermal	Hot/searing
8	Brightness	Tingling/stinging
9	Dullness	Dull/heavy
10	Sensory miscellaneous	Tender/splitting
17	—	Spreading/piercing
18	—	Tight/tearing
19	Thermal	Cool/freezing
Affective		
11	Tension	Tiring/exhausting
12	Autonomic	Sickening/suffocating
13	Fear	Fearful/terrifying
14	Punishment	Punishing/killing
15	Affective miscellaneous	Wretched/blinding
20	—	Nagging/torturing
Evaluative		
16	Evaluative	Annoying/unbearable

discriminant validity (3). When two hypothetically similar variables correlate highly with a factor, evidence for convergent validity has been found; when two presumably different variables "load on" different factors, discriminant validity is evidenced. Thus, when seemingly different variables correlate highly with the same factor, questions regarding theory and/or methodology must be asked. Consequently, factor analysis is a tool capable of placing the conceptualization of theoretical constructs on a firm foundation.

Most factor analyses performed in psychology are exploratory rather than confirmatory (9), and the studies of the MPQ are no exception. It is now possible to test, in an hypothesis-testing manner, if an hypothesized number of factors is present in a given set of data by using "maximum likelihood factor analysis." The nature of and the relationships among these factors may also be tested.

Many researchers inappropriately reject factor analysis procedures because they involve a series of subjective decisions. Perhaps worse, however, is that many investigators seek to avoid subjectivity by blindly following the standard default options provided by readily available statistical analysis packages. Decisions inherent in factor analysis may be summarized as choice of model, number of factors retained, and factor rotations involved, and are discussed below[1].

---

[1]These issues, however, are complex and beyond the scope of the present chapter. Comrey (5), Gorsuch (9), Harmon (10), and Mulaik (18) are recommended sources for elaborative information.

The first issue in factor analysis concerns the choice of a factor-analytic model. Among the major distinctions inherent in the choice of a model is the definition of variable commonalities. Commonalities represent the proportion of the variance of a variable that is to be reproduced by the factor-analytic solution. The Full Component model, for example, sets the commonalities equal to 1.00 for all variables, and thus totally reproduces item variance. Commonalities are operationally represented by the values that lie along the diagonal in the variable-by-variable (or item-by-item) matrix, and in the Full Component model are equal to 1.00. Other models set their sights lower and typically estimate commonalities as that proportion of the variance of variables accounted for by all the other variables in the study. (Hence, the reliability of a variable is the upper bound of its commonality.)

After choosing the factor-analytic model to be used and initially analyzing the data, one must subjectively determine the number of factors to retain. This decision should be based on (a) the results of the specific solution, and (b) theory. Too frequently, however, theory is not employed, in favor of the default option of the computer package used—typically, the criterion of Eigenvalue >1.00. Most factor analyses of the MPQ have employed this criterion, which should be used only when variables are clearly continuous and when their intercorrelations are high (5). The implications resulting from the necessity for continuity is that the 20 MPQ subclasses, rather than the 78 descriptors (items), should be factored. Furthermore, the use of the Eigenvalue >1.00 criterion frequently leads to too many factors being extracted (9). Future factor analyses of the MPQ should employ Cattell's Scree test to determine whether a factor is indeed nontrivial in addition to having reasonably sized Eigenvalues. Nonetheless, interpretability of factors is the most important criterion in determining the number of factors for a given solution.

The third decision involves the rotation of the initial factors to a more parsimonious solution—one that will maximize the explanatory power of the solution. Rotation may be performed to match a proposed solution or to satisfy various analytic criteria (the most commonly used of which are Thurstone's principles of "simple structure"). Factors may be left uncorrelated (orthogonal) or may be correlated (oblique), depending on how the investigator envisions the factors. Gorsuch (9) suggests that an oblique solution should be tried first. If the factors are minimally correlated, an orthogonal solution may be substituted. If the factors are moderately correlated (e.g., 0.30 to 0.60), the oblique solution may be retained. If the factors are at least moderately correlated, the factors themselves may be subjected to a second factor analysis with the solutions then interpretable on both levels (the initial factor analysis and the subsequent higher-order analysis). Prieto et al. (19) performed one such analysis, which is described below. Since rotation offers an almost infinite variety of possible solutions, the logic that guides one's choice must be clear and well explicated. Although no rotation is ever perfect, its choice ought not to rely on the fact that it is the default option on a program, or even that it is frequently used.

A final caution must be made regarding the data to be used in the factor-analytic studies. These analyses demand large sample sizes. Gorsuch (9) recommends three or four variables for each expected factor, and Comrey (5) suggests no fewer than 200 subjects per study for the factor solutions to stabilize. Otherwise, the finding that solutions do not agree becomes potentially attributable to the instability of one solution, the other, or both. Furthermore, subjects should be from similar populations. Comrey (5) demonstrated conceptually that if subjects differ markedly in their overall levels of pain, a single factor of pain will result. If, on the other hand, subjects are similar in this regard, qualitative differences in the language of pain will emerge as factors.

PERTINENT RESEARCH

Bailey and Davidson (1) were probably the first researchers to test empirically the hypothesis that intensity is the underlying dimension of variation of adjectives descriptive of pain. They used factor analysis to test this hypothesis and to find additional dimensions of pain, gathering Likert-scale rating data on 39 descriptors from two samples of 93 and 90 students. They employed a principal-axis routine on the data from the first sample, extracting each factor with an Eigenvalue >1.00, and performed a Varimax (orthogonal) rotation. They then employed similar factor-analytic procedures on the second sample, using a Procrustian rotation to ensure a solution similar to that of the first sample. Of the six factors that emerged, only the first two were interpretable. Since the latter four factors were uninterpretable and had Eigenvalues that were similar and close to 1.00, these factors should probably be perceived as trivial. Thus, it may be inferred that Bailey and Davidson found a two-factor solution, with their first and largest factor, as hypothesized, relating to pain intensity. The items that loaded most heavily on this factor were from the MPQ affective and evaluative categories. The factor, however, accounted for less of the total variance than they had expected. Furthermore, Bailey and Davidson provided evidence for the construct validity of the factor in that it was positively related to various other indices of pain intensity. Their second factor was composed primarily of adjectives from the sensory domain. Although the first two factors should be uncorrelated (given the Varimax rotation), the second factor was described as negatively related to the first factor and ratings of intensity. Thus, results from this study must be reviewed cautiously.

Crockett et al. (6) employed a more diverse sample of subjects than did Bailey and Davidson (1) and obtained dramatically different results. Crockett et al. gave the MPQ to 85 back-pain patients and 129 students who had been exposed to experimentally induced pain. Thus, the researchers were able to employ factor-analytic methodology to develop dimensions of pain and compare mean scores of the two groups over each of the resultant factors. These investigators employed a truncated component model of factor analysis (9). Their solution included five factors, which they named immediate anxiety, perception of harm, somesthetic pressure, cutaneous sensitivity, and sensory information. One limitation of their study was that they did not report the proportion of the total variation for which these five factors accounted. Their match to the tripartite model of Melzack and

Torgerson (17) was mixed. Their first and second factors were primarily affective and their fifth sensory. Surprisingly, adjectives from the sensory and evaluative categories comprised the third and fourth factors. Their conclusion that no factor appeared to represent a simple intensity dimension is an important one.

In another study, Leavitt et al. (13) administered descriptors from the MPQ in a randomized order to 131 back-pain patients and reviewed the frequency with which each adjective was selected before conducting their factor analysis. Based on low frequency of selection, 13 adjectives were deleted from the analysis. (This procedure, as well as the randomized adjective presentation, is somewhat questionable and makes interpretation of their results difficult.) They performed a principal-component analysis (truncated component model) on the remaining descriptors. Leavitt et al. extracted seven factors with Eigenvalues >1.00, accounting for approximately 76% of the total variance, and rotated these factors using a Varimax (orthogonal) rotation. The first factor was called severe emotional discomfort. It was composed largely of affective and evaluative items and appeared to represent the individual's personal emotional reaction to pain. The second factor was largely sensory in content but had loadings from all three of Melzack's categories. The remaining five factors represented pure sensory factors and related to specific kinds and extents of pain (e.g., mild skin pressure and severe throbbing pressure). Thus, this study provided generally supportive evidence for the Melzack conceptualization of pain, albeit with two exceptions. It did not provide evidence of the discriminant validity of the affective and evaluative categories, and it suggested further taxonomic work within the sensory category.

Reading (20) performed a factor analysis on MPQ data gathered from 166 dysmenorrheic patients. Although he did not state the type of factor-analytic procedure employed, it may be inferred that it was a form of common factor analysis, probably a principal-axis solution. He extracted four factors, each of which was required to have Eigenvalues >1.00 and to account for at least 10% of the common variance—two somewhat duplicative criteria. He employed a Varimax rotation but provided only minimal information regarding the resultant factors. The four factors accounted for approximately 80% of the variance (presumably of the common variance, although he reports 80% of the total variance). The first factor constituted an affective and evaluative reaction to the pain experience. The second and third factors were from the sensory dimension. The fourth factor was also affective, relating to emotionally distressing aspects of the pain experience. Thus, in accordance with previous findings (13), the sensory category items comprised relatively pure factors, but the affective and evaluative descriptors could not be distinguished.

Prieto et al. (19) employed data from 198 low-back-pain patients in a factor-analytic manner but made numerous revisions in attempting to avoid various methodological problems. For example, rather than using individual adjectives as the units of analysis forming the correlation matrix, they used the 20 descriptive sub-classes, following a procedure employed by Dubuisson and Melzack (7). Furthermore, after using the principal factor method of analysis, these researchers used both Eigenvalue >1.00 and Scree tests to remove trivial factors from consideration.

The remaining four factors were rotated using an oblique rotation, since they perceived no rationale for expecting dimensions of the pain experience to be uncorrelated. The emerging four factors accounted for 51% of the total variance and three of them closely matched Melzack's three-factor model. The first factor represented the sensory dimension and emphasized pressure aspects. The second and fourth factors corresponded to the evaluative and affective categories, respectively. The third factor was composed evenly of sensory and affective descriptors. The factor intercorrelations ranged from −0.27 to 0.58, and, following Gorsuch's (9) suggested procedures, a second- or higher-order factor analysis was performed using the factor intercorrelations as the matrix to be decomposed. A single factor emerged. This finding suggests that whereas summing over all descriptor subclasses may be an effective method of assessing generalized pain intensity, on a different level the factors are qualitatively different, although correlated, aspects of the pain experience.

The study of Prieto et al. has provided the strongest evidence to date that Melzack's model of pain is a useful one. This research team (2) also performed a second factor-analytic investigation using a similar methodology and again extracted four factors. These four included two sensory factors and two mixed factors, representing sensory–affective and evaluative–affective combinations. These results were related to those of the former factor analysis (19) using coefficients of congruence, but the results were mixed. Nonetheless, such replicatons are necessary for the advancement of research beyond the "shotgun" exploratory empirical level.

McCreary et al. (14) employed factor analysis to report pain dimensions found in 102 back-pain patients. Unfortunately, several necessary pieces of information regarding the analysis were not provided. For example, neither the type of factor analysis nor the rationale for retaining four factors was provided. However, based on their description, it may be inferred that principal-component analysis was performed, that the four factors accounted for approximately 56% of the total variance, and that the factors were rotated using a Varimax procedure. Their results support the Melzack model and are reasonably similar to the findings of Prieto et al. (19). Sensory, affective, and evaluative dimensions were represented in pure manner by three of the four factors, with the remaining factor containing a mixture of sensory and affective adjectives, probably representing a fear of bodily harm dimension.

Although interpretation of their factor-analytic results is difficult without knowing critical methodological information, McCreary et al. (14) extended their investigation beyond the factor analysis in a scientifically worthwhile way. They related various Minnesota Multiphasic Personality Inventory scales to their four pain factors and found three scales (hysteria, depression, and hypochondriasis) related to an affective component of one factor, and one scale (hysteria) related to the evaluative dimension. Since they did not report the total number of correlations computed, it is not possible to ascertain if these four significant relationships were more than would be expected by chance, or even if they were originally hypothesized. Nonetheless, this kind of construct validation is needed to interpret the meaning of the dimensions adequately.

DISCUSSION

Factor-analytic procedures for the empirical derivation of the dimensions of pain appear to be a useful approach to the MPQ. Although the research evidence is generally supportive of Melzack's tripartite conceptualization of pain (perhaps even with varying types of pain arising from different etiologies), refinements of the descriptor subclasses are needed. Leavitt et al. (13) questioned the affective–evaluative distinction proposed by Melzack and Torgerson (17). In a study by Van Buren and Kleinknecht (21), intercorrelations of the MPQ scales attained high values, bringing the discriminant validity of the scales into question. A reorganization of the descriptors may lead to refinements of the MPQ.

Reading (20), Prieto et al. (19), and McCreary et al. (14) extracted four factors in each of their studies. In each case, three of the four factors were exclusively unidimensional. In all cases, the affective factor formed part of a fourth mixed factor. Only in the Preito et al. (19) study, however, were the unidimensional factors extracted the same as those postulated by Melzack and Torgerson (17).

In accordance with Comrey's (5) suggestions, research of a factor-analytic nature on the MPQ should improve in a number of ways. One recommended change is to begin research projects of this type with hypothesized numbers of factors and their structures; Melzack and Torgerson (17) have provided a structure to be tested in this manner. Instead of exploring whatever solution emerges from computer-provided options in a given set of data, their three-factor theoretical model should be tested for its explanatory power. To date, no confirmatory factor-analytic studies have been performed on the MPQ. Approaches such as those provided by Jöreskog (11,12) are now needed to test the model in this manner. Only if the model were found lacking would it appear reasonable to explore new models.

REFERENCES

1. Bailey, C. A., and Davidson, P. O. (1976): The language of pain: Intensity. *Pain*, 2:319–324.
2. Byrne, M., Troy, A., Bradley, L. A., Marchisello, P. J., Geisinger, K. F., Van der Heide, L. H., and Prieto, E. J. (1982): Cross-validation of the factor structure of the McGill Pain Questionnaire. *Pain*, 13:193–201.
3. Campbell, D. T., and Fiske, D. W. (1959): Convergent and discriminant validation by the multitrait-multimethod matrix. *Psychol. Bull.*, 56:81–105.
4. Chapman, C. R. (1976): Measurement of pain: Problems and issues. In: *Advances in Pain Research and Therapy, Vol. 1*, edited by J. J. Bonica and D. Albe-Fessard. Raven Press, New York.
5. Comrey, A. L. (1978): Common methodological problems in factor-analytic studies. *J. Consult. Clin. Psychol.*, 46:648–659.
6. Crockett, D. J., Prkachin, K. M., and Craig, K. D. (1977): Factors of the language of pain in patient and volunteer groups. *Pain*, 4:175–182.
7. Dubuisson, D., and Melzack, R. (1976): Classification of clinical pain descriptions by multiple group discriminant analysis. *Exp. Neurol.*, 51:480–487.
8. Fox, E. J., and Melzack, R. (1976): Comparison of transcutaneous electrical stimulation and

acupuncture in the treatment of chronic pain. In: *Advances in Pain Research and Therapy, Vol.1*, edited by J. J. Bonica and D. Albe-Fessard. Raven Press, New York.

9. Gorsuch, R. L. (1974): *Factor Analysis*. W. B. Saunders Co., Philadelphia.
10. Harmon, H. H. (1976): *Modern Factor Analysis*. University of Chicago Press, Chicago.
11. Jöreskog, K. G. (1967): Testing a simple structure hypothesis in factor analysis. *Psychometrika*, 32:443–482.
12. Jöreskog, K. G. (1969): A general model to confirmatory maximum likelihood factor analysis. *Psychometrika*, 34:183–202.
13. Leavitt, F., Garron, D. C., Whisler, W. W., and Sheinkop, M. B. (1978): Affective and sensory dimensions of back pain. *Pain*, 4:273–281.
14. McCreary, C., Turner, J., and Dawson, E. (1981): Principal dimensions of the pain experience and psychological disturbance in chronic low back pain patients. *Pain*, 11:85–92.
15. Melzack, R. (1975): The McGill Pain Questionnaire: Major properties and scoring methods. *Pain*, 1:277–299.
16. Melzack, R., and Perry, C. (1975): Self-regulation of pain: The use of alpha feedback and hypnotic training for the control of chronic pain. *Exp. Neurol.*, 46:452–469.
17. Melzack, R., and Torgerson, W. S. (1971): On the language of pain. *Anesthesiology*, 34:50–59.
18. Mulaik, S. A. (1972): *The Foundations of Factor Analysis*. McGraw-Hill, New York.
19. Prieto, E. J., Hopson, L., Bradley, L. A., Byrne, M., Geisinger, K. F., Midax, D., and Marchisello, P. J. (1980): The language of low back pain: Factor structure of the McGill Pain Questionnaire. *Pain*, 8:11–19.
20. Reading, A. E. (1979): The internal structure of the McGill Pain Questionnaire in dysmenorrhoea patients. *Pain*, 7:353–358.
21. Van Buren, J., and Kleinknecht, R. A. (1979): An evaluation of the McGill Pain Questionniare for use in dental pain assessment. *Pain*, 6:23–33.

Pain Measurement and Assessment,
edited by Ronald Melzack,
Raven Press, New York © 1983.

Pain Language and Ideal Pain Assessment

Richard H. Gracely

Clinical Pain Section, Neurobiology and Anesthesiology Branch, National Institute of Dental Research, National Institutes of Health, Bethesda, Maryland 20205

Clinical and experimental assessment of pain and analgesic mechanisms depends on human verbal description of personal experience. Gracely and Dubner (5) have proposed five properties of an ideal verbal pain measure. These properties are modified and elaborated in this chapter. They reflect the goals of both clinical treatment and research on mechanisms of pain and analgesia.

FIVE PROPERTIES OF AN IDEAL PAIN MEASURE

Property 1: Sensitive Measurement Free of Biases Inherent in Different Assessment Methods

The effect of bias, the tendency to over- or underestimate the magnitude of a pain perception, has been a major focus in experimental studies assessing the effects of expectation, suggestion, social role models, placebo, and similar manipulations on responses to pain either produced experimentally or associated with clinical conditions. The clinician who encounters an overly expressive patient is also concerned with the amount of exaggeration in pain reports.

These biases are constant, tending to amplify or attenuate responses to produce a constant error. Another type of bias results from random errors. This type of bias has been called attention, noise, response variability, and psychophysical performance. Random errors can directly influence experimental measures that include variability in the analysis, such as sensory decision theory (SDT) measures of discrimination, and measures sensitive to changes in attention, such as cortical evoked potentials. Random error also degrades clinical report, reducing the statistical sensitivity of clinical trials. An ideal pain measure would be relatively free of random biases that reduce sensitivity and alter certain experimental measures, and of constant biases that reduce accuracy and validity.

Property 2: Provision of Immediate Information about the Accuracy and Reliability of the Subject's Performance in the Task

The concept of performance accuracy is related closely to the concept of response bias. Certain individuals may be more skilled than others at describing their pain experience. Groups of "good" subjects or patients may provide quality data in either experimental trials or clinical assessments. This concept is recognized in other fields of psychological assessment. For example, the L, ?, F, and K control keys of the Minnesota Multiphasic Personality Inventory assess ability to complete all the items and the validity of the resulting profile. Similar performance scales should be developed for measures of pain experience.

Property 3: Separation of the Sensory-Discriminative Aspects of the Pain Experience from Its Hedonic Qualities

The aim of separation of sensory-discriminative aspects of the pain experience from its hedonic qualities needs little elaboration. These aspects refer to sensory intensity, sensory quality, location, and duration. The hedonic properties refer to the motivational and emotional properties of pain, to feelings of aversion, distress, anxiety, and fear. The separate assessment of these dimensions of pain experience is the primary goal of many assessment methods, a task aided greatly by the use of language descriptive of these dimensions.

Property 4: Usefulness for Clinical as well as Experimental Pain Measurement, Allowing Reliable Comparisons Between These Fundamentally Different Types of Pain

Although experimental pain procedures cannot simulate either the severity or the psychological impact of clinical acute or chronic pain, they do allow a degree of control and measurement not possible with clinical pain assessment. These methods are commonly used to assess the analgesic efficacy of pharmacological and non-pharmacological treatments. The ultimate usefulness of these studies depends on their ability to predict clinical pain response. The value of experimental pain procedures, however, extends beyond the assessment of analgesic efficacy. These methods provide important information about the mechanisms of both pain perception and analgesia. Experimental methods can also enhance clinical pain assessment by procedures in which subjects match clinical pain sensations to those produced experimentally. Most pain assessment methods are specialized for either clinical or experimental pain assessment. An ideal pain measure would assess both in equivalent units, providing information about the common and uncommon factors of experimental and clinical pain experience and the analgesic modification of this experience. Common pain measures also improve the validity of pain assessments that use experimental pain matching (3,12,23).

Property 5: Absolute Measures That Increase the Validity of Pain Comparisons Between Groups and Within Groups over Time

Many psychophysical procedures and rating methods provide relative measures— they assess how stimuli compare in relation to each other. Others assess change in perceived stimulation, often following the administration of putative analgesic treatments. These methods, however, may not adequately assess differences in pain levels between groups or changes within groups that occur over long periods of time. Methods such as numerical rating scales and visual analogue scales provide valid information about immediate change in pain, but they provide information about pain level only if assumptions that a certain number or a certain part of a line represents the same level of pain for different subject groups are made. The face validity of these assumptions may be less than those of methods that anchor ratings to an absolute rather than a relative scale. Examples include verbal descriptors of pain intensity, quality, and unpleasantness and measures of psychophysical performance such as the discrimination measures of SDT or the stimulus integration or stress measures in integration tasks such as functional measurement or conjoint measurement (3,9,13,14). An ideal pain measure would anchor verbal judgments as much as possible.

VERBAL DESCRIPTOR PAIN ASSESSMENT

Almost all pain measures that use verbal descriptors involve the quantification of the magnitude of a specified dimension implied by a subset of words and the use of one or more subsets to quantify pain experience. Subjects and patients typically choose words that best describe what they feel, and the previously quantified values of these words or the numbers of words chosen are used in the data analysis. Prior to pain assessment, these procedures have been used by experimental psychologists to assess semantic relations among word groupings. For example, Cliff (2) used category rating methods to quantify the magnitude of adverb–adjective pairs such as "unusually pleasant," "quite ordinary," and "decidedly bad." These methods were applied to pain assessment in a landmark study by Melzack and Torgerson (17). They used category scaling techniques to produce 16 classes of words describing sensory, affective, and evaluative qualities of perceived pain. Each class consisted of two to six descriptors ranked in order of increasing magnitude. These investigators have each pursued this original work in separate ways. Torgerson and BenDebba *(this volume)* discuss their development of an elegant multidimensional model that uses multivariate techniques to specify the relationships among the original set of pain descriptors. Melzack *(this volume)* describes the development of the McGill Pain Questionnaire (MPQ), probably the most widely used clinical pain assessment tool. This questionnaire uses the original 16 descriptor classes scaled by Melzack and Torgerson, 4 additional miscellaneous classes, and other information such as variation in pain and pain location (16).

The MPQ emphasizes the differences among pains. The magnitudes of several scales vary with the number of qualities selected. Another complementary approach emphasizes the factors common to all pain experience. This measure is also based on psychophysical procedures used by experimental psychologists. Several psychophysicists have used category scales and direct ratio scaling methods to assess sensory modalities other than pain that have both sensory and motivational characteristics. The results of studies of thermal, odor, and taste stimuli have demonstrated that sensory intensity and hedonic quality (unpleasantness–pleasantness) have different psychophysical functions in relation to stimulus intensity, and that usually hedonic, but not sensory intensity, functions are altered by changes in internal states such as hunger or body temperature (18–20).

Tursky (24) used a sophisticated sensory psychophysical technique to rate the magnitude of intensity, sensory quality, and reaction implied by 39 descriptors, many of which are used in the MPQ. Following this example, Gracely et al. (6) used the same methodology to rate descriptors of sensory intensity (e.g., mild, moderate, intense) and unpleasantness (e.g., annoying, unpleasant, distressing), the dimensions used by sensory psychologists to assess temperature, taste, and odor stimuli. The rated words were used as response choices with experimental pain stimuli in studies that assessed the reliability and validity of the resulting functions (7). These words have been recently used to construct the Descriptor Differential Scale (4,5) in which patients assess their clinical pain by rating it in comparison to 24 subscales of sensory intensity and unpleasantness. Each subscale is anchored by a specific descriptor, and subjects indicate if their pain is greater than, less than, or equal to that implied by the descriptor.

VERBAL DESCRIPTORS AND IDEAL PAIN ASSESSMENT

Many methods used to assess clinical pain, such as simple numerical category scales and visual analogue scales, treat pain as a unitary phenomenon assessed only in terms of magnitude. These measures can assess pain in a limited number of ways, such as magnitude of present pain or pain relief. Verbal descriptor methods, in contrast, can ask an endless variety of questions about pain intensity, its unpleasantness, and its qualities of pressure, temperature, or vibration. Averaging responses from multiple measures can potentially reduce the influences of random biases that may decrease the sensitivity of pain reports, satisfying property 1 of an ideal pain measure. These multiple measures also satisfy property 3 because they specify the significant dimensions of pain experience. Considerable evidence with the MPQ (discussed in other chapters) shows that the questionnaire can distinguish among different pain syndromes and that verbal pain reports are composed of multiple independent factors.

An analysis of the response patterns in the Descriptor Differential Scale suggests that these questionnaires can also provide information about the ability of subjects to describe their pain, satisfying the requirements of property 3. For example, responses made to each Descriptor Differential subscale can be compared with the values previously determined for the descriptors that identify that subscale. Preliminary evidence shows that the correlation between these scores provides a measure of internal consistency that assesses subjects' ability to assess their pain in relation to the magnitude implied by the descriptors (4,5). Other studies that assess response patterns to the MPQ have identified patterns specific to particular pain syndromes. Additional research may reveal that scores from this questionnaire that diverge dramatically from syndrome-specific patterns indicate poor psychophysical ability.

Unlike numerical or visual analogue scales, the MPQ and the Descriptor Differential Scale provide measures anchored to the meanings of words. The results of studies (7,9,11,15,16,21,22) that assess the reliability, validity, and objectivity of these meanings suggest that these methods approach the requirements of property 5. They present relatively objective, verbally anchored scales that can be used to compare pain levels in different populations or within populations over long periods of time. The Descriptor Differential Scale, in addition, employs the same verbal descriptors used to assess experimental pain stimulation. It was designed as a research tool specifically to address property 4. It compares the common factors of experimental and clinical pain with a measure common to both pain types.

Property 4 has also been addressed by studies that use a triangular design to compare (a) verbal scales of experimental pain sensations, (b) verbal scales of clinical pain sensations, and (c) direct matches between experimental and clinical pain sensations (3,12). In the first of these three procedures, patients use verbal descriptors of sensory intensity and unpleasantness to rate sensations produced by electrical tooth pulp stimulation. This procedure produces reliable psychophysical functions that appear to satisfy property 3, the separate assessment of the sensory and motivational aspects of pain. Placebo or diazepam reduced unpleasantness but not sensory intensity responses, whereas the narcotics fentanyl and morphine reduced sensory intensity responses with variable effects on unpleasantness (3,8,26).

To complete the triangular assessment, the psychophysical function from the first procedure is plotted on a figure showing psychological magnitude of sensory intensity or unpleasantness plotted against tooth pulp stimulus intensity. The results of the second and third procedures are compared with this function. The verbal assessment of the clinical pain determines a psychological magnitude, and the direct matching determines a stimulus intensity that allows the clinical pain to be plotted on the same figure in the same units. Since any two of these three procedures theoretically predict the third, this clinical point should lie close to the psychophysical function if all three methods are reliable and valid. Thus, this method also addresses property 2, since it provides information about the ability of subjects to perform the task. Experiments using this method have shown that the clinical point does lie close to the function (3,12).

The ability of verbal methods to anchor subjective judgments (property 5) has been demonstrated with experimental pain stimulation. Wolskee and Gracely (25) showed that the pricking pain threshold to thermal stimuli applied to the skin was significantly higher in chronic pain patients than in pain-free subjects. However, when subjects used a handgrip dynamometer to assess the intensity and unpleasantness of these stimuli through a wide range of stimulus intensities, there was no difference between the groups. A verbal descriptor scaling procedure, however, showed a difference and, in addition, provided evidence for the mechanism behind the threshold difference. Verbal descriptor scaling showed that chronic pain patients found the thermal stimuli to be equally intense but significantly less unpleasant. Thus, their increased threshold probably represented a change in affective response and not a physiological change in sensory sensitivity. These results provide additional evidence that verbal descriptor procedures discriminate between the sensory and aversive aspects of pain perception (property 3) as well as provide subjective anchors permitting valid comparisons among different groups of subjects (property 5).

Since descriptors provide symbols of specific pain intensities and emotional reactions, they have also been useful in studies that integrate perceptual and linguistic information. Experiments using functional measurement integration tasks (1) have shown that subjects can average the intensity or unpleasantness of sensation evoked by electrical tooth pulp stimulation and sensations symbolized by a word (9). This method may be extremely useful for experimental pain assessment because it produces three measures: a measure of perceptual magnitude, a measure of psychophysical ability, satisfying property 2, and a measure of response bias, satisfying property 1. A recent experiment using functional measurement methods showed that the perceptual intensity of painful tooth pulp sensations was reduced after administration of a narcotic analgesic. The minor tranquilizer diazepam, however, reduced psychophysical ability without altering perceptual intensity (10).

In summary, just as measures of personality have evolved to consider rating ability, bias, and specification of unique dimensions, pain measures must also strive for a level of sophistication that considers these and other relevant factors. This chapter has presented some of the attributes of an ideal pain measure and examples of how language can help achieve the goals of ideal pain assessment.

REFERENCES

1. Anderson, H. H. (1970): Functional measurement and psychophysical judgment. *Psychol. Rev.*, 77:153–170.
2. Cliff, N. (1959): Adverbs as multipliers. *Psychol. Rev.*, 66:27–44.
3. Gracely, R. H. (1979): Psychophysical assessment of human pain. In: *Advances in Pain Research and Therapy, Vol. 3*, edited by J. J. Bonica, J. D. Liebeskind, and D. Albe-Fessard, pp. 805–824. Raven Press, New York.
4. Gracely, R. H. (1980): Clinical pain assessment: The descriptor differential scale. *Am. Pain Soc. Abstr.*, 49.
5. Gracely, R. H., and Dubner, R. (1981): Pain assessment in humans—A reply to Hall. *Pain*, 11:109–120.
6. Gracely, R. H., McGrath, P., and Dubner, R. (1978): Ratio scales of sensory and affective verbal pain descriptors. *Pain*, 5:5–18.
7. Gracely, R. H., McGrath, P., and Dubner, R. (1978): Validity and sensitivity of ratio scales of sensory and affective verbal pain descriptors: Manipulation of affect by diazepam. *Pain*, 5:19–29.
8. Gracely, R. H., McGrath, P., and Dubner, R. (1979): Narcotic analgesia: Fentanyl reduces the intensity but not the unpleasantness of painful tooth pulp sensations. *Science*, 203:1261–1263.
9. Gracely, R. H., and Wolskee, P. J. (1983): Semantic functional measurement of pain: Integrating perceptional language. *Pain (in press)*.
10. Gracely, R. H., Wolskee, P. J., Deeter, W. R., and Dubner, R. (1981): Differential effects of fentanyl and diazepam on pain sensation and psychophysical performance. *Soc. Neurosci. Abstr.*, 7:340.
11. Graham, C., Bond, S. S., Gerkovich, M. M., and Cork, M. R. (1980): Use of the McGill Pain Questionnaire in the assessment of cancer pain: Replicability and consistency. *Pain*, 8:377–387.
12. Heft, M. W., Gracely, R. H., Dubner, R., and McGrath, P. A. (1981): A validation model for verbal descriptor scaling of human clinical pain. *Pain*, 9:363–373.
13. Heft, M. W., and Parker, S. R. (1981): Perceptual scales for electrical tooth-pulp stimulation. *J. Dent. Res.*, 60(A):383.

14. Jones, B. (1980): Algebraic models for integration of painful and nonpainful electric shocks. *Percept. Psychophys.*, 28:572–576.
15. Kremer, E., and Atkinson, J. H., Jr. (1981): Pain measurement: Construct validity of the affective dimensions of the McGill Pain Questionnaire with benign pain patients. *Pain*, 11:93–100.
16. Melzack, R. (1975): The McGill Pain Questionnaire: Major properties and scoring methods. *Pain*, 1:277–299.
17. Melzack, R., and Torgerson, W. S. (1971): On the language of pain. *Anesthesiology*, 34:50–59.
18. Moskowitz, H. R., Klutzer, R. A., Westerling, J., and Jacobs, H. L. (1974): Sugar sweetness and pleasantness: Evidence for different psychological laws. *Science*, 184:583–585.
19. Mower, G. (1976): Perceived intensity of peripheral thermal stimuli is independent of internal body temperature. *J. Comp. Physiol. Psychol.*, 90:1152–1155.
20. Mower, G., Mair, R., and Engen, T. (1978): Influence of internal factors on the perception of olfactory and gustatory stimuli. In: *The Chemical Senses and Nutrition*, edited by M. Kare and O. Maller, pp. 103–121. Academic Press, New York.
21. Prieto, E. J., Hopson, L., Bradley, L. A., Byrne, M., Geisinger, K. F., and Marchisello, P. J. (1980): The language of low back pain: Factor structure of the McGill Pain Questionnaire. *Pain*, 8:11–19.
22. Reading, A. E., Everitt, B. S., and Sledmere, C. M. (1981): The McGill Pain Questionnaire: A replication of its construction. *Pain [Suppl.]*, 1:184.
23. Sternbach, R. A., Murphy, R. W., Timmermans, G., Greenhoot, J. H., and Akeson, W. H. (1974): Measuring the severity of clinical pain. In: *Advances in Neurology, Vol. 4*, edited by J. J. Bonica, pp. 281–288. Raven Press, New York.
24. Tursky, B. (1976): The development of pain perception profile: A psychophysical approach. In: *Pain: New Perspectives in Therapy and Research*, edited by M. Weisenberg and B. Tursky, pp. 171–194. Plenum Press, New York.
25. Wolskee, P. J., and Gracely, R. H. (1980): Effect of chronic pain on experimental pain response. *Am. Pain Soc. Abstr.*, 4.
26. Wolskee, P. J., and Gracely, R. H. (1980): The effects of morphine on experimental pain response in chronic pain patients. *Soc. Neurosci. Abstr.*, 6:246.

Pain Measurement and Assessment,
edited by Ronald Melzack,
Raven Press, New York © 1983.

Detecting Psychological Disturbance Using Verbal Pain Measurement: The Back Pain Classification Scale

Frank Leavitt

*Rush Medical College, Rush Presbyterian St. Luke's Medical Center,
Chicago, Illinois 60612*

Low back pain is a common medical problem and often occurs in patients who have no diagnosable medical disease or injury (9,18,19). These patients have been observed to differ from other patients with proven medical disease in their psychological status. They have more emotional disturbance as a group, with estimates as high as 80% reported (18).

The need to direct treatment in an appropriate direction for this group has led to an interest in the identification of patients whose low back pain reflects psychological disturbance. This has proved difficult for a number of reasons. Early in treatment, most cases of low back pain are managed in general medical settings, where both patient and physician emphasis is on medical features. Patients are habitually silent about psychological problems (5), and even the most astute of physicians are by their training poorly equipped to evaluate these highly complex processes with any degree of sophistication. As a result, the diagnosis of psychological disturbance is either ignored or based on the absence of evidence of organic pathology (2,10). The latter process carries significant risk for the individual patient because many cases in the undiagnosable group will prove to be false-negatives (16).

These difficulties also stem in part from the fact that few objective measures are available that are sensitive to psychological disturbance and usable by physicians. Of those available, the Minnesota Multiphasic Personality Inventory (MMPI) is the assessment instrument most frequently selected (4,7,15), but it has several major disadvantages for use in the general medical setting. In addition to being long and time consuming, MMPI questions delve into sensitive life issues, which often provokes hostility and resentment because the questions are seen as irrelevant to physical complaints, and as implying that pain is imaginary.

Our own dissatisfaction with the MMPI as well as the need to identify patients with serious emotional disturbance in the general medical setting led us to look at other measures that might be feasible for clinical application. In this process, we examined verbal descriptions of pain on which physicians ordinarily rely as part of the diagnostic process. We found that patients with psychological disturbance differed significantly from patients with psychological disturbance in the following ways (9). They used more words in their description of pain, distributed these words over more pain factors, and endorsed significantly more pain of the affective and skin pressure variety. Additional studies (11) using the same pain terms but different statistical techniques showed that description of pain sensations could be a valid tool for detecting psychological disturbance in patients reporting low back pain.

BACK PAIN CLASSIFICATION SCALE

The Back Pain Classification Scale (BPCS) (11) consists of 13 words that describe pain (Table 1), embedded in a comprehensive low back pain scale. In two studies, scores on the BPCS correctly identified 81.8% of patients with psychological disturbance and 88.8% of patients with organic disease. In the first study, we identified pain words that correctly diagnosed 62 of 63 patients (98.4%) with organic disease of the back and 27 of 32 patients (84.4%) with psychological disturbance. In the second study (a replication), the scale correctly diagnosed 105 of 125 patients (84%) with organic disease and 27 of 34 patients (79.4%) with psychological disturbance. These rates were superior to rates achieved with other measures (4).

Administration and Scoring

The BPCS presents patients with 103 pain terms listed in three columns and asks them to check those words that best describe how their pain typically feels (14). They are encouraged to check all the pain terms that describe their typical pain over the last week.

The BPCS is well received by patients because the focus is on symptoms and is therefore nonthreatening. It can be reliably administered by a secretary or nurse

TABLE 1. *Pain words and discriminant function coefficients*

Pain words	Standardized
Squeezing	0.27
Nagging	−0.34
Exhausting	0.24
Dull	−0.21
Sickening	0.25
Troublesome	0.21
Throbbing	−0.15
Tender	0.30
Intermittent	−0.19
Numb	0.33
Shooting	−0.15
Punishing	−0.52
Tiring	0.23

with a minimum of training. The test is untimed, and is completed by most reasonably literate adults in 5 to 10 min. Reading level is appropriate for most adults with more than 8 years of education. The few words that some patients may not understand can be omitted. Use of a dictionary is not allowed.

The BPCS (11) is scored according to weights (Table 1) derived from discriminant function analysis using contrasted groups of psychologically disturbed and organic patients. Endorsement of pain items with positive coefficients weights patient scores toward the functional category, whereas endorsement of pain items with negative coefficients weights patient scores toward the organic category. The group mean (centroid) for the organic group was -0.46; the group mean (centroid) for the functional group was $+0.95$. Classification function coefficients are computed for individual cases using linear combinations of the pain variables. Cases are assigned to the group for which probability of membership is highest.

Validity

The value of this brief, nonthreatening scale is enhanced by its ability to predict patient performance on generally accepted measures of psychological disturbance. Recent use (12) of the BPCS scale indicated that scale scores relate to the level of psychopathology as measured by the MMPI, a standardized instrument used to detect a wide variety of emotional disorders. Patients diagnosed as psychologically disturbed by the BPCS scale are substantially more disturbed in terms of their MMPI configurations than groups identified as free of psychological disturbance. The psychologically disturbed group as defined by BPCS admits to more somatic preoccupation and immaturity, more interpersonal and intrapsychic conflict, and more unusual and unconventional thinking in responding to the MMPI. Thus, patients diagnosed as psychologically disturbed by the BPCS scale would be diagnosed in a somewhat similar way if instruments specifically designed for the diagnosis of psychological disturbance were directly applied.

The validity of the BPCS was also confirmed in a direct comparison with the two scales traditionally used to differentiate patients with functional back pain from those with demonstrable organic disease (8). The BPCS was more accurate than either the "Conversion V" MMPI profile (Hs-Hy) or the MMPI Low Back Scale (Lb) and was the only scale to exceed base rates. In this study, the three scales were compared for accuracy in detecting psychological disturbance in 91 patients with low back pain who were classified as to the presence or absence of organic findings and psychological disturbance on the basis of objective and independent evaluations. The Lb scale correctly categorized 34 of 91 cases for an accuracy rate of 37.4%. Nineteen of 59 patients with actual psychological disturbance were correctly identified for an accuracy rate of 32.3%. Fifteen of 32 patients without psychological disturbance were correctly identified for a hit rate of 46%. The Hs-Hy MMPI profile classified only 31 cases, or 34.1%. From among these cases, 20 of 31 cases with actual psychological disturbance were correctly identified for a hit rate of 64.5%. The BPCS correctly categorized 71 of 91 cases for an accuracy rate of 78.0%. Forty-three of 59 patients with actual psychological disturbance were classified as psychologically disturbed for a hit rate of 72.9%. Twenty-eight of 32 patients without psychological disturbance were accurately classified for a hit rate of 87.5%.

Two additional validation studies (10) indicated that the BPCS might be particularly useful in assessing cases in which the medical findings are ambiguous. It is generally believed that two categories of patients make up the pain group whose disorders cannot be explained on the basis of clinical findings: patients with undiagnosed but genuine organic disease (false-negatives), and patients without organic disease whose symptoms are secondary to serious psychological disturbance. In these two studies (10), the BPCS scale identified patients free of psychological disturbance as "organic" and the psychologically disturbed patients as "functional," and showed that they resembled patient groups of organic and functional cases identified on the basis of objective and independent clinical findings.

In study 1, pretreatment pain description was compared. Patients identified as organic despite the absence of provable pathophysiology reported pain that was quite similar in both intensity and quality to that of patients with known organic disease. Patients identified as functional described their pretreatment pain differently. Their pain was significantly more diffuse and intense, and was strikingly similar to pain description given by patients with known psychological disturbance.

In study 2, response to treatment was accurately projected on the basis of BPCS classification. Since it is known that patients who are treated medically for problems that are partly or primarily psychological tend to respond poorly to conservative medical treatment (2,3), we predicted that those patients identified as organic by the BPCS would be similar to patients with known organic disease in their response to treatment; those identified as functional by the BPCS would be similar in response to patients with actual psychological disturbance. The findings supported the assumption that those identified as organic would respond better to conservative medical treatment than those identified as functional. Over a 14-week period, both groups improved, but the pattern of improvement differed. In the organic group, improvement was greater, and there was a trend for this group to continue to improve over time in contrast to patients in the functional group, in which improvement was limited to the first 6 weeks. Functional patients reported as much pain on retesting 14 weeks after the onset of treatment as the organic group did prior to treatment.

Effects of Age, Education, Race, Sex, and Religion

A recent study (6) suggests that scores on the BPCS are not affected by a patient's demographic characteristics. A stepwise multiple regression analysis showed that age accounted for only 1.3% of the variance, and that no other demographic variable accounted for as much as 1% of the variance. Thus, the BPCS can be applied in a variety of different adult clinical settings, without need for separate norms based on age, education, race, religion, or sex of the patient.

Reliability

The reliability of the BPCS was confirmed in two separate investigations. In the first, a split-half reliability of 0.89 was obtained with 158 patients hospitalized with a primary complaint of low back pain. In the second, the test-retest reliability was 0.86 after 24 hr again using a hospitalized sample with low back pain.

SUMMARY

The BPCS represents a somewhat novel approach to the assessment of psychological disturbance. Quantified verbal descriptions of pain report are used to categorize the patient as disturbed or nondisturbed. This method reduces patient resistance and irritability. Compliance is readily obtained because patients have little reason to feel defensive or conceal their pain experiences.

The BPCS will probably be found of most value among populations with back disorders that are difficult to diagnose. It is within this group that diagnoses by exclusion are frequently made (2,10). Also, dramatic and labile behaviors play important but poorly defined roles in the diagnosis of psychological disturbance. These behaviors trigger notions of conversion and often lead to the overdiagnosis of hysteria (17). Other studies suggest that patients who respond to stress with rigidity and inhibition are more likely to develop conversion patterns (13). The BPCS should help the physician to avoid mislabeling patients because it provides a more accurate method of identifying the false-negative and functional patients among the otherwise undiagnosable, and seems to identify accurately those patients who can be expected to respond favorably to conservative medical treatment.

The BPCS may also be useful among patients with proven organic findings, since the level of clinical pain in this group often does not correlate well with the level of pathology that is documentable. In a significant percentage of cases, emotional disturbance is suspected to contribute to the level and quality of pain (1,4). In one study, 40% (25/63) of the patients with organic disease were also psychologically disturbed. This suggests that it may be useful to carry out formal and independent evaluations of both the medical and psychological status of patients with low back pain.

Why this particular set of verbal pain descriptors works as discriminators and others do not is unclear from research to date. The shared variance of pain words with MMPI items is only 21%, and does not seem to fit any particular pattern in terms of the sensory and affective divisions of pain experience (6). Much research is still needed to understand the apparently heterogeneous content of the scale as it reflects some pain experience and/or personal characteristics that are as of yet not apparent.

As formulated here, the BPCS is a screening device that relies exclusively on patient language for the rapid evaluation of psychological factors in cases of low back pain. It is most useful as part of a comprehensive evaluation that includes the usual medical examinations and laboratory procedures. The information gained from it can be used in the following ways. When a thorough medical examination fails to reveal significant pathology and the psychological pain indicators are elevated, then a more thorough evaluation of the psychological component is in order. Although the BPCS indicates with a high degree of probablity that a psychological disturbance exists, it does not identify the specific nature of the emotional problems. An in-depth examination of psychological issues should provide the patient with other options in addition to conventional medical treatment. When a medical examination fails to reveal significant pathology and psychological disturbance is also not indicated, then medical reevaluation may be in order. In this instance, BPCS scores may avoid the dismissal of cases that are truly false-negatives.

REFERENCES

1. Beals, R. K., and Hickman, N. W. (1972): Industrial injuries of the back and extremities. *J. Bone Joint Surg.*, 54a:1593–1611.
2. Blumetti, A. E., and Modesti, L. C. (1976): Psychological predictors of success or failure of surgical intervention for intractable pain. In: *Advances in Pain Research and Therapy*, edited by J. J. Bonica and D. Albe-Fessard, pp. 323–325. Raven Press, New York.
3. Burke, F. D. (1976): Lumbar disc surgery, a review of a series of patients. *Br. J. Clin. Pract.*, 30:29–31.
4. Freeman, C., Calsyn, D., and Louks, J. (1976): The use of the Minnesota Multiphasic Personality Inventory with low back pain patients. *J. Clin. Psychol.*, 32:294–298.
5. Frost, H. M. (1972): Diagnosing musculoskeletal disability of psychogenic origin in orthopaedic practice. *Clin. Orthop.*, 82:108–120.
6. Garron, D. C., and Leavitt, F. (1983): Social and psychological correlates of the Back Pain Classification Scale. *J. Pers. Assess.*, 47:60–65.
7. Hanvik, L. J. (1951): MMPI profiles in patients with low back pain. *J. Consult. Psychol.*, 15:350–353.
8. Leavitt, F. (1982): Comparison of three measures for detecting psychological disturbance in patients with low back pain. *Pain*, 13:299–305.
9. Leavitt, F., and Garron, D. C. (1979): Psychological disturbance and pain report differences in both organic and non-organic low back pain patients. *Pain*, 7:187–195.
10. Leavitt, F., and Garron, D. C. (1979): Validity of a back pain classification scale among patients with low back pain not associated with demonstrable organic disease. *J. Psychosom. Res.*, 23:301–306.
11. Leavitt, F., and Garron, D. C. (1979): The detection of psychological disturbance in patients with low back pain. *J. Psychosom. Res.*, 23:149–154.
12. Leavitt, F., and Garron, D. C. (1980): Validity of a back pain classification scale for detecting psychological disturbance as measured by the MMPI. *J. Clin. Psychol.*, 36:186–189.
13. Leavitt, F., and Garron, D. C. (1982): Rorschach and pain characteristics of patients with low back pain and "conversion V" MMPI profiles. *J. Pers. Assess.*, 46:18–25.
14. Leavitt, F., Garron, D. C., Whisler, W. W., and Sheinkop, M. B. (1978): Affective and sensory dimensions of back pain. *Pain*, 4:273–281.
15. McCreary, C., Turner, J., and Dawson, E. (1977): Differences between functional versus organic low back pain. *Pain*, 4:73–78.
16. Nachemson, A. L. (1976): The lumbar spine, an orthopaedic challenge. *Spine*, 1:59–71.
17. Pilling, L. F., Brannick, T. L., and Swenson, W. M. (1967): Psychologic characteristics of psychiatric patients having pain as a presenting symptom. *Can. Med. Assoc. J.*, 97:387–394.
18. Sarno, J. E. (1977): Psychosomatic backache. *J. Family Pract.*, 5:353–357.
19. Wolkind, S. N., and Forrest, A. J. (1972): Low back pain: A psychiatric investigation. *Psychosom. Med. J.*, 48:76–79.

Pain Measurement and Assessment,
edited by Ronald Melzack,
Raven Press, New York © 1983.

Verbal Measurement in Non-English Language: The Finnish Pain Questionnaire

*P. J. Pöntinen and **Heikki Ketovuori

*Pain Clinic, Palomäentie 34, SF-33230 Tampere 23, and **Acupuncture Research Project, University of Kuopio, SF-70101 Kuopio 10, Finland

Pain as a subjective experience is difficult to quantify objectively. Simple rating indices do not reflect changes in the sensory and affective dimensions, which may be essential to understand a patient's suffering. It has been well established that the visual analogue scale is a reliable tool when quantifying acute or experimental pain (8,16), but a substantial number of patients are unable to imagine their pain as a point on a straight line (9,11,16). More complicated pain vocabularies and questionnaires [such as the McGill Pain Questionnaire (MPQ)] provide information on the quality of pain as well as on its intensity (3,6,14). But the MPQ is valid in English-speaking areas only. It is not possible to translate this kind of specialized vocabulary into other languages without losing its validity, since no dictionary contains reliable and meaningful category/intensity equivalents.

THE FINNISH PAIN QUESTIONNAIRE

We compiled a pain vocabulary in the Finnish language (9) for the reason mentioned above. The pain words were classified according to the MPQ and then rank listed. The relative intensities of the rank-listed, classified words were then estimated on a visual analogue scale. The Finnish Pain Questionnaire (FPQ) was formed of those words with numerical values differing significantly from those of other words in the same subgroup (9; Table 1).

It was found that, as with the MPQ (14), different people classified the words into distinct groups with remarkable uniformity. People with widely different backgrounds showed equally great uniformity when constructing an intensity scale. By using the visual analogue scale method, one can form a measuring system that uses a ratio-graduated scale in place of a mere sequence scale (9,18,19). That is, each group of words contains statistically significant increases in intensity when moving from one descriptor to the next. This feature permits the use of complex statistical methods. Moreover, it is possible to obtain an intensity comparison among the groups on the basis of the ratio-graduated scale.

Fifty-six words chosen on the basis of word frequencies and t-test results form the final definitive FPQ. In the FPQ word groups, A and B appear in the sensory–

TABLE 1. The McGill Pain Questionnaire (MPQ) and Finnish Pain Questionnaire (FPQ)

Classes and subclasses	MPQ[a] Pain descriptors	Rank order	FPQ[b] Pain descriptors	Mean values in visual analogue scale ± SD
Sensory				
Temporal	Flickering	1	A Aaltoileva	32.5 23.0
	Quivering	2	Kohtauksittainen	49.5 24.0
	Pulsing	3	Jatkuva	73.4 23.6
	Throbbing	4	B	
	Beating	5	Tykyttävä	40.2 24.6
	Pounding	6	Jumputtava	59.1 19.7
			Jyskyttävä	75.7 18.2
Spatial	Jumping	1	Pinnallinen	19.1 12.0
	Flashing	2	Toispuoleinen	45.0 19.3
	Shooting	3	Säteilevä	55.5 21.8
			Syvä	72.9 16.6
Punctate pressure	Pricking	1	Pistävä	44.6 24.5
	Boring	2	Lävistävä	63.4 22.9
	Drilling	3	Läpitunkeva	72.1 21.8
	Stabbing	4		
	Lancinating	5		
Incisive pressure	Sharp	1	Terävä	43.4 23.3
	Cutting	2	Vihlova	55.1 23.1
	Lacerating	3	Viiltävä	63.1 22.4
			Repivä	78.7 15.4
Constrictive pressure	Pinching	1	Vyömäinen	27.1 16.7
	Pressing	2	Puristava	45.6 21.3
	Gnawing	3	Kouristava	62.9 16.6
	Cramping	4	Tukahduttava	73.4 18.7
	Crushing	5	Musertava	82.3 14.0
Traction pressure	Tugging	1	Nykivä	30.0 20.8
	Pulling	2	Tempova	52.2 20.7
	Wrenching	3	Riuhtova	73.0 18.1

TABLE 1. *(continued)*

Classes and subclasses	MPQ[a] Pain descriptors	Rank order	FPQ[b] Pain descriptors	Mean values in visual analogue scale ± SD
Thermal	Hot	1	Kuumottava	23.0 18.4
	Burning	2	Paahtava	44.1 23.7
	Scalding	3	Polttava	63.5 18.3
	Searing	4	Tulinen	72.4 16.9
Brightness	Tingling	1	A	
	Itchy	2	Kutiseva	22.5 17.4
	Smarting	3	Syyhyävä	37.0 20.3
	Stinging	4	Kirvelevä	62.2 21.2
			B	
			Hellä	25.7 17.7
			Aristava	34.2 20.9
			Kihelmöivä	44.1 23.9
Dullness	Dull	1	Hiipivä	17.6 16.5
	Sore	2	Painava	32.7 15.0
	Hurting	3	Turruttava	56.1 24.9
	Aching	4	Jäytävä	65.1 22.3
	Heavy	5		
Affective Tension	Tiring	1	Ärsyttävä	38.6 21.5
	Exhausting	2	Ahdistava	57.6 25.4
			Tuskastuttava	73.1 19.3
Autonomic	Sickening	1	Närästävä	24.1 15.9
	Suffocating	2	Kuvottava	48.3 20.0
			Tainnuttava	76.2 21.3
Fear	Fearful	1	Pelottava	29.5 21.7
	Frightful	2	Kauhea	50.0 23.8
	Terrifying	3	Karmiva	70.9 19.7
Punishment	Punishing	1		
	Grueling	2		
	Cruel	3		

TABLE 1. (continued)

| | MPQ[a] | | FPQ[b] | |
Classes and subclasses	Pain descriptors	Rank order	Pain descriptors	Mean values in visual analogue scale ± SD
Evaluative	Vicious	4		
	Killing	5		
	Annoying	1	Lievä	9.1 7.9
	Troublesome	2	Kiusallinen	27.0 12.9
	Miserable	3	Kova	57.5 17.4
	Intense	4	Sietämätön	79.7 11.5
	Unbearable	5	Tappava	93.1 5.9
Affective–evaluative–sensory (miscellaneous)	Wretched	1		
	Blinding	2		
Supplementary				
Sensory				
Spatial pressure	Spreading	1		
	Radiating	2		
	Piercing	3		
Pressure–dullness	Tight	1		
	Numb	2		
	Drawing	3		
	Squeezing	4		
	Tearing	5		
Thermal	Cool	1	Viileä	19.1 16.5
	Cold	2	Kylmä	40.9 16.3
	Freezing	3	Hyytävä	68.4 18.3
Affective	Nagging	1		
	Nauseating	2		
	Agonizing	3		
	Dreadful	4		
	Torturing	5		

aFrom Melzack (14).
bFrom Ketovuori and Pöntinen (9).

temporal division. A and B here represent different aspects of the temporal property of pain and form clearly distinct subgroup differences. Moreover, they differ in relation to degree of intensity. The same occurs in the brightness division, which also has A and B groups. The punishment division was eliminated from the FPQ because the translated MPQ words were almost always assigned to the evaluative group. Furthermore, the FPQ absorbed the words comprising the miscellaneous subclasses in the MPQ into their original groups, except for words relating to temperature, which were divided into words indicating warmth or coldness.

For clinical purposes, a pain rating index (PRI) can be formed on the basis of the numerical values of the words included in the FPQ. In addition to the total value [PRI (T)], three other indices were created: sensory, PRI(S), affective PRI(A), and evaluative PRI (E). The FPQ has been tested under various circumstances in which pain has been the dominant factor.

CHRONIC PAIN

Low-back-pain patients answered the FPQ before and after a 3-week rehabilitation period (Fig. 1). The change in the FPQ was also compared with the evaluation performed by the physician in charge of the rehabilitation. There was a good correlation between the PRI(T) and the physician's evaluation ($t = 3.413$, $p < 0.01$, two-tailed). It is remarkable that the change in the PRI was significant in the affective subclass, but not in the evaluative and sensory subclasses (Fig. 1). To obtain the number of words chosen, (NWC) the patients were permitted to choose as many words as they wished from a single list of pain words without subgroups. The NWC should have gained more weight in this procedure. But the drawback of the method was that some patients forgot to list any of the evaluative words. We therefore

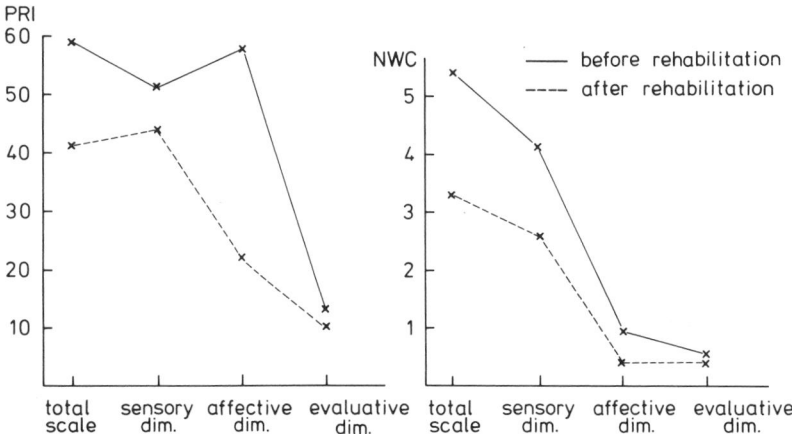

FIG. 1. Patients' estimation of pain before and after a 3-week rehabilitation period based on the pain rating index (PRI) and number of words chosen (NWC). The PRI scores are the means of the visual analogue score values of all the words chosen in each dimension (dim.) or for the total questionnaire. Similarly, the NWC scores are the means of the number of words chosen.

formed a separate list of evaluative pain words and asked patients to choose at least one word from this list in addition to the others.

In routine clinical work, we use the visual analogue scale and the FPQ concomitantly. Patients estimate their pain on the visual analogue scale before and after each treatment session, and the FPQ is checked at approximately 3-month intervals. Patients also draw their pain on a printed figure to show the pain areas, maximal pain sites, and possible radiating pain. In this context, the visual analogue scale seems to reflect primarily immediate changes, whereas the FPQ correlates better with a long-term response.

ACUTE PAIN

One may ask if a positive answer to a general question about pain is an adequate indication for the delivery of analgesics. It has been claimed that the amount of distress a patient expresses is the proper measure of postoperative pain (4). On the other hand, it has been stressed that there are two components in the treatment of postoperative pain: decrease of the patient's discomfort and pain relief per se (2). One of us (H. K.) compared postoperative distress scores and PRIs derived from the FPQ to see if drug delivery was based on distress or on pain as such. Distress score included the following variables: the presence of pain at the site of the wound and its intensity on a verbal rating scale; pain elsewhere and its intensity on a verbal rating scale; disturbances in sleeping pattern; difficulties in concentrating; several affective disturbances: depression, anxiety, crying, moaning, nervousness, anger, irritation, and dissatisfaction with medication.

The most intense pains on the day of the operation and on the first and second postoperative days were estimated on a visual analogue scale, which is useful for the measurement of postoperative pain relief (1,13). The frequency of drug delivery on the day of surgery and on the first and second postoperative days and the total frequency of delivery of analgesics were recorded and compared with the visual analogue scale values of patients with low and high distress scores. The FPQ was administered on the third postoperative day for the definition of PRIs of the most severe and the least intense pains (Figs. 2 and 3).

Despite routine analgesic medication, nearly every patient suffered from postoperative pain. They also had various affective disturbances, especially concerning sleeping pattern and ability to concentrate. It was possible to form a distress score for every patient. They were then divided into high distress and low distress groups (Table 2). The distress scores correlated highly significantly with the total drug delivery, but this correlation could not explain the pain proper measured by PRI. From the results we may conclude that the drug delivery was based more on the patient's affective behavior than on the pain the patient suffered. The distress score may, however, serve as an indicator of postoperative pain to some extent. It is probable that the distress score measures the situational and placebo factors more effectively than the pain itself. Thus, distress appears to be related to the "comfort–discomfort" component of the situation, and the PRI measures pain itself.

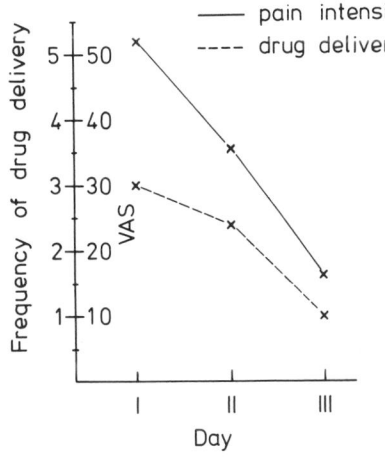

FIG. 2. Comparison of pain intensity on visual analogue score and the frequency of drug delivery on the day of operation (I) and on the first (II) and second (III) postoperative days.

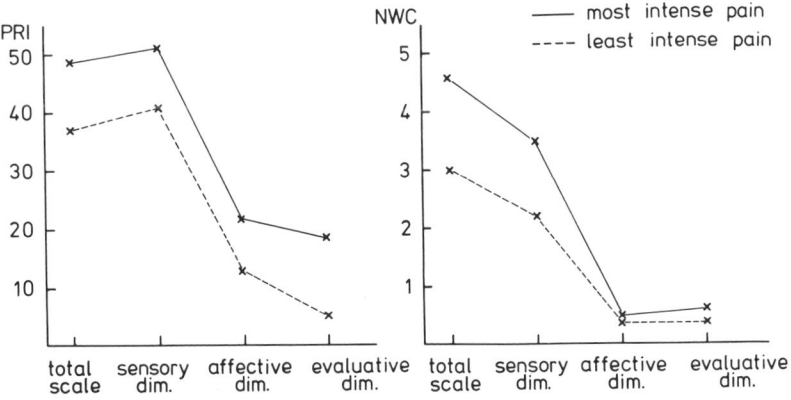

FIG. 3. The most and least intense postoperative pain indicated by the pain rating index (PRI) and the number of words chosen (NWC).

The FPQ was able to differentiate between the most and least intense pains. This difference was shown in the PRI(T), PRI(S), and PRI(E). In the affective dimension, PRI(A), there was no difference. The difference between the low and high distress groups in the most intense pain was the following: PRI(T), $p < 0.05$; PRI(S), $p < 0.01$; PRI(A), ns; and PRI(E), $p < 0.01$ (two-tailed test). For the least intense pain, there were no significant differences between the groups. The visual analogue scale and the FPQ do not exclude each other in the assessment of acute pain, but rather together provide more reliable information about its quality and intensity.

FURTHER EXPERIENCES WITH FPQ

We have long been interested in how nurses estimate postoperative pain. Nurses working in a surgical ward were asked to select those words from the FPQ that

TABLE 2. *Intercorrelations of variables*

	1	2	3	4	5
1 Distress					
2 Frequency	0.65[c]				
3 VAS on the day of operation	0.38[a]	0.40[a]			
4 VAS on the 1st postoperative day	0.44[b]	0.32	0.67[c]		
5 PRI (total) most intense	0.23	0.30	0.38[a]	0.34	

One-tailed testing: [a] $p < 0.05$; [b] $p < 0.025$; [c] $p < 0.005$.
VAS, visual analogue scale; PRI, pain rating index.

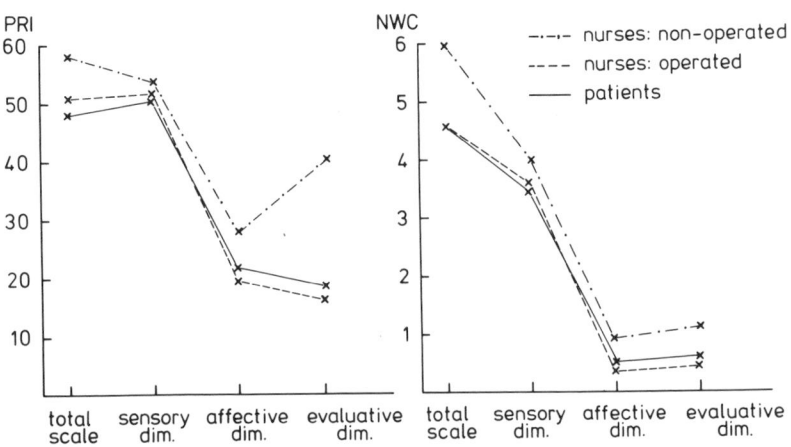

FIG. 4. Maximal postoperative pain estimated by nurses and patients on the pain rating index (PRI) and the number of words chosen (NWC).

reflected the most intense postoperative pain. Nurses who had undergone a surgical operation formed one group, nonoperated nurses another, and patients who estimated their own pain formed a control group.

Patients and operated nurses did not differ in the PRI or in NWC. To our surprise nonoperated nurses estimated postoperative pain with higher scores in the evaluative division (Fig. 4). Clearly, we may use the FPQ for teaching purposes when training nursing staff to understand patients' suffering and pain better.

DISCUSSION

It has been shown elsewhere that the MPQ can be used as a diagnostic tool and also to differentiate between organic and psychogenic pain (12,14,17). In our limited experience, the FPQ has similar properties. It would be important, however, to list the characteristic pain words of common pain syndromes and then check the validity of their differing values.

Changes in chronic pain are reflected both in the visual analogue scale and the MPQ (5,7,15), and there seems to be a good correlation between them (19). In our experience we should use the visual analogue scale and FPQ together, since the visual analogue scale reflects mainly short-term and the FPQ long-term changes. Both the visual analogue scale and the MPQ should have a permanent place in the evaluation of responses to therapy or any changes in long-lasting pain.

It is remarkable that changes in the PRI(T) are sometimes induced by changes in one subclass only--e.g., the PRI(A). How much do we measure discomfort or suffering instead of sensory pain intensity? This is another good reason to use the FPQ and the visual analogue scale concomitantly when evaluating responses to therapy.

REFERENCES

1. Andersen, H. B., Chraemmer-Jørgensen, B., and Engquist, A. (1981): Influence of epidural morphine on postoperative pain, adrenocortical and hyperglycaemic responses to surgery. A controlled study. *Pain [Suppl.]*, 1:123.
2. Beecher, H. K. (1951): Pain and some factors that modify it. *Anesthesiology*, 12:633–641.
3. BenDebba, M., Torgerson, W. S., and Long, D. M. (1981): The structure of pain descriptors. *Pain [Suppl.]*, 1:73.
4. Cohen, F. L. (1980): Postsurgical pain relief: Patients' status and nurses' medication choices. *Pain*, 9:265–274.
5. Corkin, S., and Hebben, N. (1981): Subjective estimates of chronic pain before and after psychoneurosurgery or treatment in a pain unit. *Pain [Suppl.]*, 1:150.
6. Elton, D., Burrows, G. D., and Stanley, G. V. (1979): Clinical measurement of pain. *Med. J. Aust.*, 1:109–111.
7. Gitelson, J., Ferrer-Brechner, T., and McCreary, C. (1981): Assessing treatment response for cancer pain: Use of modified form of the McGill Pain Questionnaire. *Pain [Suppl.]*, 1:150.
8. Huskisson, E. C. (1974): Measurement of pain. *Lancet*, 2:1127–1131.
9. Ketovuori, H., and Pöntinen, P. J. (1981): A pain vocabulary in Finnish—the Finnish Pain Questionnaire. *Pain*, 11:247–253.
10. Kremer, E., Atkinson, J. H., and Ignelzi, R. J. (1981): Measurement of pain: Patient preference does not confound pain measurement. *Pain*, 10:241–248.
11. Leavitt, F., and Garron, D. C. (1979): Psychological disturbance and pain report differences in both organic and non-organic low back pain patients. *Pain*, 7:187–195.
12. Løkken, P., and Skjelbred, P. (1981): Post-operative pain and swelling reduced by injection of a steroid. A controlled trial with bilateral oral surgery. *Pain [Suppl.]*, 1:95.
13. Melzack, R. (1975): The McGill Pain Questionnaire: Major properties and scoring methods. *Pain*, 1:277–299.
14. Nehemkis, A. M., Charter, R. A., Stampp, M., and Gerber, K. E. (1981): Cancer patients describe their pain: The McGill Pain Questionnaire. *Pain [Suppl.]*, 1:151.
15. Ohnhaus, E. E., and Adler, R. (1975): Methodological problems in the measurement of pain: A comparison between the verbal rating scale and the visual analogue scale. *Pain*, 1:379–384.
16. Reading, A. E. (1979): The internal structure of the McGill Pain Questionnaire in dysmenorrhoea patients. *Pain*, 7:353–358.
17. Reading, A. E., Everitt, B. S., and Sledmere, C. M. (1981): The McGill Pain Questionnaire: A replication of its construction. *Pain [Suppl.]*, 1:151.
18. Walsh, T. D., Bowman, K., and Leber, B. (1981): Measurement of chronic pain: Visual analogue scale and McGill-Melzack Pain Questionnaire compared. *Pain [Suppl.]*, 1:15.

III. RECENT RESEARCH USING VERBAL MEASUREMENT METHODS

Pain Measurement and Assessment,
edited by Ronald Melzack,
Raven Press, New York © 1983.

Chronic Headache Experience

Clare Philips

*Department of Psychiatry, Shaughnessy Hospital, Vancouver,
British Columbia, V6H 3N1, Canada*

In the clinical assessment of headache, a central role is given to the sufferer's description of his pain. In the first place, it provides the clinician with the fundamental data for assessment of the severity of the pain problem and thus establishes the basis for any therapeutic interventions. In the second place, the qualities of the pain experience aid the clinician in the diagnosis. There are considered to be two major types of nonorganically determined headache—tension and migraine—of which the former is by far the most prevalent (approximately 80% of headache sufferers; see ref. 18). Although differentiated in terms of their putative psychological basis, muscular and vascular, respectively, the working definitions (10) stress the differing sensory experiences that result from the two etiologies. Thus tension headache is characterized as producing aching, tight, pressing sensations, whereas migraine is felt to entail throbbing and pulsing ones. Physiological assessments of electromyograph (EMG) levels or arterial responses are rarely performed to confirm the headache classification. It is the patient's recall of pain experiences that contributes to the differential diagnosis.

During the last decade, psychologists have become increasingly interested in the problem of chronic pain, particularly headache (9). However, the assessment of pain experience has been circumscribed and limited in scope. Analogue or adjective scales to assess the intensity of pain have been incorporated in the daily recording of episodes in a headache diary (7). Although the self-monitoring methods have varied extensively, the aims have been similar: to provide data on the severity of the headaches and their characteristic pattern (frequency and duration). The result has been a preoccupation with the intensity of headache pain, thus implying a single sensory dimension that varies merely in severity. The limitations of this view of pain experience have been made clear in Melzack's (16) systematic exploration of the variety of stable linguistic labels available for describing distinguishable pain experiences (8). The concern for intensity alone has led to the neglect of the sensory qualities of headache pain.

There are a number of reasons why it has now become important to utilize a finer-grained analysis of pain experience, and no longer continue to rely on intensity judgments alone. (a) During the last few years, the diagnostic division of headaches into two clear-cut types has been challenged (3,20,21,28). Sustained tension in the neck, head, and shoulders has not been confirmed as the necessary and distinguishing feature of only one type of headache. A substantial proportion of so-called "tension" sufferers have no detectable muscular abnormalities (4,6,15,19,25), while high EMG levels are often found in migraine. This implies that two distinguishable pain experiences may not be produced. Bakal (2,3) has suggested that headache may be better conceived along an intensity dimension or continuum, with increasing vascular characteristics as severity increases. Were severity equated, it would follow that migraine and tension are indistinguishable with respect to pain experience and associated symptoms. (b) Intensity, frequency, and duration characteristics of an individual's pain problem have been found to be blunt assessment tools. Individuals may be equal in these respects, and yet have various physiological and behavioral correlates of their problems (23,24). But of even greater importance, equally intense pain judgments conceal different amounts and qualities of sensory, affective, and evaluative pain experiences (11). Thus the group "tension headache" is in fact a heterogeneous group of chronic pain cases. A clinician must assess the qualities of the pain experience in order to determine the nature of the problem. (c) Different psychological approaches to the treatment of tension headache have been found to produce remarkably similar effects. Biofeedback and progressive relaxation, the two most popular, appear to be equally efficacious (14,17). However, it is now unclear how these results are produced (23–27). Biofeedback appears not to operate on the basis of specific muscular retraining, and developed self-control (1,23) and nonpsychological or "nonspecific" factors seem to mediate symptom improvement. It is important to identify these psychological influences and to clarify their mode of action (that is, via behavioral change or affective pain reaction) to advance further in these studies. An adequate assessment of the qualities of pain experience will be vital in order to tackle these issues properly.

MAJOR FINDINGS

We have recently begun to take a more detailed, fine-grained approach to the experience of headache—the qualities of the pain reported by tension headache sufferers. The development of the McGill Pain Questionnaire (MPQ) (8,16) has provided the assessment instrument necessary to evaluate the pain qualities and to compare headache cases with other chronic pain groups (phantom limb, cancer, etc.).

After more sinister organic bases (such as tumor) have been ruled out, headache is considered a minor health problem. Rather like the common cold, it is seen as a periodic irritant: reversible and not life threatening. However, for anyone dealing with severe chronic pain problems—whether headache or cancer—it is evident that the problem can be far from minor, leading to profound changes in the quality of the sufferers' daily life and relationships. In headache sufferers, we have found the levels of pain experienced by severe chronic cases [MPQ pain rating index, total;

PRI (T)] to be approximately the same as those reported by Melzack (16) for cancer, phantom limb pain, and postherpetic neuralgia (11). The affective pain qualities [PRI (A)] in tension headache (from a psychiatric population) were considerably higher than in any of the severe pain groups reported (menstrual, arthritis, cancer, dental, back, phantom limb, or postherpetic neuralgia). In light of this, the therapeutic neglect of this pain in psychiatric illness is astonishing (26).

Looking at the sensory qualities of the headache experience, we have found chronic tension and migraine to be remarkably similar, whether drawn from the general population or a psychiatric group (12). The most commonly used MPQ scales were: No. 1, temporal (i.e., pulsing, beating, etc.); No. 3, punctate pressure (i.e., boring, stabbing); No. 5, constrictive pressure (i.e., pinching, pressing); No. 9, dullness (i.e., hurting, aching); No. 18 (i.e., tight, numb, etc.); and No. 20 (i.e., nagging, nauseating). The only difference between tension and migraine with respect to these sensory descriptions lay in the more frequent use of the spatial scale (No. 2, i.e., jumping, shooting) and incisive pressure scale (No. 4, i.e., sharp, cutting) by migraine cases. An analysis of specific pain descriptors showed that the previously favored discriminating sensory adjectives ("throbbing" and "tight") were used equally frequently by both tension and migraine sufferers.

Consequently, it appears that the sensory experience of headache is very similar in headache sufferers, irrespective of their medical diagnosis into tension and migraine types. Differences do emerge, however, if we look at the affective scales. Although a high proportion (approximately 80%) of both groups reported the pain as "tiring" or "exhausting" (tension scale), they responded differently on three of the affective scales: the autonomic, fear, and punishment scales. Migraine cases experienced more "sickening" and "suffocating" pain, whereas tension cases experienced more "fearful," "punishing," etc. pain. Thus, with respect to the affective qualities of the experience, the two groups are distinguishable. We are currently investigating the extent to which the affective adjectives may in fact be separable into a number of clusters. A cluster analysis has revealed distinguishable groups of adjectives suggestive of anxiety/depression and discomfort (M. Hunter, C. Philips, *in preparation*, 1982). Assessment of these ingredients of the emotional experience may be of great importance in understanding the chronic sufferer.

These studies of headache were undertaken on subjects with equally severe headache problems (on the basis of intensity, frequency, and duration). Thus, the continuum view of headache would have predicted comparable experiences to be reported by such a group. In fact, the results reviewed above are not consistent with this, in that differences were found between migraine and tension sufferers on certain scales—both sensory and affective. On the other hand, the remarkable overlap on most of the sensory scales, especially on those entailing the traditional discriminating sensations (throbbing and aching), must throw doubt on the traditional distinction between migraine and tension headache experiences. This further supports the growing evidence suggesting that our current medical view of these pain problems are inadequate (22). By clustering individuals in terms of the quality of their pain experience (M. Hunter, C. Philips, *in preparation*, 1982), we have found four distinguishable groupings, equally represented by the former migraine and tension headache types. This is a preliminary attempt to develop a psychological differentiation into subgroups on the basis of the subjective pain descriptors. Although only the first step in developing an alternative classification, it may provide a basis for selecting the appropriate treatment approach for the individual case.

It has been argued that scales such as the MPQ cannot be useful in studying pain because like all verbal reports, they are irredeemably influenced by memory distortions and personality differences. Often a sufferer does not describe a current pain, but comes to the clinician and reports on how he remembers his suffering. Jones (13), expressing a commonly held belief, asserted that pain is hard to imagine or recall. Melzack (16) advised that the MPQ be used while the sufferer is in pain, presumably to minimize inaccuracy owing to memory loss or distortions. However, this gravely limits the utility of the instrument in a clinical setting.

We recently carried out a study (12) to see if this restriction is necessary. Over a 5-day period, remarkably accurate recall of the qualities of headache pain was found. The recall was, in fact, as good for pain descriptors as for incidental cognitive material. Seventy-six percent of the cases chose exactly the same word or words for the sensory pain ratings. The correlation of the various measures between the original pain assessment and 5 days after (pain recall) was as follows: present pain intensity (PPI), 0.94; sensory qualities [PRI(S)], 0.83; and affective qualities [PRI(A)], 0.95. It is therefore clear that pain reports, at least over short periods, have a reassuring accuracy and reliability. The qualities of the experience are remembered just as accurately as the overall rating of the remembered PPI. This study was carried out on neurologically induced headache (post-air-encephalograms, lumbar puncture, etc.), and the recall is likely to be even greater in chronic pain cases in which repeated experience would be expected to benefit memory storage.

The other source of error in verbal reports of pain experience is often claimed to be a function of the personality differences of sufferers. The neurotic, extroverted pain cases tend to complain more readily of their problem (5), and it is feasible that the MPQ may become a measure of these personality differences rather than an independent assessment instrument. In fact, we have found no correlation between any of the MPQ indices and the Eysenck Personality Questionnaire assessment of personality (11). Affective pain qualities [PRI(A)] did not correlate with neuroticism. This suggests that these pain responses are not associated with trait measures. Their relationship with current emotional (depression and/or anxiety) state is, however, an area that will need careful future study. Our data (11) have shown strong significant relationships between both PPI and affective pain qualities [PRI(A)], as well as an assessment of depression (Wakefield Depression Scale; see ref. 29).

CONCLUSION AND SUMMARY

There has been a reluctance among headache researchers to assess in detail the qualities of the pain experience, despite the fact that this information is of particular importance to the clinician. Several investigations of chronic headache have introduced the MPQ in order to extend the evaluation from an intensity dimension alone to the varied sensory and affective aspects of the pain.

Headache as a chronic pain problem appears as severe to sufferers as that of phantom limb or cancer. This fact helps explain the extent of behavioral disruption and the emotional problems that so often accompany the headache symptom in severe cases (25). Also, it is an important reminder that the suffering of these individuals should not be underestimated. Chronic pain is too often assumed to be an expression of depression, and its active role in producing a state of helplessness and depression is ignored. The association of affective pain qualities and depression makes it important to consider these issues in more detail in future studies.

The expected sensory differentiation of tension and migraine headache (in terms of throbbing and aching sensation) has not been confirmed, thus supporting the growing evidence that there are not two clear-cut physiological causes of these disorders. However, certain sensory and affective descriptors have emerged that have not been focused on before. It is possible that these scales may be of use in differential diagnosis of tension and migraine. If such distinctions prove to have implications for the choice of treatment, pain quality assessment could prove useful to the clinician. At present, the distinction of tension and migraine appears to make little difference to the choice of a psychological treatment (14,17), but it is still considered relevant in the selection of an appropriate drug regimen.

Analysis of the pain experience has not supported a continuum view of headache, nor has it entirely supported the prevailing medical model. Future studies will have to assess severe and mild cases of both tension and migraine to clarify this issue further.

Our current studies (M. Hunter, C. Philips, *in preparation*, 1982) on pain qualities suggest that an alternative approach may be more fruitful. Ignoring the division into migraine and tension, it has been possible, using a cluster analysis, to group headache sufferers in terms of the psychological qualities of their pain experience. Four separable clusters emerged that discriminate between subjects more adequately than the migraine—tension diagnosis. Future work must investigate to what extent these clusters have implications for treatment and management.

Finally, the pronounced affective pain qualities in the experience of tension headache in a psychiatric group are likely to have implications for treatment choice. Progressive relaxation treatment has been shown to be remarkably powerful for a group of severe cases (24), whereas biofeedback had no effect on their pain problem (23). The power of relaxation training may lie in the specific effect it has on the affective aspect of pain experience, and may be the treatment of choice when this aspect of experience is pronounced. In future work it is hoped to assess the changes in pain experience during successful treatment in order to clarify the manner in which the therapeutic change is achieved.

The assessment of the qualities of headache pain has been fruitful. It has provided important information about the type of distress and discomfort experienced by sufferers of one of the most prevalent chronic pain problems. In planning clinical and research studies, it will be useful to assess individual differences in pain qualities in order to select appropriate psychological treatments, to monitor headache improvement, and to illuminate how such changes are produced.

REFERENCES

1. Andrasik, F., and Holroyd, K. A. (1980): A test of specific and non specific biofeedback treatment of tension headache. *J. Consult. Clin. Psychol.*, 48:575–586.
2. Bakal, D. A. (1979): *Psychology and Medicine: Psychological Dimension of Health and Illness.* Springer, New York.
3. Bakal, D. A. (1980): Headache. In: *Encyclopedia of Clinical Assessment*, edited by R. H. Wood, pp. 308–318. Jossey Bass, San Francisco.
4. Bakal, D. A., and Kaganov, J. A. (1977): Muscle contraction and migraine headache: A psychophysiological comparison. *Headache*, 5:208–216.
5. Bond, M. R., and Pilowsky, I. (1966): Subjective assessment of pain and its relationship to the administration of analgesics in patients with advanced cancer. *J. Psychosom. Res.*, 10:203–208.
6. Boxtel, Van A., and Van der Ven, J. R. (1978): Different EMG activity in subjects with muscle contraction headaches related to mental effort. *Headache*, 17:233–237.
7. Collins, F. L., and Thompson, J. K. (1979): Reliability and standardization in the assessment of self-reported headache pain. *J. Behav. Assess.*, 1:73–86.
8. Dubuisson, D., and Melzack, R. (1976): Classification of clinical pain descriptions by multiple group discriminant analysis. *Exp. Neurol.*, 51:480–487.
9. Dunnell, K., and Cartwright, A. (1972): *Medicine Takers, Prescribers, and Hoarders.* Routledge & Kegan Paul, London.
10. Friedman, A. P. (1962): 'Ad Hoc' Committee on Classification of Headache: Classification of headache. *JAMA*, 179:717–718.
11. Hunter, M., and Philips, C. (1981): The experience of headache—Assessment of the qualities of tension headache pain. *Pain*, 10:209–219.
12. Hunter, M., Philips, C., and Rachman, S. (1979): Memory for pain. *Pain*, 6:35–46.
13. Jones, E. (1977): Pain. *Int. J. Psychoanal.*, 38:255.
14. Martin, P. R. (1981): Behavioral management of headaches: A review of evidence. *Int. J. Ment. Health*, 9:88–110.
15. Martin, P. R., and Mathews, A. M. (1978): Tension headaches: A psychophysiological investigation. *J. Psychosom. Res.*, 22:389–399.
16. Melzack, R. (1975): The McGill Pain Questionnaire: Major properties and scoring methods. *Pain*, 1:277–299.
17. Neuchterlein, K. H., and Holroyd, J. C. (1980): Biofeedback in treatment of tension headache. *Arch. Gen. Psychiatry*, 37:866–873.
18. Ostfeld, A. M. (1962): *The Common Headache Syndromes: Biochemistry, Pathophysiology, Therapy.* Charles C Thomas, Springfield.
19. Philips, C. (1977): A psychological analysis of tension headache. In: *Contributions to Medical Psychology, Vol. 1*, edited by S. Rachman, pp. 91–113. Pergamon Press, Oxford.
20. Philips, C. (1978): Tension headache: Theoretical problems. *Behav. Res. Ther.*, 16:249–261.
21. Philips, C. (1980): Recent developments in tension headache research: Implications for understanding and management of the disorder. In: *Contributions to Medical Psychology, Vol. 2*, edited by S. Rachman, pp. 113–130. Pergamon Press, Oxford.
22. Philips, C. (1982): The nature and treatment of chronic tension headache. Banff International Conference on Behavioral Sciences. March, 1982.
23. Philips, C., and Hunter, M. (1981): The treatment of tension headache: I. Muscular abnormality and biofeedback. *Behav. Res. Ther.*, 19:485–498.
24. Philips, C., and Hunter, M. (1982): The treatment of tension headache: II. EMG 'normality' and relaxation. *Behav. Res. Ther.*, 19:494–507.
25. Philips, C., and Hunter, M. (1982): Pain behavior in headache sufferers. *Behav. Anal. Mod.*, 4:257–266.
26. Philips, C., and Hunter, M. (1982): Headache in a psychiatric population. *J. Nerv. Ment. Dis.*, 170:34.

27. Philips, C., and Hunter, M. (1982): A psychophysiological investigation of tension headache. *Headache*, 22 *(in press).*
28. Raskin, N. M., and Appenzeller, O. (1980): *Headache*, pp. 172–185. W. B. Saunders, Philadelphia.
29. Snaith, R. P., Ahmed, S. N., Mehta, M. C., and Hamilton, M. (1971): Assessment of severity of primary depressive illness. *Psychol. Med.*, 1:143–149.

Pain Measurement and Assessment,
edited by Ronald Melzack,
Raven Press, New York © 1983.

Laboratory-Induced and Acute Iatrogenic Pain

Robert K. Klepac and Elizabeth Lander[1]

*Programs in Health and Behavior, Department of Psychology,
North Dakota State University, Fargo, North Dakota 58105*

An almost universally accepted typology of pain has grown out of the two divergent perspectives of the psychophysiological laboratory and the medical/pharmacological clinic. "Laboratory pain" and "clinical pain" are usually discussed as if they are inherently different, albeit remotely related, phenomena (e.g., 15). A brief consideration of acute iatrogenic pain—the kind that might be encountered during dental restoration or bone marrow aspiration—hints at some of the difficulties involved in this assumed typology. Such pain is similar to clinical pain in that it is often emotionally charged, involves the subjective risk of tissue damage, and can induce suffering. On the other hand, it is like laboratory pain in its brief duration, situational dependency, and identifiable external source. Problems in placing particular pain phenomena into their appropriate categories (16) have led the International Association for the Study of Pain to form a committee to develop a nosology of pain types, and has led some investigators to search for a "pure" pain element common to all forms of pain (e.g., 14).

Given the state of knowledge in the area of pain, both of these efforts should be lauded and pursued. It is possible, however, that neither of these strategies will prove adequate. Pain phenomena may neither sort themselves into discrete categories, nor share a single characteristic central enough to each of the specific phenomena to be useful in furthering our understanding of the "puzzle of pain." It is too soon to tell. There is room, then, for a third strategy in addressing specificity and generality among pain phenomena: seeking dimensions along which similarities and differences among kinds of pain might be plotted. Pursuing dimensions of similarity and difference across a wide range of pain phenomena requires common measures that are applicable across this same range. Such measures have not been a prime focus of pain research and theory. Our "lab versus clinic" typology has led researchers within each of these areas to develop and use measures most appropriate to the settings in which they work. Although such a strategy is quite

---

[1]Drs. Klepac and Lander are now at the Department of Psychology, Florida State University, Tallahassee, Florida 32306.

understandable, it leads to a certain irony, wherein continued use of setting-specific measures reinforces the distinction made between experimental and clinical pain and further lessens the likelihood of generating data directly relevant to the empirical search for similarities and differences across our assumed "types."

Richard Gracely (2) has pointed out that common measures that allow comparison between the common and uncommon factors of clinical pain and pain produced in the laboratory would increase the reliability and validity of these methods. Common measures would also provide researcher and clinician with an index of generalizability and thereby streamline the process of adapting laboratory-developed pain reduction techniques for use in the clinic. In short, convenient measures that can be applied across the range of pain phenomena would be a desirable addition in both scientific and clinical applications.

THE McGILL PAIN QUESTIONNAIRE AND LABORATORY PAIN

Based heavily on the traditions of psychophysics and sensation, an elegant armamentarium of measurement strategies has evolved in the pain laboratory (15). Verbal descriptors, like the clinically derived McGill Pain Questionnaire (MPQ), have not yet found a firm place in that armamentarium, despite their widespread use in clinical research and treatment.

Gracely has reported a series of investigations that present a compelling case for the use of verbal descriptors in the search for measures common to both laboratory and clinic (2–5). His data argue that such measures are not only acceptable, but more powerful and sensitive than more complex and sophisticated psychophysiological strategies like cross-modality matching.

For his research, Gracely devised his own set of descriptors and form of administration on the assumption that laboratory pain would lead to too few word choices on the MPQ. However, with the increasing popularity of the MPQ in both clinical and research applications, it is reasonable to ask whether the MPQ might, in fact, be useful as one measure applicable across research settings. The verbal descriptor portion of the MPQ provides a standard and carefully scaled set of descriptors, which, like Gracely's scales, can be scored for more than simple pain intensity (10,11). Relative to many other assessment strategies, the MPQ is convenient and economical to use, and it requires only minimal modifications from its original form to be rendered useful in the laboratory: instructions must include as a referent "the most intense experience during this session" rather than "pain right now"; and a "no pain" or "zero" category should be added to present pain intensity (PPI) and other direct ratings to permit subjects in studies of acute iatrogenic pain to report experiences as nonpainful. These changes are trivial, but the addition of a zero rating category would be expected to lead to slightly lower ratings than the original format.

Data that examine the use of the MPQ within the confines of the pain laboratory are beginning to appear. One factor-analytic study of the MPQ (1) included groups describing threshold or tolerance levels of laboratory pain. The study employed factor analysis to derive novel scoring categories rather than employing the categories originally devised by Melzack. Of these five unique factor scores, threshold and tolerance levels of stimulation led to a difference on only one score; in that single case, threshold stimulation was associated with higher scores than tolerance. These data, although not supportive of the use of the MPQ with laboratory pain, have been challenged on the basis of the factor-analytic procedures employed in deriving the novel scoring categories (12).

In another study of laboratory pain, the MPQ was completed by subjects to describe either pain threshold or tolerance levels of either shock to the forearm or cold pressor pain (7). Standard scoring categories suggested by Melzack were employed. Tolerance levels of stimulation were associated with higher scores than threshold levels on the sensory and evaluative dimensions (but not the affective) and on the miscellaneous items; the same relationship was observed on the overall pain rating index (PRI) and on the PPI rating, but not on the count of number of words chosen. Interestingly, differences in the quality of the pain stimulus being described were reflected in higher scores associated with cold pressor pain on all of the derived scores and in some of the specific words and word groups frequently chosen.

Data from this study support inferences drawn from the clinical application of the MPQ that differences in scores and descriptors reflect differences in intensity and quality of pain experience. More to the point here, they also support the utility of the instrument in laboratory (and possibly acute iatrogenic) pain measurement.

CONVENIENCE OF ADMINISTRATION

In designing the MPQ as a clinical assessment tool, Melzack argued that it should be administered in an interview format, by a trained assessor who could answer questions, provide definitions if needed, and note nonverbal aspects of the patient's behavior during the session (10). Compared with more complex procedures like cross-modality matching, one of the attractive features of using the MPQ in the clinic is its relative ease of administration. Nonetheless, the use of the MPQ in large-scale research programs would be facilitated if paper-and-pencil administration were possible. Such administration might, in fact, encourage research that otherwise would not be done. For example, paper-and-pencil administration would permit subjects to complete the MPQ periodically at home to document changes in pain over time that might be associated with drug action or the healing process itself.

Van Buren and Kleinknecht (13) employed a paper-and-pencil administration of the MPQ in just such an application, demonstrating interesting relationships between MPQ scores and measures of state anxiety during recovery from oral surgery. Although that study suggests that a paper-and-pencil MPQ yields reasonable and roughly predictable scores, it was not intended to address the issue of possible differences between the two modes of administration.

Graham et al. (6) compared data gathered in a paper-and-pencil administration with those from an earlier study of the same clinical population gathered in an interview format. Since the two studies yielded similar data, the authors argued that mode of administration may have no effect on MPQ scores. Although these data are suggestive, they do not offer the strong support that would stem from a direct comparison of the two modes of administration within the same sample of subjects. In one such direct comparison (9), subjects used the MPQ to describe either pain threshold or tolerance levels of cold pressor pain, with half of the subjects in each condition completing the MPQ on paper and half in a clinical interview. As in an earlier study (7), tolerance level stimulation was associated with higher scores on five of six scores derived from the MPQ. In contrast to the findings of Graham et al. with clinical pain patients (6), interview administration led to higher scores than paper-and-pencil administration on five of the scoring categories, with only the straightforward PPI ratings failing to differentiate reliably between the two modes of administration. These differences could not be accounted for by the opportunity to request definitions among the interviewed subjects. Thirty-five definitions were requested, eight of which were subsequently chosen, for a mean of 0.2 words per subject. Interviewed subjects actually chose a mean of 2.85 more words than subjects that received the paper-and-pencil administration.

The factors responsible for differences in MPQ scores associated with mode of administration are not apparent. The lack of any reliable interactions between mode of administration and intensity of pain being described offers a bit of support to the internal validity of studies employing either mode of administration. Comparisons across studies or across individual patients with differing modes of administration, however, can be made only at some risk. Whether or not these same differences would emerge in a study of clinical pain patients like those examined by Graham et al. (6) is a question currently under study.

COMPARING LABORATORY AND CLINICAL PAIN

Two studies have employed the MPQ in direct comparisons of laboratory and nonlaboratory pain. The first of these (1) factor analyzed MPQ descriptors gathered from low-back-pain patients and from volunteer subjects describing pain threshold or tolerance levels of cutaneous electrical stimulation. This analysis yielded five factors that overlapped (but were not identical to) the scoring categories originally devised by Melzack. The authors then tested for differences among the three subject groups along these five dimensions. Although potentially interesting patterns of similarity and difference were found, the meaning of those patterns is unclear, and the study has been criticized on the basis of the factor-analytic methods employed (12).

The second attempt at comparing clinical and experimental pain (8) was aimed at the evaluation of the pain of routine dental treatment. MPQ scores of patients describing just-completed dental treatment were compared with age-matched subjects describing tolerance levels of either cutaneous shock or electrical tooth pulp stimulation. Dental patients' scores were lower than one or both of the laboratory pain subjects' scores on PPI, total PRI, and sums of the sensory and miscellaneous items. Unpublished pilot data from that same laboratory suggest a similar pattern when subjects were asked simply to rate the pain experienced during tolerance levels of laboratory pain and their recollection of the pain experienced in their most recent dental treatments. At this stage it is not possible to state categorically that the use of the MPQ permits meaningful comparisons of laboratory and clinical pain, but the available data are promising and suggest that further study along these lines would be a worthwhile endeavor.

CONCLUSIONS AND IMPLICATIONS

The MPQ is responsive to differences in pain threshold and tolerance levels of laboratory pain of various types, and yields differences among qualitatively different laboratory stressors. The MPQ, therefore, appears to be useful in the experimental pain laboratory. On other issues discussed in this chapter, conclusions are less clear.

Data suggest that paper-and-pencil administration of the MPQ can be employed in laboratory pain studies, but that the resulting data may not be comparable with those gathered in a clinical interview. The differences resulting from mode of administration do not appear to derive from the opportunity to seek clarification of meanings of the MPQ descriptors, and it is not known if the same results would be found among clinical pain patients. Studies that compare clinical and experimental pain with the MPQ are few, suggestive, and in need of replication and extension.

Although much more work is needed, it is probably safe to predict that the MPQ will prove to be useful as one measure that can be meaningfully applied across types of laboratory and experimental pain; others are needed as well. Too many assumptions have been made about critical differences among pain phenomena in the face of too few data. Measures like the MPQ may allow the delineation of dimensions along which pain phenomena may be grouped, whether those phenomena derive from the experimenter's laboratory, the physician's or dentist's healing efforts, or the exigencies of life and health. At this state of our knowledge, such an effort provides a reasonable complement to attempts to create a demonstrably useful typology and efforts to find the common element among all pain types. It is hoped that sound data will dictate which one or which combinations of these approaches will prove most productive in testing and refining our assumptions about pain.

ACKNOWLEDGMENTS

Preparation of this article was supported in part by PHS grant #DE-04976 awarded to the first author by the National Institute of Dental Research. The advice of Drs. Charles Klemz of Fargo and Ronald Kleinknecht of Western Washington University is gratefully acknowledged.

REFERENCES

1. Crockett, D. C., Prkachin, K. M., and Craig, K. D. (1977): Factors in the language of pain in patient and volunteer groups. *Pain*, 4:175–182.
2. Gracely, R. H. (1979): Psychophysical assessment of human pain. In: *Advances in Pain Research and Therapy, Vol. 3*, edited by J. J. Bonica, J. D. Leibeskind, and D. Abel-Fessard, pp. 805–824. Raven Press, New York.
3. Gracely, R. H., Dubner, R., McGrath, P., and Heft, M. (1978): New methods of pain measurement and their application to pain control. *Int. Dent. J.*, 28:52–65.
4. Gracely, R. H., McGrath, P., and Dubner, R. (1978): Ratio scales of sensory and affective verbal pain descriptors. *Pain*, 5:5–18.
5. Gracely, R. H., McGrath, P., and Dubner, R. (1978): Validity and sensitivity of ratio scales of sensory and affective verbal pain descriptors: Manipulation of affect by diazepam. *Pain*, 5:19–29.
6. Graham, C., Bond, S. S., Gerkovich, M. M., and Cook, M. R. (1980): Use of the McGill Pain Questionnaire in the assessment of cancer pain: Replicability and consistency. *Pain*, 8:377–387.
7. Klepac, R. K., Dowling, J., and Hauge, G. (1980): Sensitivity of the McGill Pain Questionnaire to intensity and quality of laboratory pain. *Pain*, 10:199–207.
8. Klepac, R. K., Dowling, J., Hauge, G., and McDonald, M. (1980): Reports of pain after dental treatment, electrical tooth pulp stimulation, and cutaneous shock. *J. Am. Dent. Assoc.*, 100:692–695.
9. Klepac, R. K., Dowling, J., Rokke, P., Dodge, L., and Schafer, L. (1981): Interview vs. paper-and-pencil administration of the McGill Pain Questionnaire. *Pain*, 11:241–246.
10. Melzack, R. (1975): The McGill Pain Questionnaire: Major properties and scoring methods. *Pain*, 1:277–299.
11. Melzack, R., and Torgerson, W. S. (1971): On the language of pain. *Anesthesiology*, 34:50–59.
12. Prieto, E. J., Hopson, L., Bradley, L. A., Byrne, M., Geisinger, K. F., Midax, D., and Marchisello, P. J. (1980): The language of low back pain: Factor structure of the McGill Pain Questionnaire. *Pain*, 8:11–19.
13. Van Buren, J., and Kleinknecht, R. A. (1979): An evaluation of the use of the McGill Pain Questionnaire for use in dental pain. *Pain*, 6:23–33.
14. Wolff, B. B. (1971): Factor analysis of human pain responses: Pain endurance as a specific pain factor. *J. Abnorm. Psychol.*, 78:292–298.
15. Wolff, B. B. (1978): Behavioural measures of human pain. In: *The Psychology of Pain*, edited by R. A. Sternbach, pp. 129–168. Raven Press, New York.
16. Zimmerman, M. (1980): Recurrent persistent pain: Mechanisms and models (group report). In: *Pain and Society*, edited by H. W. Kosterlitz and L. Y. Terenius, pp. 367–382. Verlag Chemie, Weinheim.

Pain Measurement and Assessment,
edited by Ronald Melzack,
Raven Press, New York © 1983.

Postoperative Pain: Relationships Among Measures of Pain, Mood, and Narcotic Requirements

Paul Taenzer

Pain Management Program, Tulsa Rehabilitation Center, Hillcrest Medical Center, Tulsa, Oklahoma 74104

Few studies have directly investigated postoperative pain after Beecher's classic work in the 1950s (3). Various versions of Beecher's verbal rating scale (6,10) continue to be used extensively (5), but verbal rating scales that offer patients only four to six choices to rate their pain have been criticized for their lack of sensitivity in estimating pain relief (8,15). New measurement techniques that are worthy of consideration have recently been developed. As part of a larger study of psychological control of postoperative pain, several pain measurement scales and psychological tests were administered. These data permitted evaluation of the properties of these scales and comparisons between measurement systems.

METHODS

A sample of 40 patients (28 females and 12 males) who underwent routine elective gallbladder surgery were studied. The mean age was 47 years with a range of 20 to 65 years. All patients provided informed consent prior to their operation.

During the first 3 postoperative days, pain measurement scales were administered at 9 a.m. and 4 p.m. These included the McGill Pain Questionnaire (MPQ) and visual analogue scales. The MPQ (12) contains a verbal rating scale—the present pain index (PPI)—and a series of adjective descriptors. Multidimensional scaling procedures were used to separate the descriptors into 20 distinct categories (13). The summed rank values of the adjectives within each category comprise the pain rating index (PRI), which can be expressed as separate scores for sensory [PRI(S)], affective [PRI(A)], evaluative [PRI(E)], and miscellaneous [PRI(M)] words, in addition to a total score [PRI(T)].

Two visual analogue scales were constructed in the manner described by Aitken (1) using horizontal 10-cm lines to measure: pain intensity [VAS(P)], using "no pain" and "worst pain possible" as verbal anchors; and distress [VAS(D)] using "no distress" and "severe distress" as anchors.

During the afternoon data collection period, the State-Trait Anxiety Inventory-State form (STAI-S) of Speilberger et al. (18) and a short form of the Beck Depression Inventory (BDI) (2) were also administered. The number of doses of narcotic analgesics administered on the first 3 postoperative days was also recorded. All tests were readministered during the morning of the sixth postoperative day.

RESULTS

The means and standard deviations for each measure are displayed in Table 1, which shows a steady decline of all measures across the postoperative period. Exceptions are PRI(M) and VAS(P) which showed a slight rise in scores on day 2. The increase in standard deviations of pain scores across the data collection period appears to reflect the well-known variability in the course of postoperative pain.

Figure 1 displays the mean PRI(T) values for each data collection period. In order to compare the intensity of postcholecystectomy pain with other clinical pains, the mean PRI(T) scores for other acute and chronic pains are also indicated in this figure (12). Although it is inappropriate to use these data as a precise comparison of overall intensity of clinical pain syndromes, they do indicate that during the first 2 postoperative days, postcholecystectomy pain, treated with routine narcotic analgesia, is in the range of other forms of clinical pain previously measured with the MPQ.

While most methods of pain assessment require the patient to rate his experience along an abstract intensity dimension, the MPQ has the advantage of using the richness and subtlety of the language to describe the precise phenomena experienced by the patient. One benefit of this approach is that it is then possible to describe the collective experience of persons experiencing the same pain problem in a precise

TABLE 1. *Means (and SD) of pain, mood, and analgesic usage measures*

| | Day 1 | | Day 2 | | Day 3 | | Day 6 |
	a.m.	p.m.	a.m.	p.m.	a.m.	p.m.	a.m.
PPI	2.5(0.9)	2.1(0.7)	2.0(0.7)	1.9(0.7)	1.6(0.81)	1.4(0.81)	1.0(0.9)
PRI(S)	17(7)	15(7)	14(7.6)	13(6)	10(6.3)	8.1(6.5)	5.1(6.1)
PRI(A)	3.0(2.1)	2.3(1.8)	2.0(2.0)	1.9(2.0)	1.5(1.8)	0.95(1.6)	0.43(.90)
PRI(E)	2.1(1.2)	2.0(1.2)	1.6(1.2)	1.6(1.1)	1.2(1.1)	1.0(1.1)	0.55(.85)
PRI(M)	5.9(2.9)	4.6(2.7)	3.0(2.3)	3.6(2.7)	2.7(2.7)	2.0(2.1)	1.0(2.0)
PRI(T)	28(11)	24(11)	21(11)	20(11)	16(10)	12(10)	7.0(8.9)
VAS(P)	55(19)	50(21)	42(20)	44(21)	35(22)	28(19)	17(18)
VAS(D)	50(23)	46(21)	41(21)	40(21)	33(23)	27(21)	15(18)
STAI-S	—	39(8.7)	—	38(9.6)	—	34(12)	28(6.9)
BDI	—	3.6(3.2)	—	2.9(3.2)	—	2.1(2.8)	1.9(2.0)
Doses of narcotics	—	3.4(1.3)	—	2.1(1.3)	—	1.2(1.4)	—

For abbreviations see text.

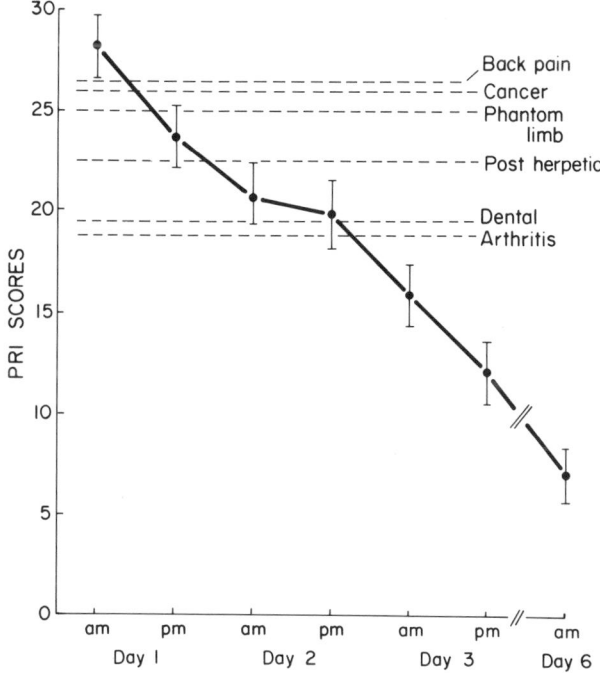

FIG. 1. Mean PRI(T) scores recorded at each data collection point during the postoperative recovery period. Mean scores for several pain syndromes recorded in an outpatient pain clinic are included for comparison (13).

qualitative manner. The descriptive words chosen by more than 30% of the subjects at one or more data collection point are displayed in Fig. 2. Thirteen descriptors fulfill this criterion. Overall, these data suggest a pattern of relatively higher-intensity descriptors (e.g., stabbing, exhausting, throbbing) being used predominantly on the first postoperative day and diminishing in frequency rapidly across days 2 and 3. Relatively lower-intensity descriptors (e.g., pulling, nagging, tight, tender, sore) show a more consistent pattern through the data collection period.

Intercorrelations among the postoperative outcome measures averaged across the postoperative period are displayed in Table 2. The correlations on the left of the table represent the interrelationships among the MPQ indices. All correlations except that between PPI and PRI(A) have p values less than 0.001.[1] The exceptionally high correlations between PRI(T) and its three major components, PRI(S), PRI(A), and PRI(M), are worthy of special attention. They suggest that whereas PRI(T) is perhaps the best overall measure by virtue of being the sum of the other PRI measures, it is clearly redundant when presented along with its components. Overall, the levels of the correlation coefficients are similar to those previously reported with a chronic pain population (12).

---

[1] All significance levels are based on one-tailed tests.

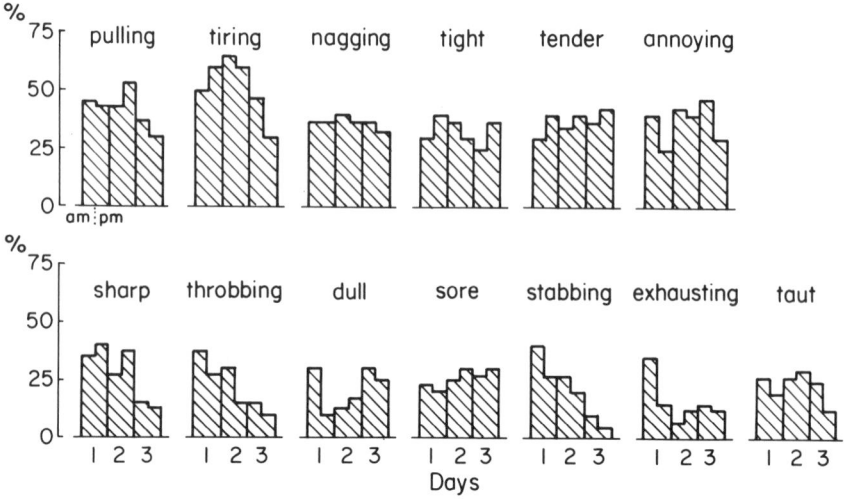

FIG. 2. MPQ adjectives used by more than 30% of patients to describe postcholecystectomy pain at one or more data collection points. Each section of the histogram represents one postoperative day. These are divided into a.m. and p.m. sections, as indicated.

TABLE 2. *Intercorrelations among dependent measures N = 40*

	PPI	PRI(S)	PRI(A)	PRI(E)	PRI(M)	PRI(T)	VAS(P)	VAS(D)	STAI-S	BDI	Analgesics
PPI	0.66	0.36	0.54	0.65	0.66	0.65	0.65	0.28	0.17	0.34	
PRI(S)		0.71	0.62	0.79	0.97	0.62	0.60	0.51	0.18	0.35	
PRI(A)			0.48	0.65	0.80	0.50	0.53	0.50	0.43	0.06	
PRI(E)				0.71	0.72	0.53	0.49	0.40	0.34	0.24	
PRI(M)					0.88	0.59	0.64	0.39	0.28	0.34	
PRI(T)						0.65	0.64	0.43	0.27	0.32	
VAS(P)							0.88	0.42	0.20	0.22	
VAS(D)								0.51	0.26	0.28	
STAI-S									0.61	0.44	
BDI										0.30	
Analgesics											

For abbreviations see text.
$p(0.05) = 0.25$; $p(0.01) = 0.35$; $p(0.001) = 0.45$.

Inspection of the correlations between the MPQ indices and the visual analogue scales reveals highly significant correlations ($p < 0.001$). The mean of those correlations is 0.59, implying that the two systems of pain measurement are highly related and yet not redundant. On the other hand, the correlation between the two visual analogue scales is so high, $r = 0.88$, that, clearly, little additional information is gained from using two rather than one scale for the measurement of postcholecystectomy pain.

The correlations between the pain measures and postoperative anxiety are all statistically significant, confirming the expected relationship between situational anxiety and pain experiences. The relationship between the pain measures and postoperative depression scores are on the whole weaker than those for postoperative anxiety (average $r = 0.26$). However, five of the eight pain measures are significantly correlated with postoperative depression.

The total number of narcotics administered during the postoperative course is significantly correlated with five of the eight pain measures (average $r = 0.27$) as well as with postoperative anxiety and depression. It is interesting that whereas narcotics are administered to relieve pain, the relationship between the measures of pain and total number of doses is relatively weak. There is, however, a stronger relationship between analgesic requirement and situational anxiety ($r = 0.44$, $p < 0.01$).

By measuring pain seven times during the postoperative course, it was possible to describe accurately the average course of the postcholecystectomy pain experience (see Fig. 1). These data are also valuable in so far as they can be used to address the following question: how many samplings are sufficient to represent accurately the total course of postoperative pain?

For each pain measure, Pearson correlations were calculated: (a) between scores for the individual sampling point and the average for the remaining samplings (Table 3, columns 1 through 7); and (b) between two sampling points on days 2 and 3 and the remaining five data collection points (columns 8 and 9). Inspection of these results for the single sampling points on days 1 through 3 reveals high average correlations (across pain measures) but also high variability for individual measures. The day 6 correlations are both less and highly variable. Correlations for the two sampling points on days 2 and 3, on the other hand, are consistently high for all pain measures (mean = 0.77, range = 0.68–0.87 for the afternoon ratings of days 2 and 3). This suggests that measuring pain at these two time periods provides an

TABLE 3. *Pearson correlations between average pain scores and those measured at individual points during the postoperative course*

Pain measure		Day 1 a.m.	p.m.	Day 2 a.m.	p.m.	Day 3 a.m.	p.m.	Day 6	Days 2,3 a.m.	Days 2,3 p.m.
PRI:	Sensory	0.60	056	0.64	0.73	0.74	0.50	0.33	0.76	0.75
	Affective	0.60	0.30	0.77	0.71	0.69	0.65	0.14	0.69	0.80
	Evaluative	0.60	0.38	0.59	0.57	0.66	0.46	0.30	0.70	0.68
	Misc.	0.45	0.30	0.55	0.54	0.53	0.49	0.10	0.62	0.70
	Total	0.67	0.49	0.67	0.72	0.78	0.54	0.30	0.76	0.79
PPI		0.67	0.72	0.39	0.55	0.62	0.56	0.50	0.68	0.76
VAS:	Pain	0.76	0.62	0.56	0.71	0.78	0.70	0.57	0.76	0.87
	Distress	0.53	0.47	0.59	0.61	0.85	0.73	0.67	0.78	0.82
Mean ($\bar{X}$)		0.61	0.48	0.60	0.64	0.70	0.58	0.36	0.72	.77

For abbreviations see text.

adequate estimation of the total course of postcholecystectomy pain for any of the pain indices used in this study.

DISCUSSION

The present study examined the interrelations between the MPQ and visual analogue scale pain rating methods, in addition to examining the effects of anxiety, depression, and narcotic requirements. These results indicate that both the pain and affect measures showed the clinically expected pattern of decreasing scores across the postoperative period. Highly significant intercorrelations among the MPQ indices support the internal consistency of this measure for this population. Significant correlations between the MPQ and visual analogue scale measures indicate that they are indeed measuring a common dimension. The correlation between the visual analogue scale and the PPI, a simple verbal rating scale included in the MPQ, equaled 0.65. This is in the range of correlations reported by Reading (16) who studied the correspondence between the PPI and visual analogue scale with a postepisiotomy pain population [$r = 0.29$ (day 1); $= 0.71$ (day 2)]. Other studies (11,15,22) that compared similar scales with chronic pain populations reported correlations ranging from 0.64 to 0.87.

This is the first study that reports the relationship between the PRI scales of the MPQ and visual analogue scale scores. These correlations ranged from 0.49 to 0.65. The highest correlations were between PRI scales, which are most heavily loaded with sensory descriptors [PRI(S), (M), and (T)]. For these scales the range was 0.59 to 0.65.

Analysis of the pattern of scores across the postoperative period suggests that measuring pain at two time periods during the postoperative course, the afternoons of days 2 and 3, provides an adequate approximation for the average pain experienced across the postcholecystectomy recovery period. If this result can be replicated by future research, it suggests that subsequent studies with this population can be less intrusive for the convalescing patient while maintaining methodological rigor. One would expect this pattern to change for different operative procedures.

Although it has become popular to use independent scales to measure pain and distress (9), the data presented here suggest that this practice is a redundancy for the postcholecystectomy population.

The advantages of the visual analogue scale for measuring clinical pain have been reviewed previously (7,11). These reports have also indicated that the visual analogue scale method is inappropriate for some 7 to 11% of patients who are unable to use the scale to rate their pain. This problem was not encountered in the present study. This may be due to the instructions the patients received. The visual analogue scale was compared to measuring temperature with a thermometer, having the freezing and boiling points of water as verbal anchors.

The significant correlations found between pain scores and situational anxiety are consistent with many previous reports [see Weisenberg (21) and Sternbach (20) for reviews]. Depressive effect has not received much attention from researchers studying acute pain states (19). The low yet significant correlations between BDI scores and five of the eight pain measures suggest that this area may be worthy of further consideration. The relatively low correlations between pain scores and narcotic requirements are somewhat puzzling. It may be in part explained by pain being rated on a fixed schedule and analgesics being administered on a PRN basis. It is likely, therefore, that some patients who were in severe pain had been medicated shortly before pain was assessed. The higher correlation between anxiety and analgesic requirements is consistent with previous reports that have indicated that the decision to administer a narcotic is related to many factors that may not be directly related to pain levels (4,21).

Taken together, these results indicate that the MPQ and the visual analogue scale are valid and appropriate indices for assessing postoperative pain. Both appear to reflect the clinical course of postoperative pain and reflect the patient's affective state. Both have shown adequate test–retest reliability in previous research (12,17). The visual analogue scale has the advantage of simplicity and brevity. Previously reported difficulties involving a subset of patients not able to complete the visual analogue scale appear to have been solved through a modification of the instructions presented. The MPQ, on the other hand, while being somewhat more complex and time consuming, has the advantage of measuring three phenomenologically and statistically distinct dimensions of pain experience. Additionally, it has been demonstrated to be sensitive to diagnostically distinct pain syndromes as well as to pain therapies that have a differential effect on the pain dimensions it purports to measure (13). A choice between the MPQ and visual analogue scale can be based on these considerations.

ACKNOWLEDGMENTS

It is a pleasure to thank Dr. Ronald Melzack, Dr. Mary Ellen Jeans, Dr. Campbell Perry, and the physicians and nurses of the General Surgery Service of the Montreal General Hospital for their advice and support. This study was supported by grant A7891 to Dr. Ronald Melzack from the Natural Sciences and Engineering Research Council of Canada.

REFERENCES

1. Aitken, R. C. B. (1969): A growing edge of measurement of feelings. *Proc. R. Soc. Med.*, 62:989–996.
2. Beck, A. T., and Beck, R. W. (1972): Screening depressed patients in family practice: A rapid technique. *Postgrad. Med.*, 52:81–85.
3. Beecher, H. K. (1959): *Measurement of Subjective Responses.* Oxford University Press, New York.
4. Cohen, F. L. (1980): Postsurgical pain relief. Patient's status nurses' medication choices. *Pain*, 9:265–274.
5. Cooper, S. A., and Beaver, W. T. (1976): A model to evaluate mild analgesics in oral surgery outpatients. *Clin. Pharmacol. Ther.*, 20:241–250.
6. Houde, R. W., and Wallenstein, S. L. (1953): A method for evaluating analgesics in patients with chronic pain. *Bull. Drug Addic. Narcot.*, Appendix F:660.
7. Huskisson, E. C. (1974): Measurement of pain. *Lancet*, 9:1127–1131.

8. Huskisson, E. C., Shenfield, G. M., Taylor, R. T., and Hart, F. D. (1970): A new look at Ibuprofen. *Rheumatol. Phys. Med.*, 10[*Suppl.*] pp. 88–98.
9. Johnson, J. E., Rice, V. H., Fuller, S. S., and Endress, M. P. (1978): Sensory information, instructions in a coping strategy and recovery from surgery. *Res. Nurs. Health*, 1:4–17.
10. Keele, K. D. (1968): Pain complaint threshold in relation to pain of cardiac infarction. *Br. Med. J.*, 1:670–673.
11. Kremer, E., Atkinson, J. H., and Ignelzi, R. J. (1981): Measurement of pain: Patient preference does not confound pain measurement. *Pain*, 10:241–248.
12. Melzack, R. (1975): The McGill Pain Questionnaire: Major properties and scoring methods. *Pain*, 1:277–299.
13. Melzack, R., Taenzer, P., Feldman, P., and Kinch, R. A. (1981): Labour is still painful after prepared childbirth training. *Can. Med. Assoc. J.*, 125:357–363.
14. Melzack, R., and Torgerson, W. S. (1971): On the language of pain. *Anesthesiology*, 34:50–59.
15. Ohnhaus, E. E., and Adler, R. (1975): Methodological problems in the measurement of pain: A comparison between the verbal rating scale and the visual analogue scale. *Pain*, 1:385–390.
16. Reading, A. E. (1981): A comparison of pain rating scales. *J. Psychosom. Res.*, 24:119–124.
17. Revill, S. I., Robinson, J. O., Rosen, M., and Hogg, I. J. (1976): The reliability of a linear analogue for evaluating pain. *Anaesthesia*, 31:1191–1198.
18. Spielberger, C. D., Gorsuch, R. L., and Luschene, R. E. (1970): *Manual for the State Trait Anxiety Inventory*. Consulting Psychologists Press, Palo Alto.
19. Sternbach, R. A. (1974): *Pain Patients: Traits and Treatments*. Academic Press, New York.
20. Sternbach, R. A. (1978): Clinical aspects of pain. In: *The Psychology of Pain*, edited by R. A. Sternbach, pp. 241–264. Raven Press, New York.
21. Weisenberg, M. (1977): Pain and pain control. *Psychol. Bull.*, 84:1008–1044.
22. Woodforde, J. M., and Merskey, H. (1972): Some relationships between subjective measures of pain. *J. Psychosom. Res.*, 16:173–178.

Pain Measurement and Assessment,
edited by Ronald Melzack,
Raven Press, New York © 1983.

Pain Language as a Measure of Affect in Chronic Pain Patients

Edwin F. Kremer and J. Hampton Atkinson, Jr.

*Department of Psychiatry, University of California at San Diego Medical School,
La Jolla, California 92093*

Although systematic efforts to understand the relationship between pain experience and its verbal description have a long history (6,28), it is only recently that an empirically derived standard vocabulary for pain has become available. In their seminal work, Melzack and Torgerson (25) and Melzack (23) cast pain experience as a multidimensional phenomenon consisting of sensory, affective, and evaluative qualities. The McGill Pain Questionnaire (MPQ) (23) introduced a standardized vocabulary ranked for pain intensity that allowed quantitative assessment of the dimensions of pain complaint and permitted estimation of the relative contribution of each category to the pain communication. Subsequent studies of experimentally induced and of acute and chronic pathological pain indicated that the MPQ is reliable, valid, and responsive to treatment of somatic or affective disturbances. Melzack (23) and Graham et al. (12) demonstrated that patients reliably selected the same descriptors to characterize their pain experience over assessment intervals, and Klepac et al. (16) reported that different laboratory-induced pain stimuli (cold pressor or electrical tooth pulp stimulation) resulted in reliably different MPQ-derived scores and word patterns. Dubuisson and Melzack (8) found that 77% of a sample of patients in predominantly acute pain could be correctly identified by computer analysis using only sensory descriptors chosen by the patients. Similarly, Hunter and Philips (14) were able to differentiate tension from migraine headache patients on the basis of pain descriptors used in the MPQ.

Finally, Kremer and Atkinson (17) reported that the affective dimension of the MPQ was systematically related to an independent measure of affective distress [Brief Symptom Inventory (BSI)] in chronic pain patients. The treatment responsiveness of the instrument was noted by Melzack and Perry (24), who found that the language of the MPQ allowed for reliable discrimination among groups of chronic pain patients treated with modalities of differential effectiveness. In addition, Gracely et al. (11), using experimentally induced pain in normal subjects, found that an antianxiety drug, diazepam (Valium®), reduced affective but not sensory descriptors.

Although these data are important in demonstrating that language assessment, and in particular the MPQ, may be a valid and reliable means of measuring some types of pain, it is uncertain if the technique is generally applicable to chronic pain syndromes. For example, chronic pain populations are characterized by a high incidence of anxiety and depression (see 27), and the disruptive effect of affective distress on cognitive tasks pertinent to responding to the MPQ is well documented (see 9). This review summarizes recent work addressing the interplay of affective disturbance and pain language; it (a) reviews selected variables confounding pain language; (b) describes the behavior of affective language in relation to different chronic pain syndromes, to psychopathological states, and to the sensory dimension of pain language; and (c) delineates a role for affective language in clinical practice. A review of the literature on language and pain suggests that affective distress influences pain language in a systematic fashion, and that the MPQ is a reliable, valid, and unobtrusive measure of emotional disorder in chronic pain patients.

VARIABLES THAT CONFOUND PAIN REPORT

The task of assigning adjectival descriptors to pain experience is a complex interaction of affective and cognitive operations. First, the patient must discriminate the sensory effects of pain from similar sensory effects that commonly accompany mood states, such as pounding, throbbing, tingling, cold, and hot. Indeed, Agnew and Merskey (2) found that patients who complained of headache were no more likely to use descriptors such as throbbing, beating, and pounding than patients with anxiety but without headache. Second, the patient must endorse the appropriate descriptors presented in the MPQ. Obviously, this task is more or less difficult as a function of the emotional distress the patient is experiencing. For example, Lindsay and Wyckoff (22) found that 85% of chronic pain patients suffer clinically significant depression, and Weingartner et al. (31) have shown that depressed patients suffer identifiable defects in cognitive operations that make any psychophysical task involving subtle discriminations among sensory events most difficult. Finally, the patient must select a verbal label for sensory effects that are often vague and fluctuating over time. Thus, the patient might not only experience difficulty in finding an appropriate label, but might be forced to rely on the memory of some aspect of the pain experience. The behavior of memory effects on pain language is difficult to assess. On the one hand, Hunter et al. (15) have shown that memory for pain is very reliable over long periods of time. Nevertheless, memory deficits are a common symptom of depression, and depression frequently accompanies chronic pain (22).

A major task for the student of pain language, then, is to determine how these various factors confound pain report. The hypothesis adopted here is that affective distress causes diffusion of pain language. It follows that both sensory and affective descriptors reflect affective distress but do not reliably indicate the sensory phenomena of pain. In some populations, then, pain language assessment such as the MPQ might better serve as a measure of affect. This argument is based on three lines of evidence. One demonstrates that pain language is more diffuse in psychiatric populations relative to medical populations, given that affective distress is greater in psychiatric groups. Next, studies that directly measure affective distress find a systematic relationship between affective distress and pain language. Finally, comparison of affective language in diagnostic categories in which the meaning of pain is likely to be differentially distressing (cancer versus benign) demonstrates greater use of affective language in cancer patients than in benign pain patients. These studies will be discussed below.

PAIN LANGUAGE IN MEDICAL AND PSYCHIATRIC POPULATIONS

Four studies addressing different populations reveal that language diffusion increases with psychiatric disorder. Veilleux and Melzack (30) compared responses on the MPQ for psychotic patients and patients in seven medical diagnostic categories, and found that psychotic patients used more words to describe their pain and on the average complained of more intense pain. Although patients in some medical diagnostic categories (cancer, phantom limb) used more sensory descriptors than did psychotic patients, the psychotic patients on the average used many more affective descriptors, more evaluative descriptors, and more combined sensory–affective descriptors. Interestingly, in comparing psychotic patients with and without pain complaints, there was a marked difference in the use of sensory descriptors (6.6 versus 2.4) but no difference in affective descriptors (3.0 versus 2.6). Thus, when a psychotic patient describes how he is feeling using the language of the MPQ, the presence or absence of pain appears to be irrelevant to the affective language outcome.

In a study of less psychologically disturbed subjects, Devine and Merskey (7) compared the complexity of spontaneous pain description in outpatients referred for psychiatric or medical consultation. Controlling for severity of pain complaint and sex, these investigators found that the complexity of the pain complaint was significantly greater for the psychiatric referrals than for the medical referrals. Complexity was defined by use of a greater number of words and descriptors that were either "bizarre or markedly unusual." Thirteen of the sixteen patients using the most complex level of language were psychiatric patients. There was no indication whether this increased complexity consisted of sensory or affective descriptors. These investigators also found that within the medical referrals, complexity increased significantly as pain severity increased. Thus, elaboration of pain complaint is influenced both by diagnostic category (psychiatric versus medical) and perceived intensity of pain. Although no attempt was made to determine the relative strength of these two variables, it is interesting that the psychiatric patients complained of significantly more intense pain than the medical referrals.

Hunter and Philips (14) studied the pain language (MPQ) of headache patients, some of whom were from a psychiatric population and some of whom were free of psychiatric illness. These researchers found that the psychiatric group used a greater number of affective descriptors than the nonpsychiatric group. These groups did not appear to differ in their use of sensory descriptors. Leavitt et al. (21), using their Low Back Classification Scale (LBCS), found that patients classified as having "functional pain" were significantly more variable than "organic" patients in the characterization of their pain; they described a more diffuse pain and reported greater pain intensity. In a second series of studies, Leavitt and Garron (20) demonstrated that low-back-pain patients without demonstrable medical etiology for pain responded with significantly higher scores on each of the seven subscales of the LBCS than a group with organic findings. Importantly, they were able to use this verbal descriptor scale, which was derived from the MPQ, to discriminate between patients with so-called "functional" pain and patients complaining of low back pain but with no identifiable psychiatric or organic pathology. Because low back pain can be attributed to undiagnosed abnormalities of the spine (13), they reasoned that patients who did not receive a medical diagnosis but who characterized their pain in a manner similar to patients with a medical diagnosis would respond to conservative treatment. Conversely, patients with a diagnosis of functional pain would fail to respond to medical intervention. This reasoning relies on the observation that patients treated medically for psychiatric problems typically fail to improve (4). Assessment of these patients at 6 and 14 weeks post-treatment indicated that the functional patients failed to improve, whereas the undiagnosed pain patients showed significant improvement.

The studies reviewed above used a range of psychiatric disturbance and were consistent in finding that pain language in psychiatric patients is typically more diffuse than that of normal pain patients. In some studies, at least, this diffusion invades both sensory and affective descriptors. Thus, for some patients, it would appear that sensory descriptors are influenced not only by the sensory experience per se but also by the patient's affective distress.

STUDIES THAT MEASURE AFFECTIVE DISTRESS

There are investigations of both acute and chronic pain that measure affective distress. In a study of acute pain, Van Buren and Kleinknecht (29) studied the relationship between pain language (MPQ) and anxiety (state anxiety on a semantic differential) in 60 surgery patients. A correlation analysis of anxiety and pain language after oral surgery indicated that sensory, affective, and evaluative pain language all were highly correlated ($r = 0.22–0.44$) with level of anxiety. In fact, and as these authors noted, the more consistent relationship was between anxiety and sensory and evaluative adjectives rather than with affective descriptors. As present pain intensity (PPI) was also highly correlated with anxiety and pain language, and the MPQ is scaled for intensity, it is possible that this effect of anxiety is mediated by differences in perceived PPI. That more psychologically distressed patients report greater PPI is not an uncommon finding in the literature (e.g., 7).

Kremer and Atkinson (17) studied consecutive admissions to a chronic pain clinic. Each patient completed the MPQ, the BSI, and the Sickness Impact Profile. Grouping patients based on their use of affective descriptors, these investigators found that patients who reported a high affective component to their pain (indicated by a greater use of affective descriptors) were significantly more depressed and anxious and complained of significantly greater physical and psychosocial disability and reliably more intense pain. Importantly, the group that used greater affective language also used significantly more sensory and evaluative descriptors, even though the incidence of medical and psychiatric diagnosis did not differ between the groups.

Finally, Hunter and Philips (14) used the Wakefield Depression Scale to measure depression in chronic tension headache patients recruited from a psychiatric population. Pain intensity, affective language, and evaluative language were significantly correlated with level of depression.

Although these studies are consistent in showing that pain language becomes more diffuse as affective distress increases, the precise nature of this diffusion is unclear. Since descriptors in the MPQ are ranked for intensity, and affectively distressed patients complain of more intense pain, it is possible that language diffusion occurs primarily along the intensive dimension. That is, patients use no greater number of descriptors but simply elect descriptors with a high rank of intensity. Atkinson et al. (3) attempted to clarify this issue by examining the number of sensory and affective descriptors used by groups of chronic pain patients that differed in degree of affective distress as measured by the General Symptom Index on the BSI. Differences in pain intensity and pain involvement were controlled by using these two factors as covariates in separate analyses of covariance. Between-group differences were tested for the number of sensory and the number of affective words used to describe the pain complaint. A pain involvement measure was derived by measuring the total surface area identified as painful by the patient on the figure provided on the MPQ and then dividing by the number of anatomical sites involved. The results of these analyses indicated that even when intensity and pain involvement were controlled, affectively distressed patients used a significantly greater number of both sensory and affective descriptors to characterize their pain complaint. Additional analysis revealed that distressed patients matched on pain intensity with nondistressed patients also reliably selected descriptors with a higher intensity ranking. Thus, a series of investigations of acute and chronic pain note that diffusion of pain language mediated by affective distress involves the sensory, affective, and intensive dimensions of pain.

COMPARISON OF PAIN LANGUAGE IN CANCER AND BENIGN PAIN PATIENTS

Only a few studies have compared cancer and benign pain populations. Kremer et al. (18) compared responses to the MPQ for patients suffering chronic pain secondary to malignancy and patients with chronic benign pain. These groups were further divided by sex and by pain intensity report (high versus low) on a scale of 0 to 100. This comparison indicated that cancer pain patients who complained of low-intensity pain used more affective language to describe their pain than their counterparts with benign pain of the same intensity. Patients complaining of high-intensity pain did not differ by diagnostic category in their use of affective language, but did use reliably more affective language than patients complaining of low-intensity pain. Finally, women tended to use greater affective and evaluative language than men, but as sex was balanced between diagnostic categories, this effect did not confound interpretation of the diagnostic category effect. There was some suggestion that the affective distress of pain secondary to cancer might be reflected in sensory language, but the evidence was slight. Men with cancer complaining of low-intensity pain had higher sensory dimension scores than their same-sex benign counterparts. These observations are consistent with the diffusion of pain language across sensory and affective descriptors.

To our knowledge there is only one other comparison of language used for cancer pain with that of other diagnostic categories. These data were first reported by Melzack (23) and subsequently employed by Dubuisson and Melzack (8) and Graham et al. (12). This work suggests less affective and sensory language in cancer than in some other illnesses like disc disease. It is important to note, however, that there was no control for differences in pain intensity and the number of subjects was small. Obviously, considerably more study is needed in this area. Important variables such as expected survival time and type and level of medication have not been addressed, and it is very likely these factors influence descriptions of cancer pain.

This review of the literature suggests that affective distress influences pain language in a systematic fashion. It appears that when intensity is controlled, patients with high levels of affective distress select more pain descriptors and spread their choices among more word categories than less disturbed individuals. Given this finding, the role of pain language in clinical care can now be addressed.

IMPLICATIONS OF PAIN LANGUAGE DIFFUSION FOR DIAGNOSIS

Patients' descriptions of pain are often considered a dependable and useful adjunct (1) in the diagnosis and treatment of disease. Such an assertion assumes that certain illnesses elicit unique sensations: thus, the pain of angina is characterized as "squeezing," "crushing," or "choking"; duodenal ulcer is "gnawing" and "burning"; bone pain is "aching"; nerve root compression is "sharp" and "stabbing"; and pain of abdominal viscera and nerve plexus is "sickening."

Alternatively, affective descriptors might be useful in communicating the patient's urgency in desiring relief but are of little use in identifying the likely etiology of the pain. But since pain patients are distressed, it is not likely that pain language would be of much assistance in formulating a medical diagnosis. Although some studies have demonstrated that diagnostic groups can be discriminated on the basis of the pain descriptors used by patients, the preponderance of the data fails to support the usefulness of pain language in this area.

Dubuisson and Melzack (8) were able to correctly categorize patients into eight diagnostic categories using a discriminant analysis of sensory descriptors from the MPQ. Similarly, Hunter and Philips (14) found that although tension and migraine headache patients had much pain language in common, there were some descriptors unique to each diagnostic category. Finally, Leavitt and Garron (20) have developed a pain language questionnaire (LBCS) that can reliably discriminate between organic and "functional" low back pain. There is no evidence to date, however, that this scale can discriminate among back pains of different organic etiology. Thus, in the strict sense, the LBPS allows only discrimination between psychiatric and medical diagnostic categories.

In contrast to the above findings, Fordyce et al. (10) failed to detect any systematic relationship between medical diagnostic category and pain language, and suggested the possibility that pain language could be influenced by so many variables that it is likely to be highly idiosyncratic. Similarly, Agnew and Merskey (2) failed to find any pattern of pain descriptors that discriminated among pain etiologies. In a rigorous effort to examine this question, Atkinson et al. (3) studied the pain language of 126 chronic pain patients. This population included benign pain patients, patients suffering pain secondary to malignancy, and patients complaining of pain secondary to chronic renal failure. These patients were diagnosed by both disease (benign, cancer, renal) and by pathological mechanism (nerve compression, bone pain, psychiatric, etc.). Analysis of pain language using multiple discriminate analyses failed to distinguish differences in language among these various diagnostic categories. A separate analysis of patients who complained of low-intensity pain and who might be expected to have more orderly language also failed to yield any discriminate function for the different diagnostic categories. In a separate study, Kremer et al. (19) examined the language of patients in the same diagnostic categories as used in the above study. Pain descriptors from the MPQ were subjected to a principal-component factor analysis, which affords greater opportunities for discrimination. This procedure revealed considerable overlap among diagnostic categories. At the same time, however, clustering did occur as a function of level of affective distress.

Although there is clearly a need for additional work on this question, the conclusion from the available literature must be that pain language cannot discriminate among medical diagnostic categories. There is some evidence that pain language can distinguish between medical and psychiatric diagnoses (e.g., 20) but even here one must be cautious, because the discrimination is based on diffusion of pain language by patients with functional pain. Such observations are consistent with the diffusion model outlined above so long as patients with functional pain are assumed to suffer consistently greater affective distress than patients with identifiable organic pathology. This is not a good assumption, however, as a number of workers (e.g., 5,32) have found that pain patients with a medical diagnosis suffer as much affective distress as patients without identifiable organic etiology for their pain. Because language diffuses as a function of affective distress, it would appear unlikely that consistent discrimination between medical and psychiatric diagnosis is possible. The most reliable use of pain language, then, might be as an index of affective distress.

THE MPQ AS A MEASURE OF AFFECTIVE DISTRESS

A patient suffering unremitting pain need not also be psychiatrically ill to experience a high level of affective distress. In addition to its other properties, the MPQ could serve as an important clinical measure in assessing the degree of affective distress that the pain patient is suffering. As Morgan et al. (26) noted, chronic pain patients are often sensitive to any implied psychogenicity to their pain complaint. Obviously, instruments that are blatantly psychological in nature could evoke defensiveness and perhaps hostility in the patient. Consequently, the patient would fail to respond to the psychological test in an open and honest manner, and, if hostile, might also fail to comply with any treatment regimen. The MPQ has been demonstrated to be a sensitive and reliable measure of affective distress, and, at the same time, is constructed in such a fashion as not to alienate the patient.

There are several important tasks for future research. One is to determine if the MPQ is specific in terms of the categories of affective distress it measures. For example, is the language used more sensitive to the symptomatology of anxiety as opposed to signs and symptoms of depression? Furthermore, the clinical usefulness of the MPQ will be enhanced with the publication of normative data involving diverse diagnostic categories of benign and cancer-related pain.

ACKNOWLEDGMENTS

This work was supported in part by Contract RFP No. NO1-CN-85417-06 from the National Cancer Institute.

REFERENCES

1. Adams, R. D. (1980): Pain: General considerations. In: *Harrisons Principles of Internal Medicine*, edited by K. J. Isselbacher, R. D. Adams, E. Braunwald, R. G. Petersdorf, and J. D. Wilson, pp. 12–18. McGraw-Hill, New York.
2. Agnew, D. C., and Merskey, H. (1976): Words of chronic pain. *Pain*, 2:73–81.
3. Atkinson, J. H., Kremer, E. F., and Ignelzi, R. J. (1982): Diffusion of pain language with affective disturbance confounds differential diagnosis. *Pain*, 12:375–384.
4. Blumetti, A. E., and Modesti, L. C. (1976): Psychological predictors of success or failure of surgical intervention for intractable pain. In: *Advances in Pain Research and Therapy*, edited by J. J. Bonica and D. Albe-Fessard, pp. 323–325. Raven Press, New York.
5. Bond, M. R. (1973): Personality studies in patients with pain secondary to organic disease. *J. Psychosom. Res.*, 17:257–263.
6. Dana, C. L. (1911): The interpretation of pain and the dysaesthesias. *JAMA*, 56:787–791.
7. Devine, R., and Merskey, H. (1965): The description of pain in psychiatric and general medical patients. *J. Psychosom. Res.*, 9:311–316.
8. Dubuisson, D., and Melzack, R. (1976): Classification of clinical pain descriptions by multiple group discriminant analysis. *Exp. Neurol.*, 51:480–487.
9. Ellis, H. C. (1978): *Fundamentals of Human Learning, Memory and Cognition*. Wm. Brown Co., Dubuque.
10. Fordyce, W. E., Brena, S. F., Holcomb, R. J., De Lateur, B. J., and Loeser, J. D. (1978): Relationship of patient semantic pain descriptions to physician judgments, activity level measures and MMPI. *Pain*, 5:293–303.
11. Gracely, R. H., McGrath, P., and Dubner, R. (1978): Validity and sensitivity of ratio scales of sensory and affective verbal pain descriptors manipulation of affect by diazepam. *Pain*, 5:19–29.
12. Graham, C., Bond, S. S., Gerkovich, M. M., and Cook, M. R. (1980): Use of the McGill Pain Questionnaire in the assessment of cancer pain: Replicability and consistency. *Pain*, 8:377–387.

13. Gunn, C. C., and Milbrandt, W. E. (1978): Early and subtle signs of low back sprain. *Spine*, 3:267.
14. Hunter, M., and Philips, C. (1981): The experience of headache—An assessment of the qualities of tension headache pain. *Pain*, 10:209–219.
15. Hunter, M., Philips, C., and Rachman, S. (1979): Memory for pain. *Pain*, 6:35–46.
16. Klepac, R., Dowling, J., and Hauge, G. (1981): Sensitivity of the McGill Pain Questionnaire to intensity and quality of laboratory pain. *Pain*, 10:199–207.
17. Kremer, E. F., and Atkinson, J. H. (1981): Pain measurement: Construct validity of the affective dimension of the McGill Pain Questionnaire with chronic benign pain patients. *Pain*, 11:93–100.
18. Kremer, E. F., Atkinson, J. H., and Ignelzi, R. J. (1982): Pain measurement: The affective dimensional measure of the McGill Pain Questionnaire with a cancer pain population. *Pain*, 12:153–163.
19. Kremer, E. F., Atkinson, J. H., and Ignelzi, R. J. (1982): Analysis of pain language in different diagnostic categories. *J. Psychosom. Res. (in press).*
20. Leavitt, F., and Garron, D. C. (1979): Validity of a back pain classification scale among patients with low back pain not associated with demonstrable organic disease. *J. Psychosom. Res.*, 23:301–306.
21. Leavitt, F., Garron, D. C., D'Angelo, C. M., and McNeill, T. W. (1979): Low back pain in patients with and without demonstrable organic disease. *Pain*, 6:191–200.
22. Lindsay, P. G., and Wyckoff, M. (1981): The depression-pain syndrome and its response to antidepressants. *Psychosomatics*, 22:571–577.
23. Melzack, R. (1975): The McGill Pain Questionnaire: Major properties and scoring methods. *Pain*, 1:277–299.
24. Melzack, R., and Perry, C. (1975): Self-regulation of pain: The use of alpha-feedback and hypnotic training for the control of chronic pain. *Exp. Neurol.*, 46:452–469.
25. Melzack, R., and Torgerson, W. S. (1971): On the language of pain. *Anesthesiology*, 34:50–59.
26. Morgan, C. D., Kremer, E. F., and Gaylor, M. (1979): The behavioral medicine unit: A new facility. *Compr. Psychiatry*, 20:79–89.
27. Sternbach, R. A. (1974): *Pain Patients: Traits and Treatment.* Academic Press, New York.
28. Titchener, E. B. (1920): Notes from the psychological laboratory of Cornell University. *Am. J. Psychol.*, 31:212.
29. Van Buren, J., and Kleinknecht, R. (1979): An evaluation of the McGill Pain Questionnaire for use in dental pain assessment. *Pain*, 6:23–33.
30. Veilleux, S., and Melzack, R. (1976): Pain in psychotic patients. *Exp. Neurol.*, 52:535–543.
31. Weingartner, H., Cohen, R. M., Murphy, D. L., Martello, J., and Gerdt, C. (1981): Cognitive processes in depression. *Arch. Gen. Psychiatry*, 38:42–47.
32. Woodforde, J. M., and Merskey, H. (1972): Personality traits of patients with chronic pain. *J. Psychosom. Res.*, 16:167–172.

Pain Measurement and Assessment,
edited by Ronald Melzack,
Raven Press, New York © 1983.

Relationships Between the MMPI and the McGill Pain Questionnaire

Laurence A. Bradley

*Section on Medical Psychology, Bowman Gray School of Medicine,
Wake Forest University, Winston-Salem, North Carolina 27103*

Many studies have appeared during the last 15 years concerning the utility of various psychometric instruments for the assessment of the cognitive and affective responses of chronic pain patients (5,14). With regard to patients' cognitive responses, the McGill Pain Questionnaire (MPQ) (20) represents a major advance in the measurement of pain experience. Several investigators have provided evidence for the reliability (12) and objectivity (10) of the MPQ. Other investigators have produced positive data regarding the construct validity of the MPQ using various procedures such as factor analysis (8,21), univariate correlational designs (13,17), and laboratory analogue techniques (16). Indeed, the MPQ is probably the most frequently used self-report pain measure in studies of chronic pain (14).

The Minnesota Multiphasic Personality Inventory (MMPI) is the instrument most often used to evaluate the affective responses of chronic pain patients (5). A great deal of effort was devoted to the delineation of an MMPI "personality profile" of chronic pain patients during the late 1960s and early 1970s (see 5,24). These attempts were eventually abandoned, as it became clear that numerous demographic and situational factors influenced patient responses to the MMPI (5). Recently, investigators have examined the feasibility of using the MMPI to differentiate patients with "organic" pain from those with "functional" or "mixed" pain (9), and predict patient responses to behavioral (15) and medical interventions (25). The results of these research efforts have not been consistent. The inconsistency has been due to the numerous methodological flaws associated with the majority of the investigations performed to date (see 4,5,14), such as the use of clinical outcome judgments with no reliability checks and the use of heterogeneous patient samples and treatment interventions.

MULTIVARIATE ANALYSES OF MMPI PROFILES

Bradley and his colleagues (5,22) have advocated the use of multivariate procedures, such as cluster analysis, to analyze the MMPI profiles of chronic pain patients and to delineate homogeneous patient subgroups that may show different behavioral and self-report correlates with respect to pain behavior, subjective pain estimates, or demographic variables (such as the duration of pain, number of previous surgeries or hospitalizations). As noted by Watson and Kendall (27), the delineation of patient subgroups may allow investigators more accurately to predict treatment outcome for individual patients than would the derivation of the linear relationships between a small number of MMPI scales and various measures of outcome (25). Two recent MMPI investigations by Bradley, Prokop, and their colleagues have used hierarchical clustering procedures to delineate replicable, homogeneous subgroups within independent samples of low-back-pain (6) and multiple-pain (23) patients of both sexes. The predictive power of the clustering approach was demonstrated by Turner and her colleagues (26). These investigators categorized the presurgery (laminectomy, discectomy, and/or fusion) MMPI profiles of 69 chronic low-back-pain patients on the basis of the four subgroups originally identified by Bradley et al. (6). The patients were examined and interviewed by an orthopedic surgeon 1 to 11 years after surgery and evaluated on several variables including overall outcome. It was found that patient subgroup membership was significantly associated with the overall outcome of surgery at long-term follow-up. Thus, preliminary evidence suggests that the MMPI profile clustering procedures used by Bradley and his colleagues eventually may allow clinicians and investigators to develop reliable and valid predictions concerning chronic pain patients' outcomes.

VALIDATION OF CLUSTER ANALYSES OF MMPI PROFILES

Several investigators have commented on the methodological difficulties associated with the use of multivariate methods to empirically delineate patient subgroups. These difficulties include the need for large patient samples in order to meet the criterion of a subject-to-variable ratio of at least 5:1 (22,27); the need to demonstrate the reliability of any derived cluster solution by means of replication across parallel data sets, different cluster analytic methods, or different variables (3,11,22); and the need to demonstrate the validity of any cluster solution by examining the relationships between the derived subgroups and external variables (3,22).

Both Bradley et al. (6) and Prokop et al. (23) used sufficiently large sample sizes and demonstrated the reliability of the derived subgroups across parallel data sets. Two additional teams of investigators, Armentrout et al. (1) and McGill et al. (19), have replicated the Bradley et al. (6) subgroups among male and female low-back-pain patients (19) and male patients with pain of diverse etiologies (1). In addition, Bernstein and Garbin (2) have replicated the female subgroups originally identified by Prokop et al. (23) among a sample of female patients with chronic pain of diverse etiologies.

Armentrout et al. (1) and McGill et al. (19) have also provided evidence regarding the validity of the patient subgroups derived by Bradley et al. (6). Both investigations indicated that the subgroups differed significantly from one another on variables such as duration of pain and number of hospitalizations (19) as well as degree of physical activity restriction and deterioration in marital communication and social relationships (1).

THE MMPI AND THE MPQ

The most recent investigation of the validity of empirically derived subgroups among chronic pain patients was performed by Bradley et al. (7). Unlike the studies described above (1,2,6,19,23) that were performed with patient samples drawn from relatively rural populations in the southeastern, southwestern, and midwestern United States, the Bradley et al. (7) study used patients (N = 96 males and 218 females) attending a public back-pain clinic in a large city in the northeastern United States. This investigation also provided the first examination of the relationships among various subgroups found among chronic back-pain patients and patients' responses to the revised McGill Pain Assessment Questionnaire (20; MPAQ) and the MPQ. Table 1 shows that two male and two female subgroups that previously were identified among back-pain patients in other investigations were derived (1,6,19). The two male subgroups were characterized by elevations on scales hypochondriasis (Hs), depression (D), hysteria (Hy) (the "neurotic triad") and schizophrenia (Sc) (subgroup 3), and scores on scales Hs, D, and Hy that approached 70 (subgroup 4). The two female subgroups were marked by elevations on scales Hs, D, and Hy (subgroup 1) and Hs, D, Hy, psychopathic deviancy (Pd), and Sc (subgroup 3). The relatively novel male subgroups were characterized by elevations on scales D, Pd, psychasthenia (Pt), and Sc (subgroup 1), and no elevations on any clinical scale (subgroup 2). The novel female subgroups were distinguished by no elevations on any clinical scale (subgroup 2), and a nearly significant elevation on scale D (subgroup 4).

Table 2 shows the results of a series of one-way analyses of variance on male patients' responses to the continuous variables on the MPAQ and MPQ as a function of subgroup membership. An examination of the table reveals that patients in subgroup 3 (elevations on Hs, D, Hy, and Sc) showed significantly higher pain rating index (PRI) scores on the affective dimension of the MPQ than did patients in other subgroups. The patients in subgroup 3 also chose a significantly greater number of affective verbal descriptors than did the patients in subgroups 2 and 4 with relatively unelevated MMPI profiles. The subgroup 3 patients also tended to rely on a greater number of analgesic and hypnosedative medications as well as report histories of greater reliance on health professionals than did patients in the other subgroups. A series of chi-square analyses of patients' responses to the dichotomous MPAQ variables showed that, relative to other subgroup patients, those in subgroup 3 more often reported mood change, sleep disturbance, increases in pain intensity following sleeping and lying down, and decreases in pain following alcohol ingestion.

Table 3 shows the results of a series of one-way analyses of variance on female patients' responses to the continuous variables on the MPAQ and MPQ as a function of subgroup membership. There were no differences among the female patient subgroups with respect to the affective dimension of the pain experience as measured by the MPQ. However, the patients in subgroup 1 (elevations on Hs, D, and Hy) consistently showed higher present pain intensity (PPI) and evaluative PRI scores

TABLE 1. *MMPI T-score means (K corrected) for male and female patient subgroups*

| | Male | | | |
| | Subgroup | | | |
MMPI scale	1	2	3	4
L	50.00	53.18	52.93	58.68
F	70.43	53.00	61.64	53.00
K	43.29	56.84	52.57	59.16
Hs	67.00	57.39	80.43	66.32
D	83.78	59.32	74.43	66.64
Hy	62.43	59.72	74.43	63.72
Pd	72.57	60.84	62.29	52.52
Mf	68.43	63.25	68.93	58.60
Pa	69.14	53.09	61.00	49.92
Pt	73.71	53.34	69.57	55.16
Sc	81.29	55.02	72.86	53.96
Ma	62.57	60.68	67.50	47.40
Si	66.71	47.77	52.79	53.52

| | Female | | | |
| | Subgroup | | | |
MMPI scale	1	2	3	4
L	63.06	55.06	48.91	49.87
F	58.88	52.03	68.65	57.42
K	65.00	56.26	47.20	48.58
Hs	79.94	57.42	73.50	60.66
D	70.56	52.87	72.87	67.82
Hy	80.06	59.25	73.17	59.66
Pd	69.22	56.19	71.76	58.63
Mf	52.88	50.33	49.98	47.76
Pa	60.78	52.52	64.74	55.71
Pt	65.00	49.66	68.04	60.79
Sc	67.31	52.38	74.43	58.00
Ma	53.34	56.97	67.61	49.76
Si	53.88	48.34	57.67	64.13

MMPI symbols and scale names: L, lie; F, frequency; K, correction; Hs, hypochondriasis; D, depression; Hy, hysteria; Pd, psychopathic deviancy; Mf, masculinity–femininity; Pa, paranoia; Pt, psychasthenia; Sc, schizophrenia; Ma, hypomania; Si, social introversion–extroversion.

than did patients in other subgroups. The subgroup 1 patients also tended to report greater reliance on health professionals than did patients in other subgroups, particularly those with no elevations on any of the clinical scales (subgroups 2 and 4). A series of chi-square analyses of patients' responses to the dichotomous MPAQ variables revealed that, relative to other subgroup patients, those in subgroup 1 more often reported unemployment owing to pain, retirement, or other reasons,

TABLE 2. One-way analyses of variance on male patient subgroup scores on the MPAQ and MPQ

Variable	Subgroup mean				F ratio[a]	p
	1	2	3	4		
Pain right now (PPI)	1.64	1.60	2.00	1.72	0.48	
Pain at worst	3.36	3.81	4.26	4.08	2.00	
Pain at least	1.50	1.28	1.64	1.32	0.95	
NWC sensory	6.57	5.67	7.71	6.13	1.05	
NWC affective	2.57	1.95	3.79	2.00	3.59[b]	<0.02
PRI sensory	13.93	13.26	19.64	14.76	1.31	
PRI affective	3.85	3.21	7.21	3.36	4.23[c]	<0.008
PRI evaluative	1.57	1.67	2.64	2.00	1.45	
Number present drugs	0.50	0.61	1.36	0.56	4.15[c]	<0.009
Number past back surgeries	0.07	0.28	0.21	0.16	0.71	
Number past other surgeries	1.00	1.44	2.14	1.56	1.65	
Number past treatments	2.29	1.60	2.57	1.16	2.78[d]	<0.05
Number past health professionals	6.71	4.77	7.71	4.00	4.07[e]	<0.01
Average hours sleep	7.43	6.66	6.57	6.42	1.46	

[a]df = 3, 92.
[b]Subgroup 3 > subgroups 2, 4.
[c]Subgroup 3 > subgroups 1, 2, 4.
[d]Subgroup 3 > subgroup 4.
[e]Subgroups 1, 3 > subgroup 4.
Duncan's multiple range test was used to test all pairwise comparisons. NWC, number of words chosen.

sleep disturbance, loss of all sexual desire, food intake changes, and continuous pain.

SUMMARY AND CONCLUSIONS

The results of the study by Bradley et al. (7) indicate that male and female chronic back-pain patients with MMPI profiles characterized primarily by elevations on scales Hs, D, and Hy (the neurotic triad scales) showed greater pain-related disturbances in their daily activities than did patients with relatively unelevated profiles or those with profiles characterized by elevations on the neurotic triad scales as well as scales Pd and Sc. The male patient subgroups with elevations primarily on the neurotic triad scales showed relatively higher scores on the affective dimension of the MPQ than did the other male patient subgroups; the female patient subgroups with elevations on the neurotic triad scales showed relatively higher scores on the evaluative dimension of the MPQ than did their female counterparts in other subgroups. It may be hypothesized that chronic back-pain patients who produce MMPI profiles defined primarily by elevations on the neurotic triad scales suffer more intense pain (especially females) or emotionally arousing pain (especially males) than do patients with other types of MMPI profiles. Those patients with MMPI profiles marked by elevations on the neurotic triad scales as well as scales Pd and Sc may suffer greater

TABLE 3. *One-way analyses of variance on female patient subgroup scores on the MPAQ and MPQ*

Variable	Subgroup mean				F ratio[a]	p
	1	2	3	4		
Pain right now (PPI)	2.65	1.50	2.00	1.69	9.11[b]	<0.0001
Pain at worst	4.28	4.06	4.21	4.21	0.53	
Pain at least	1.94	1.42	1.47	1.21	5.55[c]	<0.002
NWC sensory	7.63	6.01	7.02	7.23	1.75	
NWC affective	2.63	2.30	2.84	2.77	0.97	
PRI sensory	20.00	14.87	18.02	17.95	2.07	
PRI affective	4.81	3.84	4.90	5.54	1.53	
PRI evaluative	2.59	1.84	2.47	2.36	2.62[d]	0.05
Number present drugs	0.94	0.92	1.18	0.87	1.04	
Number past back surgeries	0.41	0.16	0.26	0.21	1.50	
Number past other surgeries	3.25	2.36	2.65	2.44	0.81	
Number past treatments	2.28	1.59	2.07	1.69	1.69	
Number past health professionals	8.28	6.00	7.27	5.87	3.28[e]	<0.03
Average hours sleep	6.07	6.90	6.42	6.71	2.02	

[a]df = 3, 214.
[b]Subgroup 1 > subgroups 2, 3, 4; subgroup 3 > subgroup 2.
[c]Subgroup 1 > subgroups 2, 3, 4.
[d]Subgroups 1, 3 > subgroup 2.
[e]Subgroup 1 > subgroups 2, 4.
Duncan's multiple range test was used to test all pairwise comparisons.

premorbid characterological disturbances than patients in other subgroups. These patients, therefore, may report pain ratings similar to those of patients with relatively unelevated MMPI profiles, but suffer somewhat greater pain-related disabilities owing to adaptation to the chronic invalid lifestyle.

The results discussed above are generally consistent with those of McCreary et al. (18), who found that a sample of male and female patients attending an outpatient back clinic produced affective MPQ responses that were significantly associated in a linear fashion with their scores on each of the neurotic triad scales of the MMPI. Similarly, Kremer and Atkinson (17) have reported significant linear relationships between affective PRI scores and scores on measures of emotional disturbance and functional disability produced by a sample of male and female pain clinic inpatients. McCreary et al. (18) did not independently examine the MMPI and MPQ scores of their male and female patients. Thus, further research must be performed to determine whether the sex difference reported by Bradley et al. (7) with regard to the MPQ responses of patient subgroups characterized by elevations on the neurotic triad scales was an artifact of the patient sample or the clustering procedure employed, or representative of a true population difference. Nonetheless, the results reported by Bradley et al. (7) as well as those reported by McCreary et al. (18) strongly suggest that there are important relationships between chronic pain patients' MMPI responses and their responses to the MPQ and pain-related disabilities. It is hoped that further investigations using both linear and hierarchical clustering approaches to the evaluation of MMPI profiles will clarify the nature of these relationships.

REFERENCES

1. Armentrout, D. P., Moore, J. E., Parker, J. C., Hewett, J. E., and Feltz, C. (1982): Pain-patient MMPI subgroups: The psychological dimensions of pain. *J. Behav. Med.*, 5:201–211.
2. Bernstein, I. H., and Garbin, C. P. (1982): Hierarchical clustering of the MMPI profiles of pain patients: A replication of Prokop, Bradley, Margolis, and Gentry. University of Texas-Arlington Press, Arlington.
3. Blashfield, R. K. (1980): Propositions regarding the use of cluster analysis in clinical research. *J. Consult. Clin. Psychol.*, 48:456–459.
4. Bradley, L. A., and Prokop, C. K. (1982): Research methods in contemporary medical psychology. In: *Handbook of Research Methods in Clinical Psychology*, edited by P. C. Kendall and J. N. Butcher, pp. 591–649. John Wiley, New York.
5. Bradley, L. A., Prokop, C. K., Gentry, W. D., Van der Heide, L. H., and Prieto, E. J. (1981): Assessment of chronic pain. In: *Medical Psychology: Contributions to Behavioral Medicine*, edited by C. K. Prokop and L. A. Bradley, pp. 91–117. Academic Press, New York.
6. Bradley, L. A., Prokop, C. K., Margolis, R., and Gentry, W. D. (1978): Multivariate analyses of the MMPI profiles of low back pain patients. *J. Behav. Med.*, 1:253–272.
7. Bradley, L. A., Van der Heide, L. H., Byrne, M., Troy, A., Prieto, E. J., and Marchisello, P. J. (1981): Pain-related correlates of MMPI profile subgroups among back pain patients. Paper presented at the Third World Congress on Pain, Edinburgh, Scotland.
8. Byrne, M., Troy, A., Bradley, L. A., Marchisello, P. J., Geisinger, K. F., Van der Heide, L. H., and Prieto, E. J. (1982): Cross-validation of the factor structure of the McGill Pain Questionnaire. *Pain*, 13:193–201.
9. Calsyn, D. A., Louks, J., and Freeman, C. W. (1976): The use of the MMPI with chronic low back pain patients with a mixed diagnosis. *J. Clin. Psychol.*, 32:532–536.
10. Dubuisson, D., and Melzack, R. (1976): Classification of clinical pain descriptions by multiple group discriminant analysis. *Exp. Neurol.*, 51:480–487.
11. Garside, R. F., and Roth, M. (1978): Multivariate statistical methods and problems of classification in psychiatry. *Br. J. Psychiatry*, 133:53–67.
12. Graham, C., Bond, S. S., Gerkovich, M. M., and Cook, M. R. (1980): Use of the McGill Pain Questionnaire in the assessment of cancer pain: Replicability and consistency. *Pain*, 8:377–387.
13. Hunter, M., and Philips, C. (1981): The experience of headache: An assessment of the qualities of tension headache pain. *Pain*, 10:209–219.
14. Keefe, F. J. (1982): Behavioral assessment and treatment of chronic pain: Current status and future directions. *J. Consult. Clin. Psychol.*, 50:896–911.
15. Keefe, F. J., Block, A. R., Williams, R. B., and Surwit, R. S. (1981): Behavioral treatment of chronic low back pain: Clinical outcome and individual differences in pain relief. *Pain*, 11:221–231.
16. Klepac, R. K., Dowling, J., and Hauge, G. (1981): Sensitivity of the McGill Pain Questionnaire to intensity and quality of laboratory pain. *Pain*, 10:199–207.
17. Kremer, E., and Atkinson, J. H. (1981): Pain measurement: Construct validity of the affective dimension of the McGill Pain Questionnaire with chronic benign pain patients. *Pain*, 11:93–100.
18. McCreary, C., Turner, J., and Dawson, E. (1981): Principal dimensions of the pain experience and psychological disturbance in chronic low back pain patients. *Pain*, 11:85–92.
19. McGill, J., Lawlis, F., Selby, D., Mooney, V., and McCoy, C. E. (1982): The relationship of MMPI profile clusters to pain behaviors. *J. Behav. Med., (in press)*.
20. Melzack, R. (1975): The McGill Pain Questionnaire: Major properties and scoring methods. *Pain*, 1:277–299.
21. Prieto, E. J., Hopson, L., Bradley, L. A., Byrne, M., Geisinger, K. F., Midax, D., and Marchisello, P. J. (1980): The language of low back pain: Factor structure of the McGill Pain Questionnaire. *Pain*, 8:11–19.
22. Prokop, C. K., and Bradley, L. A. (1981): Methodological issues in medical psychology and behavioral medicine research. In: *Medical Psychology: Contributions to Behavioral Medicine*, edited by C. K. Prokop and L. A. Bradley, pp. 485–496. Academic Press, New York.

23. Prokop, C. K., Bradley, L. A., Margolis, R., and Gentry, W. D. (1980): Multivariate analyses of the MMPI profiles of patients with multiple pain complaints. *J. Pers. Assess.*, 44:246–252.
24. Sternbach, R. A. (1974): *Pain Patients: Traits and Treatment.* Academic Press, New York.
25. Strassberg, D. S., Reimherr, F., Ward, M., Russell, S., and Cole, A. (1981): The MMPI and chronic pain. *J. Consult. Clin. Psychol.*, 49:220–226.
26. Turner, J. A., Herron, L. D., and Pheasant, H. C. (1981): MMPI prediction of outcome following back surgery. Paper presented at the Third World Congress on Pain, Edinburgh, Scotland.
27. Watson, D., and Kendall, P. C. (1983): Methodological issues in research on coping with chronic disease. In: *Coping with Chronic Disease: Research and Applications*, edited by T. G. Burish and L. A. Bradley. Academic Press, New York.

Pain Measurement and Assessment,
edited by Ronald Melzack,
Raven Press, New York © 1983.

Pain Description and Personality Disturbance

Charles McCreary

*Department of Psychiatry and Biobehavioral Sciences, University of California at
Los Angeles School of Medicine, Los Angeles, California 90024*

The description of pain can provide important information for the diagnosis of illness or injury. However, pain description is a complex process, and there is no simple linear relationship between degree of tissue damage and amount of pain experienced by a patient. Melzack and Torgerson (11), criticizing the current emphasis on a single intensity dimension of pain experience, proposed a new approach to the problem of description and measurement of pain in humans. They found that pain descriptors could be reliably organized into classes and subclasses involving sensory, affective, and evaluative dimensions. Melzack (10) developed the McGill Pain Questionnaire (MPQ) as a systematic, quantifiable procedure to measure these components of the pain experience. The development of the MPQ fostered a more systematic examination of the relationship between pain experience and psychological disturbance. This chapter reviews the possibility that the evaluative and affective descriptors reflect the complicated motivational and emotional processes of pain patients, whereas the sensory descriptors reflect factors more specifically related to particular disease processes.

There has been little systematic research on the relationship between pain description and particular pain syndromes. Dubuisson and Melzack (3) report that each of the eight pain syndromes they examined could be characterized by a distinctive pattern of verbal descriptors. There is some evidence that clinical and experimental pain syndromes differ in pain description (2). Furthermore, Reading (12) found that patients with acute clinical pain described pain differently from patients with chronic pain.

PAIN DESCRIPTION AND EMOTIONAL DISTURBANCE

The first study to focus directly on the relationship between pain experience and emotional disturbance examined differences in pain description among chronic pain patients with psychiatric and organic diagnoses (1). In this study, patients were interviewed, and the interviewer noted how the pain experience was described. The authors found that patients with organic diagnoses tended to use sensory–thermal words more often than patients with psychiatric diagnoses. Unfortunately, the authors did not use a systematic pain descriptor scale to measure the pain experience,

137

relying on clinical impressions from the same interview to diagnose the etiology of pain. However, this study prompted other researchers to pursue the question in a more systematic fashion.

Several recent studies have examined the relationship between direct measures of variables reflecting emotional disturbance and quantitative scales of verbal pain description. Leavitt and Garron (6) studied the association between pain expression and psychological disturbance in low-back-pain patients with and without organic disease. They found that patients with versus those without psychological disturbance portrayed their pain in a more extreme fashion in terms of both sensory as well as affective pain descriptors. Similarly, Kremer and Atkinson (5) studied a population of chronic benign pain patients and examined the relationship between scores on the affective dimension of the MPQ and measures of psychosocial disturbance. They found that patients who reported high affective dimensional scores were significantly more depressed and anxious and showed more somatic concern than patients who reported low affective scores. The authors suggested that the affective dimension score from the MPQ may serve as a useful index of the overall affective status of pain patients, thus providing important information for appropriate selection of treatments.

PAIN DESCRIPTION AND EMOTIONAL DISTURBANCE: MMPI STUDIES

The Minnesota Multiphasic Personality Inventory (MMPI) is frequently used to assess emotional disturbance in chronic pain patients since it has demonstrated validity in documenting psychosocial difficulties in a variety of populations, including patients with chronic pain. However, the MMPI has been criticized for use with medical patients because of its excessive length and threatening content. In fact, Leavitt *(this volume)* suggests that the MMPI probes into sensitive life issues, often provoking hostility and resentment in pain patients because many questions are seen as irrelevant to physical complaints and as implying that pain is imaginary. Leavitt therefore describes a procedure based on verbal pain description to assess serious emotional disturbance in pain patients. Several studies have related the MMPI to verbal pain descriptor scales, and these studies are reviewed below.

Fordyce et al. (4) investigated the relationship between 25 pain descriptors and 26 scales based on the MMPI. Only three of the pain descriptors produced seven significant correlations with the MMPI scales. Since the number of significant correlations did not exceed chance expectation, the authors concluded that there was little basis for inferring that pain descriptors are related to signs of emotional disturbance reflected by MMPI scores of pain patients. However, Fordyce did not use the MPQ to quantify pain description and did not factor analyze his pain descriptor items. It is not possible to assess whether a synthesis of his pain descriptors into sensory and affective scales would have produced a significant relationship with certain MMPI scales.

Another study by Leavitt and Garron (7) examined the relationship between the Back Pain Classification Scale (BPCS), derived from verbal pain descriptor adjectives, and psychological disturbance measured by the MMPI. Patients were categorized as either functional or organic based on their BPCS scores. The group of patients identified as functional (psychologically disturbed) by the BPCS produced significantly higher scores on the following clinical scales of the MMPI: hypochondriasis (Hs), depression (D), hysteria (Hy), psychopathic deviant (Pd), paranoia (Pa), psychasthemia (Pt), and schizophrenia (Sc). This group scored well within the abnormal range on the Hs and Hy scales. Leavitt and Garron did not separately analyze affective and sensory descriptors in relation to MMPI scale scores.

MMPI AND AFFECTIVE–EVALUATIVE VERSUS SENSORY DESCRIPTORS

The present author has carried out two studies examining the relationship between verbal pain descriptor scales and measures of emotional disturbance based on the MMPI in samples of patients with chronic low back pain. The first study (8) factor analyzed the MPQ, revealing dimensions of the pain experience that reflect sensory, affective, and evaluative components. Patients with high scores on the MMPI Hs scale portrayed their pain as more intense and as high in terms of affective and evaluative descriptors on the MPQ. Patients with high scores on the D and Hy scales portrayed their pain as more intense and as high in terms of the affective descriptor dimension. The evaluative descriptor dimension was highly related to ratings of the overall intensity of the pain experience. In fact, regression analysis revealed that the MMPI scales did not increase the efficiency of intensity alone in predicting the evaluative dimension, whereas the Hs, D, and Hy scales did contribute to the prediction of the affective dimension beyond the effects of intensity alone. Three sensory dimensions also derived from factor analysis of the MPQ were not significantly related to MMPI scale scores.

The second study (9) used a modification of the MPQ to assess verbal pain portrayal. An attempt was made to simplify the MPQ, because patients in the previous study appeared to require considerable individual attention in completing the original version of the MPQ and at times had difficulty understanding the meaning of some of the words. The simplified version was designed to be appropriate for mailing to patients in a package of screening instruments. It was developed by selecting one adjective from each of the sensory and affective subgroups of the MPQ and two adjectives from the evaluation category. No adjectives were selected from the miscellaneous categories. In this way, 15 words were selected (9 sensory, 4 affective, and 2 evaluative). Care was taken to eliminate unusual words and to include words that Melzack and Torgerson (11) found to be consistently categorized into one of three dimensions. The following words were selected: throbbing, shooting, stabbing, cutting, cramping, pulling, burning, stinging, aching, tiring, sickening, terrifying, punishing, annoying, and unbearable. The patients were asked to describe their pain on an 8-point scale for each adjective, with 0 indicating none, 1 reflecting very little, and 7 representing very much of the attribute.

Factor analysis of the simplified version of the MPQ produced four major dimensions. The first factor, accounting for 16% of the total variance, contained one sensory (aching), one affective (tiring), and two evaluative (annoying and unbearable) descriptors according to the original Melzack and Torgerson classifications. This factor appeared to reflect the overall burdensomeness of the pain experience. The second factor accounted for an additional 15% of the variance and contained items in the Melzack and Torgerson sensory classifications (shooting, stabbing, and cutting) that seemed to reflect intermittent pain sensations of short duration. The third factor contributed another 15% of the variance and contained two more items originally classified as sensory by Melzack and Torgerson: burning and stinging. This factor appeared to describe continuous pain sensations of relatively long duration. The fourth factor accounted for an additional 14% of the variance and contained words originally classified by Melzack and Torgerson as affective: sickening, terrifying, and punishing. This factor seemed to reflect fear of bodily harm associated with the pain experience. The four factors accounted for over 60% of the total variance.

There was evidence that MMPI scales were more highly related to the affective and evaluative dimensions of the pain experience than they were to the sensory dimensions. The MMPI scales showing the strongest relationship with pain dimensions were the hypochondriasis and hysteria scales, which correlated most highly with the affective and evaluative dimensions. However, these scales also correlated significantly with the two sensory dimensions. The paranoia and hypomania scales showed significant correlations with the evaluative and affective dimensions and not with the two sensory dimensions. The depression and anxiety scales did not show significant correlations with the affective dimension and did not differentially separate the sensory from the affective or evaluative dimensions.

CONCLUSIONS

There seems to be clear evidence that verbal descriptor scales can reliably portray the affective, evaluative, and sensory components of the pain experience. Studies of different clinical pain populations reveal that the sensory dimensions vary in item content across populations, and that these dimensions may reflect particular features of specific pain problems. On the other hand, the affective dimensions are more uniform in item content across different populations, and, especially when the samples are patients with chronic pain problems, a single dimension typically emerges from factor analysis that seems to reflect fear of bodily harm. This single affective dimension contains descriptors such as fearful, terrifying, punishing, torturing, and sickening.

There is some evidence that an affective dimension of verbal pain description is significantly related to independent measures of psychosocial disturbance (5,8). However, there is contradictory evidence concerning the relation of pain description to indices of depression and anxiety. Kremer et al. (5) found a positive relationship, whereas two other studies (8,9) found a weak relationship at best. Kremer et al.

approached depression and anxiety as states reflecting current functioning, whereas McCreary et al. (8) and McCreary and Turner (9) utilized the MMPI, which seems to measure depression and anxiety as traits. More research is needed to clarify how affective pain description may be related to state or trait measures of anxiety and depression. The BPCS developed by Leavitt and his colleagues seems to be highly related to psychosocial disturbance, but this scale contains both affective as well as sensory items.

There is clearly a need to refine the MPQ and to relate derived measures to treatment outcome variables. One of the advantages of the MPQ seems to be its relative lack of confounding by response set problems. The simplified version of the MPQ developed by McCreary and Turner (9) may have been confounded by a response set tendency to describe pain in a more extreme fashion, since it asks patients to use a numerical system in which higher numbers reflect more pain on each descriptive adjective. On the other hand, the MPQ asks patients to chose a word within each of 20 clusters of descriptors without overt cues that certain words reflect more intense pain. It should be noted that McCreary and Turner (9), using the simplified MPQ, reported a relationship between measures of emotional disturbance and sensory descriptors, whereas the earlier study (8) using the original MPQ did not reveal such a relationship. More research is needed to assess the complex relationships among portrayal of pain as frightening, response set tendencies to dramatize difficulties and measures of psychosocial disturbance. It is important to know which of these processes most effectively identifies patients who will respond poorly to medical treatment and are therefore in need of specialized psychological intervention.

REFERENCES

1. Agnew, D. C., and Merskey, H. (1976): Words of chronic pain. *Pain*, 2:73–81.
2. Crockett, D. J., Prkachin, K. M., and Craig, K. (1977): Factors of the language of pain in patient and volunteer groups. *Pain*, 4:175–182.
3. Dubuisson, D., and Melzack, R. (1976): Classification of clinical pain descriptors by multiple group discriminant analysis. *Exp. Neurol.*, 51:480–487.
4. Fordyce, W. E., Brena, S. F., Holcomb, R. J., DeLateur, B. J., and Loeser, J. D. (1978): Relationship of patient semantic pain descriptions to physician diagnostic judgments, activity level measures and MMPI. *Pain*, 5:293–303.
5. Kremer, E., and Atkinson, J. (1981): Pain measurement: Construct validity of the affective dimension of the McGill Pain Questionnaire with chronic benign pain patients. *Pain*, 11:93–100.
6. Leavitt, F., and Garron, D. (1979): Psychological disturbance and pain report differences in both organic and non-organic low back pain patients. *Pain*, 7:187–196.
7. Leavitt, F., and Garron, D. (1980): Validity of a back pain classification scale for detecting psychological disturbance as measured by the MMPI. *J. Clin. Psychol.*, 36:186–189.
8. McCreary, C., Turner, J., and Dawson, E. (1981): Principal dimensions of the pain experience and psychological disturbance in chronic low back pain patients. *Pain*, 11:85–92.
9. McCreary, C., and Turner, J. (1983): Psychological disorder and pain description. *Health Psychology*, 2:1–10.
10. Melzack, R. (1975): The McGill Pain Questionnaire: Major properties and scoring methods. *Pain*, 1:277–299.
11. Melzack, R., and Torgerson, W. S. (1971): On the language of pain. *Anesthesiology*, 34:50–59.
12. Reading, A. A comparison of the McGill Pain Questionnaire in chronic and acute pain. *Pain*, 13:185–192.

IV. ASSESSMENT OF PAIN BEHAVIOR

Pain Measurement and Assessment,
edited by Ronald Melzack,
Raven Press, New York © 1983.

The Validity of Pain Behavior Measurement

Wilbert E. Fordyce

*Department of Rehabilitation Medicine, University of Washington School of Medicine,
Seattle, Washington 98195*

This chapter will focus on behavioral measurement in the context of clinical pain—particularly chronic clinical pain. Lazarus (6) once said, "Of course, nearly everyone, apart from ESP enthusiasts, will agree that the only way we can know anything about another person is through his or her behavior. . . . " This is no less true of chronic pain than other matters.

Strictly speaking, clinical pain is a private matter. It exists only because someone says he or she has a pain problem. The nature of the pain, its intensity, impact, and even its very existence are discernible only by something the suffering person says or does: pain behavior. This reliance on the behavior of the suffering person is to be distinguished from the situation in experimental pain, in which a stimulus of known characteristics is applied in a certain way at a certain point on the body, for a specified period of time, and with a specified level of intensity. None of these stimulus characteristics is consistently present in clinical pain. The first critical issue, then, in considering chronic clinical pain is to recognize that the phenomena under study necessarily come to be known only by the behavior of the person who has the pain and not by reliance on information about physical findings.

The second critical issue is to distinguish between acute (or recent onset) and chronic pain. With chronicity there is increasing opportunity for factors independent of the originating injury (e.g., contingent consequences) to exert influence on pain behaviors. It is now adequately documented that pain behaviors that occur for one set of reasons at the time of onset may persist for a different set of reasons (1,2,4,9,11,12,14,15; W. Fordyce, D. Lansky, D. Calsyn, J. Shelton, W. Stolov, D. Rock, *unpublished data*, 1982). It follows that pain measurement strategy based on assessment of the alleged nociceptive stimulus is bound to go astray when attempting to cope with chronic pain.

Clinical pain measurement must of necessity rely on either some aspect of patient behavior or an empirically based analogue of it. One approach, and a conceptually sound one, is to use the McGill Pain Questionnaire (MPQ), an empirically developed analogue of patient behavior, to measure the nature of the pain problem or of changes across time in that problem. Since the MPQ is dealt with extensively elsewhere in this book, our only additional comment is that the MPQ need assume nothing more than that there are demonstrable empirical relationships between MPQ "values" and other characteristics of the person with the pain problem, his/her medical history and status, or other issues of interest.

There are many possible approaches to sampling a suffering person's behavior in order to obtain relevant and valid measures of the nature of the pain problem or changes in its status. Verbal report intensity measures have often been used, as in pain intensity rating scales. An alternative approach has been to attempt to bypass some of the hazards of reliance on verbal report by resorting to a different modality, as in visual analogue scales (7). Tactile analogue scales have also been used (8), along with kinesthetic scales, as in asking the person to match experienced pain intensity by squeezing a dynamometer. These approaches, in effect, ask the person to "say" something about the pain problem, whether "say" be in the form of oral expression, visual analogue, or whatever. Conceptually, such approaches are similar to pain-related measurements that ask the person to rate or express not only the degree or intensity of pain but also the extent to which it interferes with activity (5). One might, for example, ask a suffering person to indicate in some fashion whether pain influences sitting tolerance or the performance of daily tasks. The response might be in the form of a rating or simply a narrative statement. In either case, it is still asking the person to say something about the pain problem and/or its consequences. This brings us to the next crucial issue in pain measurement: the distinction between what people say and what they do.

The distinction between say and do behavior is not always easy to draw. Both are behavior. Both are operants and, as such, are sensitive to influence by the social consequences they encounter; hence, they are subject to systematic distortion. Nonetheless, as will be shown below, seemingly useful and valid distinctions can be drawn between say and do behavior in the context of chronic pain. These distinctions form the core of this chapter.

A brief illustration of the say–do distinction may help to clarify it further. It is commonplace to hear veteran smokers voice the resolve to quit smoking, or overeaters to vow to go on a diet and lose weight. It is also common to observe, subsequently, a divergence between what they say and what they do. The smoker's say behavior, and that of the overeater, may continue in the vein of resolve to reduce the frequency of the behavior in question, but do behavior may not concur. They may continue to smoke or may remain on a diet for only a short time. It is not necessary here to consider the reasons for that divergence between say and do, except to note that say and do behaviors usually encounter quite different consequences in the environment and thus are subjected to different conditioning effects. Thus, say and do are somewhat free to diverge, without it being necessary to attribute the divergence to loss of candor or veracity by the person. One implication of this is that the difficulties in obtaining "valid" (in this instance, honest) ratings or statements about a pain problem may rest in part on failure of the measurement system to recognize the distinction between say and do behavior. Many pain measurement methods have struggled to make the say behavior more honest and accurate. Instead of struggling to obtain honest or accurate statements from the person in the form of visual analogue, pain ratings, etc., perhaps it is better to look at the do behavior of the person.

A continuum of behavioral measurement can be erected from say behavior at one end to direct observation of activity or body movement on the other. At the say end, as shown in Fig. 1, are ratings either of pain intensity or of factors likely or allegedly influenced by the pain problem—for example, sitting tolerance, ability to continue to work, ability to lift.

At the behavioral observation end of the continuum are the data revealed by skilled and precise observation of the patient's activities. This might be accomplished by videotaping the performance of a prescribed set of physical activities or counting the number of steps a person takes or the size of the lawn mowed. These methods obviously promise more valid samples of patient behavior, but they suffer from both ethical and logistical disadvantages. The ethical limitations come to bear in instances in which the veracity of the patient's account is challenged and secret observations are carried out. Some insurance companies and workers compensation programs have been reported to have sent out agents secretly to make movies of allegedly disabled pain patients performing various tasks. The logistical problems are obvious. It is expensive, time consuming, and laborious to obtain direct observations, *in vivo*, of a person functioning in a complex environment. It is at least as time consuming and laborious to reduce the data from the observations to manageable form.

There is a middle ground between these two extremes that is often overlooked. One can obtain from the patient a kind of say behavior other than ratings or descriptive statements about the pain or its effects. The person can be asked to indicate the frequency with which specified activities were performed or engaged in during a specified time period, such as the immediately preceding 7 days. In a sense, this approach uses the medium of say behavior to obtain information about do behavior. The distinction can perhaps be further clarified by noting that a person may report that the pain problem limits sitting to approximately 30 min, but report on a diary form having attended a 2-hr movie or spending many hours sitting and watching TV. Similarly, a person may say he/she can tolerate riding in a car for only a few minutes, but record on a diary form driving for a 3-hour car trip. A person may report that walking is extremely painful and must be sharply curtailed, and record on an activity frequency count checklist taking walks several times daily or going stream fishing twice weekly.

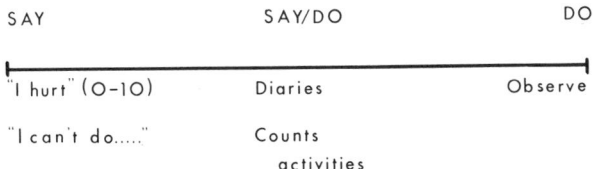

FIG. 1. Performance–observation gradient for measuring pain behavior.

If one were to rely on behavioral observations as a basic part of the data of pain measurement, obviously the preferred course would be to make direct observations. To make such observations in the patient's natural environment has, as noted, many ethical and logistical limitations. Another alternative is to make observations of the patient under structured conditions in the health care setting. This, of course, has long been the practice, although sometimes with questionable measurement precision, as in such procedures as the straight leg-raising test in the medical evaluation of a problem of back pain. This strategy of developing standardized samples of patient behavior is also represented by the work of Waddell et al. (13). Patients are put through a specified set of body maneuvers, and observations are made by the clinician. These observations form the basis of important diagnostic distinctions. Validity studies thus far reported are very promising.

There are yet other behavioral samples that could and should be standardized to strengthen measurement of pain behaviors. Seres and Newman (11) have used certain body position measures as a criterion of change in treatment. It seems plausible that, as one example, chronic low-back-pain patients whose pain problem has come under social control as a consequence of conditioning effects might be expected to show discernible differences in performance of a specified set of physical therapy exercises compared with low-back-pain patients in whom the originating tissue damage persists or the effects of surgeries have produced new sources of nociception.

Another behaviorally based approach has been followed in a number of the evaluation and treatment programs derived from a behavioral science technology (4,9,11). We shall focus here on work done by the author and colleagues (W. Fordyce, D. Lansky, D. Calsyn, J. Shelton, W. Stolov, D. Rock, *unpublished data*, 1982).

There are two measurement problems: evaluation or identification of the problem (i.e., diagnosis), and evaluation or measurement of change (progress or outcome). The parameters to be studied can be grouped as follows:

Pain behaviors. Visible or audible indicators of suffering or limited functions.

Functional impairment. Indicators of alteration or limitation in performance of life demands; for example, reduced performance vocationally or as a homemaker, reduced or altered leisure/recreational activities, reduced or altered sexual activity.

Health care utilization. Medication consumption, hospitalizations, physician visits, surgeries, emergency room visits, etc.

Associated or "ripple effect" problems. Depression, toxicity, and cognitive deficits from protracted heavy analgesic consumption, receipt of wage replacement funding because of inability to work, award of disability status, marital discord.

Each of these four aspects of clinical pain measurement can be sampled by devising forms or procedures that record patient-reported (say behavior) frequencies of what they do (do behavior). In a sense, as distinguished from say behavior at one extreme of the hypothetical continuum and do at the other, this approach lies in between, and might be termed say/do behavior.

Having provided a conceptual rationale for focusing on behavioral measures and a listing of behavioral domains of obvious interest in pain management, we must now address the question of whether or not there is adequate empirical support for this approach.

A recently completed study (D. Lansky et al., *unpublished data*, 1982) addressed directly the question of the relationship between pain ratings (say behavior) and patient-recorded frequencies of a variety of pain-related do behaviors. The study was based on data from 150 chronic pain patients referred to a multidisciplinary pain clinic for evaluation. Prior to being seen, patients completed 2 weeks of diary forms on which they recorded for each hour of the day when they were sitting, standing or walking, or reclining. In addition, diary forms provided for recording medication consumption and pain ratings on a scale of 0–10. Patients were divided according to their mean pain ratings into three subgroups: high, medium, and low. They were then compared on two kinds of data. One was a set of questionnaire items recording variations of say or self-ratings regarding the extent to which the pain problem interfered with activities: sitting tolerance, frequency of being awakened by pain, extent to which a specified set of daily activities were reduced in frequency by the pain problem. The data indicated these various say behaviors tended to intercorrelate positively. That is, analyses of variance comparing the high, medium, and low pain rating subgroups showed significant differences in the expected direction. Patients reporting more pain also reported more interference in activities, less sitting tolerance, and so forth.

The second data analyzed in this study were a variety of measures of say/do behavior. These can be categorized into three subgroupings. One was made up of patient-reported responses on a questionnaire asking health care utilization questions and of the medication consumption data reported on diary forms. The second subgrouping was the activity and body position data reported on the diary forms; that is, how much the person was sitting, standing/walking, or reclining. The third subgrouping was patient-reported frequencies of engaging in the week prior to completing the form in a 63-item set of commonplace activities. This form is known as the Activity Pattern Indicator (API).

A sampling of the results is shown in Tables 1, 2, and 3. Table 1 shows the tendency for the various say behaviors about severity of the pain problem to relate positively. Table 2 shows the lack of relationship between those say behaviors and health care utilization do behaviors. The data on medication consumption are not shown. These data also showed virtually no relationship between claimed pain severity and pain-related medication consumption.

Table 3 shows the findings derived from patient recordings of body position on the diary form. Here again, no significant relationship was found between amounts of time spent sitting, standing/walking, or reclining and reported pain severity. Those who said they hurt more reported no more or less sitting, standing/walking, or reclining. The one difference that emerged was that the high pain raters are more likely to display pain behaviors (reclining) when there are others around; a form

TABLE 1. Claimed amount of pain and limitation by pain rating subgroups

| | Pain rating subgroups | | | | | | | |
| | Low (N = 27) | | Medium (N = 96) | | High (N = 26) | | | |
Variable	Mean	SD	Mean	SD	Mean	SD	F	p
Mean pain rating	2.26	0.88	4.81	1.2	7.36	1.1	135.95	0.0000[a]
No. nights awakened by pain[b]	2.53	2.8	4.05	2.7	4.96	2.6	4.45	0.014
Min able to sit	108.95	130.95	62.95	45.8	55.65	37.0	4.42	0.014
Impairment index[c]								
Original values	1.46	1.0	1.62	0.98	2.27	0.27	6.40	0.002
Mean ranks[d]	65.06		71.55		101.08		(χ^2 = 11.48	0.003)[d]

[a]Tautological finding, as this variable was the basis for grouping S's.
[b]Week prior to being evaluated.
[c]Claimed amount of activities limited by pain. See text for details.
[d]Kruskal-Wallis one-way analysis of variance of mean ranks.

of "recredentialling" the pain problem relating to social consequences contingent on emission of pain behavior.

Scores obtained from the API yielded comparable results. High pain raters showed no significant differences in frequency of performing the activities listed on the API than those with medium or low pain ratings.

The results of this study suggest that the distinction between say and do behavior is a valid one, and that the strategy of sampling say/do behavior is promising.

There is a second validity issue to be addressed. For example, does a diary form that shows a particular number of hours per day of standing/walking mean the person actually stood or walked approximately that amount of time? Sanders (10) has compared diary recordings with mechanical devices recording actual body movement and found only a low power relationship. On the other hand, Wenck (14) compared diary-recorded activities with API-recorded activities. Where activities could be directly compared, significant correlations were found. These two concurrent validity studies yielded results suggesting that diary forms are not precise measures of what a person actually does. On the other hand, there appear to be significant correlations between two samples of activity.

A second kind of validation approach, criterion validity, has been studied, although the data are not yet complete. Fordyce and Loeser (unpublished data, 1982) have compared API data from four criterion groups: acute orofacial pain, chronic orofacial pain, acute back pain, and chronic back pain. Of 30 1 × 4 analyses of variance (15 on males, 15 on females), 28 showed significant differences among the four types of pain patients, 20 beyond the 0.001 level. In the case of the acute

TABLE 2. *Health care utilization by pain rating subgroups*

| | Pain rating subgroups | | | | | | | |
| | Low (N = 27) | | Medium (N = 96) | | High (N = 26) | | | |
Variable	Mean	SD	Mean	SD	Mean	SD	F	p
Years of pain Rx	6.74	6.1	5.94	5.0	7.50	5.5	0.83	0.44
No. clinics	6.44	5.2	8.17	7.7	9.42	7.6	0.87	0.42
Months since onset								
Original values	68.86	73.1	55.85	50.2	84.46	118.0	1.58	0.21
Mean ranks[a]	65.36		64.17		62.38		($\chi^2 = 0.08$	0.96)[a]
No. pain surgeries								
Original values	1.32	2.6	1.41	1.9	2.12	3.0	1.00	0.37
Transformed[b]	0.232	0.305	0.285	0.279	0.362	0.331	1.11	0.33
No. hospitalizations								
Original values	6.53	11.6	5.17	7.0	7.77	8.4	0.99	0.37
Transformed[b]	0.600	0.464	0.622	0.369	0.782	0.397	1.80	0.17
No. emergency room visits								
Original values	7.50	9.4	4.73	7.4	8.62	11.8	2.09	0.13
Transformed[b]	0.611	0.579	0.460	0.497	0.690	0.532	2.09	0.13

[a]Kruskal-Wallis analysis of variance of mean ranks.
[b]Log-10 transformation.

TABLE 3. *Diary-recorded activity levels by pain rating subgroups*

| | Pain rating subgroups | | | | | | | |
| | Low | | Medium | | High | | | |
Variable	Mean	SD	Mean	SD	Mean	SD	F	p
Sitting	28.64	10.7	28.96	11.3	28.65	13.3	0.01	0.90
Standing								
Original values	20.92	8.9	19.12	8.8	17.90	11.4	0.72	0.49
Transformed[b]	1.285	0.291	1.245	0.252	1.203	0.263	0.64	0.53
Reclining	46.42	8.6	47.92	13.4	49.45	16.96	0.31	0.72
Resting								
Original values	13.10	8.6	17.18	12.7	24.89	18.1	5.57	0.005
Transformed[b]	1.038	0.370	1.129	0.382	1.246	0.461	1.865	0.16
Sleeping								
Original values	33.33	5.0	30.74	7.4	24.56	7.8	11.20	0.000
Mean ranks[c]	95.59		77.80		46.04		$(\chi^2 = 18.00$	$0.000)$[c]

[a]Mean number of $\frac{1}{4}$-hr units/day.
[b]Log-10 transformation.
[c]Kruskal-Wallis analysis of variance of mean ranks.

patients, API data were based on the preceding week, during most of which there was no pain problem, since most acute patients had onset within 24 to 36 hr of being evaluated. Thus, API data on acute patients sampled activity patterns during periods in which no pain problem existed. This was not true of the chronic pain patients, whose problems had existed a minimum of 6 months. One would expect back pain to interfere more with a range of activities than orofacial pain. Indeed that was the case. In all 30 analyses of variance, the group with the lowest amount of activity was chronic back-pain patients. However, in addition, on 10 analyses of variance, there were also significant differences between acute versus chronic orofacial or acute orofacial versus acute back-pain patients. Sufficient data are not yet available from which to assess the sensitivity of the API to changes as a consequence of pain treatment, although studies are underway.

Measures of changes in health care utilization, medication consumption, etc., have been reported in a number of studies of pain treatment programs (3,9,11,12), which need no further comment here.

SUMMARY

The major points stressed in this chapter are:

In clinical pain, one cannot measure "pain." One can measure only pain behavior or analogues thereof.

In chronic pain, pain behavior is subject to influence by a variety of factors, some of which are unrelated to the tissue damage from which the pain problem originated. It follows that measurements of pain behavior cannot be relied on to characterize physical or neurophysiological characteristics of an alleged pain stimulus or nociception.

A distinction should be drawn between what people say about their pain and what they do. Moreover, a basis has been provided for relying more on what they do as a pain measure than on what they say.

ACKNOWLEDGMENT

This study was supported in part by Research Grant #G008003029 from the National Institute of Handicapped Research, Department of Education, Washington, D.C. 20202.

REFERENCES

1. Block, A. R. (1982): Multidisciplinary treatment of chronic low back pain: A review. *Rehab. Psychol.*, 27:51–63.
2. Cairns, D., Thomas, L., Mooney, V., and Pace, J. (1976): A comprehensive treatment approach to chronic low back pain. *Pain*, 2:32–36.
3. Corley, M., Owens, M., Russell, S., and Zlutnick, S. (1980): Program evaluation of a pain clinic. Paper presented at American Psychology Association meeting, Montreal.
4. Fordyce, W., Fowler, R., Lehmann, J., de Lateur, B., Sand, P., and Trieschmann, R. (1973): Operant conditioning in the treatment of chronic pain. *Arch. Phys. Med.*, 54:399–408.
5. Keefe, F., and Brown, C. (1982): Behavioral assessment of chronic low back pain. In: *Assessment Strategies in Behavioral Medicine*, edited by F. Keefe and Blumenthal. Grune and Stratton, New York *(in press)*.
6. Lazarus, A. (1977): Has behavior therapy outlived its usefulness? *Am. Psychol.*, 32:552.
7. Ohnhaus, E., and Adler, R. (1975): Methodological problems in the measurement of pain: A comparison between the verbal rating scale and the visual analogue scale. *Pain*, 1:379–384.
8. Petrie, A. (1960): Some psychological aspects of pain on the relief of suffering. *Ann. N.Y. Acad. Sci.*, 86:13–27.
9. Roberts, A., and Reinhardt, L. (1980): The behavioral management of chronic pain: Long-term follow-up with comparison groups. *Pain*, 5:151–162.
10. Sanders, S. H. (1980): Toward a practical instrument system for the automatic-measurement of up-time in chronic pain patients. *Pain*, 1:103–109.
11. Seres, J., and Newman, R. (1976): Results of treatment of low back pain at the Portland Pain Center. *J. Neurosurg.*, 45:32–36.
12. Swanson, D., Swenson, W., Maruta, T., and McPhee, M. (1976): Program for managing chronic pain. 1. Program description and characteristics of patients. *Mayo Clin. Proc.*, 51:401–408.
13. Waddell, G., McCulloch, J., Kummel, E., and Venner, R. (1980): Nonorganic physical signs in low back pain. *Spine*, 5:117–125.
14. Wenck, M. E. (1981): Activity pattern indicators: Correlation with activity diaries in chronic pain patients. Master's thesis. University of Washington, Seattle, Washington.

Pain Measurement and Assessment,
edited by Ronald Melzack,
Raven Press, New York © 1983.

Assessment of Chronic Headache Behavior

Clare Philips

*Department of Psychiatry, Shaughnessy Hospital, Vancouver,
British Columbia, V6H 3N1, Canada*

Any clinician who assesses a chronic pain sufferer is aware of the complex changes that have occurred in the sufferer's emotional state, cognitions, and behavior patterns (22). These changes are not incidental but form an integral part of the sufferer's pain problem and may even contribute to its self-perpetuation (23,24). This chapter will focus on the assessment of these pain behaviors and their relationship to the subjective experience of pain—a subject that has been given remarkably little attention in the past.

When acute injury occurs, the resultant tissue damage is associated with anxiety and pain (25). The pain appears to serve an important function, motivating a whole set of behaviors that promote tissue healing and recuperation. The individual rests, sleeps, withdraws from his normal routines, and appears disinterested in his environment. These behaviors motivated by pain can thus be seen as serving a rather special function. They actively influence recovery and are associated over time with pain diminution. Bolles and Fanselow (2) have called this aspect of the traumatic injury the "recuperative phase," functioning to promote healing.

A somewhat different situation is evident in an individual with a chronic pain problem such as headache, backache, or facial pains. The same types of behaviors can be detected, but in this case they persist and are elaborated extensively, even though no tissue damage is evident. But more importantly, the pain recovery system appears to be disordered, in that the behaviors occur without any pain decrease. There is no recuperation, and pain does not gradually reduce. Over longer periods, these behaviors increasingly replace and disrupt normal activities so that the behavior can be seen only as unadaptive and may actively delay recovery.

The possible negative role of chronic pain behavior has not yet been considered. It has long been thought that the behavior of those in pain is simply and directly a result of the intensity of their subjective experience. Thus, clinical assessments have focused on the subjective reports of sufferers concerning the severity of their pain, and from this the extent of behavioral disruption is predicted. The greater the pain experienced, the more extensive this pain behavior is presumed to be. The belief underlying this clinical approach is the existence of a 1:1:1 linkage among the major aspects of a pain problem: the physiological, the subjective, and the behavioral. In fact, over the last decade, the inadequacy of this belief has repeatedly been made evident, particularly in chronic headache (1,5,9,11,13,15,16). It is thus important to assess the behavioral aspect of a chronic pain problem in its own right in order to establish the extent of the behavioral incapacities.

In the past this has been done in two different ways. The first, and least satisfactory, has been to obtain a count of the rate of medication for pain. This single behavioral measure has been particularly popular in the headache treatment literature (3,4,14) and has been used as the valid spokesman of the myriad of pain behaviors that in fact occurs. Unfortunately, pharmacological aids are used only by sufferers with certain attitudes to drugs—attitudes that are often independent of the severity of their pain (17). Thus, this measure has proved a blunt and inadequate single measure of pain behavior.

The second method of measuring pain behavior has been in terms of activity and complaint levels. This method has been used almost exclusively by those involved in operant treatment of chronic pain (6–8), who are engaged in demonstrating the potency of environmental rewards on motivating rehabilitation. Although they have undoubtedly been able to demonstrate how reinforcement can increase general activity levels, they have not been interested in itemizing the type of behaviors manifested by an individual. The assumption made is that a homogeneous state of inactivity/withdrawal adequately represents the pain behaviors. The type and range of an individual's behavioral responses have not been relevant to the operant therapeutic approach. Consequently, although clear evidence of increased general activity and decreased complaining has been found (7,26), the functional role of particular pain behaviors in nociception and pain experience has not been investigated.

If pain behavior is considered as one expressive aspect, or component, of a complex pain problem (15), it is important for the clinician to have at his disposal an assessment instrument allowing him to evaluate the type and extent of behavioral disruption associated with a chronic pain problem. As well as giving a better characterization of the individual's problem, it would allow an evaluation of the effects of any treatment regimen, including pharmacological, behavioral, and cognitive treatments. Finally, such an instrument would permit the investigation of the functional role of such pain behavior in perpetuating the chronic pain problem.

RECENT RESULTS

While studying one of the most common chronic pain problems—headache—it became evident (17) that sufferers indulged in a wide range of activities directly motivated by pain episodes, but that these behaviors also occurred when the sufferer was pain-free. The latter occurred in anticipation or expectation that pain would result under certain conditions, unless certain behaviors were indulged in; such conditions include giving up work, refraining from going to films, and so on. Early treatment studies, using medication rate to predict pain behavior, proved to be inadequate measures of these varied behaviors, and it became necessary to devise a more systematic and objective technique to monitor the behavioral component of the problem.

The result has been the development of a checklist inventory made up of three major types of behavior that had been observed in chronic sufferers (17). The first type is avoidance behaviors, in which the individual withdraws from or minimizes contact with certain identifiable stimuli such as noise, lights, and so on. The second type is complaint behaviors that include both verbal and nonverbal complaining. The third is self-help or ameliorative behaviors that are part of the patient's attempt to cope with his problem (self-medication, seeing specialists, etc.).

The inventory was given to a group of chronic severe headache sufferers, and the results indicated a wide selection of behaviors irrespective of headache diagnoses (tension or migraine). The most commonly chosen behaviors can be seen in Table 1. Both avoidance and complaint were found to be frequent accompaniments of chronic headache. Medicating—doctor- or self-prescribed—was in fact an infrequent strategy, selected by less than 50% of the cases, thus confirming the inadequacy of medication rate as an index of pain behavior. As the headaches become more chronic, the behavioral scores increase, suggesting an enlarging behavioral repertoire as the problem persists. A more comprehensive version of this inventory has since been given to a group of chronic back-pain sufferers (27) who also found the items (derived from headache cases) relevant to their problem. It may be that chronic pain produces a stereotyped set of behaviors, irrespective of locus, rather than certain idiosyncratic pain responses. Future research will have to investigate this possibility.

The types of behavior, although significantly correlated (Table 2), in fact demonstrate a measure of independence. The correlation of avoidance and complaint behavior was $r = 0.38$ ($p < 0.004$), with only 14% of variance in common. When individual data were assessed, it was found that 33% of the cases showed a discordance between avoidance and complaint behavior. This evidence of individual differences in behavioral responses to chronic pain is an important fact for the clinician in planning treatment (16).

TABLE 1. *Percentage of behavior checklist items most commonly chosen by tension and migraine cases*

Behavior checklist items reported	Percentage of cases	
	Tension (*N* = 45)	Migraine (*N* = 10)
Avoid/reduce loud noise	82.2	100
Tell someone	80	80
Hold, press head, neck, temples	80	80
Close eyes	68.8	90
Avoid/minimize physical activity	68.8	90
Avoid/reduce bright lights	57.7	90
Avoid/reduce social contacts	68.8	80
Try to release pain by massage, etc.	60	90

TABLE 2. Correlation matrix of behavioral and subjective measures of tension headache pain (N = 45)

| | Behavioral measures | | | | | Subjective measures | | | |
| | | | | | | Headache diary | | MPQ measures | |
	Complaint	Avoidance	Behavior total	Medication measure	Intensity estimates	Frequency	Duration	Sensory	Affective
Complaint	—	0.38(0.004)	0.84(0.001)	ns	ns	ns	ns	0.39(0.003)	0.39(0.003)
Avoidance			0.69(0.001)	ns	ns	ns	ns	ns	0.32(0.01)
Behavior total				ns	ns	ns	ns	0.38(0.004)	0.39(0.009)
Medication				—	ns	0.31(0.01)	ns	0.27(0.03)	ns

The relationship between the types of pain behavior and the subjective experience of pain is evident in Table 2. No significant associations were found between the pain behaviors and the usual averaged diary assessment of headache intensity, frequency, and duration (see Philips, *this volume*). This confirms the inadequacy of predictions of pain behavior on the basis of subjective estimates of pain intensity. The clinician cannot determine the extent or type of behavioral response to pain on the basis of the sufferer's report of his pain intensity pattern. However, correlating the types of behavior with the fine-grained subjective assessment using the McGill Pain Questionnaire (MPQ) (12) produced some interesting results. The amount of complaining (verbal and nonverbal) was positively related to both the sensory and the affective qualities of the pain. Avoidance behavior, on the other hand, was related only to the pain's affective qualities. In a comparable study of low back pain, Zarkowska has shown that these associations between behavior and subjective experience gradually tighten as the problem persists over time or becomes increasingly "chronic."

The avoidance behaviors that form such a dominant aspect of the chronic pain problem are in fact the type of behavior commonly observed in anxiety neurotics and in the neurotic depressed. Certainly a persistent, unrelenting pain problem over many years would be likely to produce a state of learned helplessness, which has recently been shown to share much in common with depression (20). The depressive-like nature of this pain behavior may have contributed to the tendency of doctors to treat chronic tension headache as masked depression. In the group of severe cases we have evaluated, Wakefield Depression scores (21) did correlate significantly with avoidance behaviors ($r = 0.35$, $p < 0.009$).

Avoidance behavior, so common in fear and phobia, has been found to play an important role in perpetuating and often increasing fear reaction (19). Increased exposure under optimal conditions, however, leads to a diminution of anxiety and avoidance. It is possible that avoidance behavior in chronic pain may function in a comparable way, increasing the affective pain qualities that form an important part of the chronic headache pain experience (see Philips, *this volume*). Chronic pain has a number of features found in phobia: avoidance behavior, affective and sensory reactions, deleterious effects of high arousal, and so forth. Future progress may be made by careful manipulation of avoidance behavior in order to establish how instrumental it is in perpetuating the problem. Graded exposure may prove as useful a therapeutic technique for chronic pain as it has for chronic fear problems.

The checklist method of assessment is a quick, systematic, and easily repeatable tool for evaluating pain behavior. It is hoped that future investigations (currently underway) will both replicate and extend the work by allowing a factor analysis of these types of behavior. It will then provide a useful clinical instrument to define the nature and extent of the behavior motivated by a pain problem.

The major problem with such a measure of behavior is that it is derived from the subject's report. As with any subjective report, one is faced with error due to memory distortions, response biases, and so on. A more accurate assessment of behavior would be achieved if a laboratory assessment were made of an individual's behavioral responses to a potent exacerbating stimulus (18). Because of the degree of agreement on the effects of noise in the previously discussed checklist survey, a noise stimulus was used to assess headache sufferers' sensitivity to and tendency to avoid such stimulation. It was hoped in this way to develop an objective technique to evaluate avoidance behavior that could be used in assessing chronic pain behavior.

For ethical and practical reasons, the assessment technique had to be one that did not depend on pain induction or the presence of pain when the subject was assessed. In fact, the technique we evolved works on the prepain or subpain sensations evoked by noise. It seems likely that these sensations provide the cues the subject uses for determining exposure time and regulating active avoidance.

Subjects were asked to listen to an auditory stimulus (10,000 Hz) that gradually increased from an indiscriminable level to a possible maximum of 95 db. They were asked to calibrate the stimulus at three distinct levels on the basis of how the stimulus felt to them. The three calibrated levels were "comfortable," "uncomfortable," and "definitely unpleasant." The amplification levels were noted for each of these judgment points. Repeating this calibration procedure later in the same session showed the procedure to be highly reliable ($p < 0.001$).

Using the third judgment level of stimulation (definitely unpleasant), the subjects were asked to listen to the tone for 2 min, but were given the option of actively avoiding the stimulus if they found the exposure too long for them. An avoidance time could thus be calculated in terms of the length of time a subject exposed himself to this noise stimulus, up to a maximum of 2 min.

This technique has now been used on a group of chronic headache sufferers in pain, but also on a second occasion when pain-free. A nonheadache control group was also investigated to provide comparative data.

TABLE 3. *Auditory stimulus sensitivity*[a]

	Auditory stimulus		
	Comfortable	Uncomfortable	Definitely unpleasant
Control subjects (headache-free) N = 20	2.1 (1.9)	4.9 (2.6)	8.6 (2.1)
Headache sufferers (no pain) N = 15	1.3 (1.3)	3.1 (2.5)	5.5 (3.2)
Headache sufferers (in pain) N = 15	0.7 (0.07)	2.3 (1.6)	3.9 (2.8)

[a]Units linearly related to D.B. level (S.D.)

The results have revealed that as a group, headache sufferers are differentiated from controls on the basis of their clear and marked oversensitivity to the stimulus (Table 3). In fact, this sensitivity can be objectively detected in headache cases, whether or not they happen to be in pain during the assessment. They tolerate a narrow range of sound stimuli, calibrating a relatively low level of tone as definitely unpleasant. Not surprisingly, when they are in pain, the hypersensitivity is even more marked. Thus, a group differentiation of headache-prone and control subjects can be made merely on the basis of their sensitivity to auditory stimuli in the laboratory. This may be the consequence of a growing caution about exposing themselves to stimuli that may bring on, or exacerbate, their problem. On the other hand, it is possible that these individuals suffer from a vulnerability to certain types of stimuli that have been instrumental in the etiology of their chronic pain problem.

In addition to the group differentiation, this method also resulted in a state differentiation in terms of avoidance times. The worse the pain experience, the shorter the endurance of the stimulus, that is, the faster the avoidance. The avoidance time successfully differentiated those in pain from those who were pain-free (Table 4).

It is, of course, important that this laboratory assessment correlate with the sufferers' pain-motivated behavior outside the laboratory, thus giving the method criterion validity. A start has been made in a small study of chronic headache patients ($N = 23$). Sensitivity levels to definitely unpleasant stimuli were shown to correlate significantly with the checklist avoidance behavior total ($r = -0.32$, $p < 0.04$). These results are encouraging, and a replication of the study is now in progress.

Thus it appears that a simple, quick laboratory test can reliably quantify the well-known stimulus sensitivity of headache sufferers. This hypersensitivity can be detected independently of the current pain state. The withdrawal from such a stimulus was related to current state, but did not in fact occur as a consequence of increases in pain ratings. Avoidance behavior was associated with discomfort rating increases, but prior to pain increments, implying that the avoidance behavior was not directly pain motivated.

This fact raises a number of issues concerning avoidance behavior. It is possible that such behavior patterns are, in fact, evolved in anticipation of pain rather than as a direct consequence of it. We are currently investigating the extent to which

TABLE 4. *Avoidance time*[a]

	Auditory stimulus
Control subjects	115'' (14.4)
Headache sufferers (no pain)	104.6'' (35.9)
Headache sufferers (in pain)	91.8'' (38.8)

[a]Seconds (S.D.)

this anticipatory avoidance may play an active role in increasing subsequent sensitivity and affective pain qualities.

CONCLUSION

Little attention has been paid to the type of behaviors that develop as a consequence of a chronic pain problem. For the most part, clinicians have focused their assessment on subjective pain reports, and presumed that the behavioral patterns are directly proportional to the intensity of the pain report. In fact, the chronic pain problem presents a range of behavior patterns that are an integral part of the problem. Adequate assessment of these behaviors in the clinical evaluation of a pain sufferer is important in defining the nature of an individual's problem as well as monitoring the effects of any therapeutic intervention. The persistence of pain behaviors in chronic sufferers, in spite of the lack of recuperative power of the behaviors, makes it important to consider what role they may play in maintaining the pain problem.

In this chapter, two methods of evaluating pain-motivated behavior have been reviewed. The first is a behavioral checklist that is filled in by the pain sufferer. It reveals a wide range of behaviors associated with the problem. This instrument allows the clinician to obtain an indication of the extent of the behavioral response as well as the kind of activities that characterize an individual's problem. It is hoped that this checklist will be useful in organizing and evaluating treatment approaches.

The second method is to evaluate in the laboratory one major type of pain behavior: avoidance behavior. It has been possible to do this using a commonly avoided stimulus—noise—that can be manipulated experimentally. At this stage it is not clear how useful such a technique may be to all chronic pain groups. It may be that this sensory sensitivity is a more general characteristic of pain patients rather than being unique to head-pain patients. A replication with different chronic pain groups will be important in order to evaluate how useful this assessment tool may be. It is possible that each pain group will have to be evaluated with a relevant aversive stimulus. However, the exposure paradigm would appear to have wide application.

Future research and clinical attention must be directed to the issue of the functional role of pain behaviors in maintaining the pain experience. The significant relationship between avoidance behaviors and the affective pain qualities suggests that a fruitful line of enquiry may well be in exploring this relationship further. It is possible that the tendency to avoid stimuli actually supports and strengthens the affective pain response, much as avoidance behavior strengthens anxiety in phobic patients. The laboratory pain behavior technique will be an excellent format for systematic exploration of the functional role of avoidance behavior in chronic pain problems. It is hoped that future work on chronic pain will assess not merely the subjective and physiological aspects of the problem, but will also incorporate a concern for the behavior motivated directly or indirectly by a chronic pain problem.

REFERENCES

1. Andrasik, F., and Holroyd, K. A. (1980): A test of specific and non specific effects in biofeedback treatment of tension headache. *J. Consult. Clin. Psychol.*, 8:575–586.
2. Bolles, R. C., and Fanselow, M. S. (1980): A perceptual-defensive-recuperative model of fear and pain. *Behav. Brain Sci.*, 3:291–323.
3. Budzynski, T. H., Stoyva, J. M., and Adler, C. (1973): EMG biofeedback and tension headache: A controlled outcome study. *Psychosom. Med.*, 35:484–496.
4. Cox, D. J., Freudlich, A., and Meyer, R. G. (1975): Differential effectiveness of EMG feedback, verbal relaxation instructions and medication placebo with tension headaches. *J. Consult. Clin. Psychol.*, 43:892–898.
5. Epstein, L. H., and Abel, G. G. (1977): An analysis of biofeedback training effects for tension headache patients. *Behav. Ther.*, 8:37–47.
6. Fordyce, W. E. (1976): *Behavioral Methods for Chronic Pain and Illness.* C. V. Mosley, St. Louis.
7. Fordyce, W. E. (1978): Learning processes in pain. In: *The Psychology of Pain*, edited by R. A. Sternbach, pp. 49–72. Raven Press, New York.
8. Fordyce, W. E., Fowler, R. S., and De Lateur, B. (1968): Case history: An application of behavior modification techniques to a problem of chronic pain. *Behav. Res. Ther.*, 6:105–107.
9. Haynes, S. N., Moseley, D., and McGowan, W. T. (1975): EMG biofeedback and relaxation instruction in the treatment of muscular contraction headache. *Behav. Ther.*, 6:672–678.
10. Hunter, M., and Philips, C. (1981): The experience of headache—An assessment of the qualities of tension headache pain. *Pain*, 10:209–219.
11. Martin, P. R., and Mathews, A. M. (1978): Tension headaches: A psychophysiological investigation. *J. Psychosom. Res.*, 22:389–399.
12. Melzack, R. (1975): The McGill Pain Questionnaire: Major properties and scoring methods. *Pain*, 1:277–299.
13. Philips, C. (1977): A psychological analysis of tension headache. In: *Contributions to Medical Psychology, Vol. 1*, edited by S. Rachman, pp. 91–113. Pergamon Press, Oxford.
14. Philips, C. (1977): Modification of tension headache pain using EMG biofeedback. *Behav. Res. Ther.*, 15:119–129.
15. Philips, C. (1980): Recent developments in tension headache research: Implications for understanding and management of the disorder. In: *Contributions to Medical Psychology, Vol. 2*, pp. 113–130. Pergamon Press, Oxford.
16. Philips, C. (1982): The nature and treatment of chronic tension headache. Paper delivered at Banff International Conference on Behavioral Sciences, March, 1982.
17. Philips, C., and Hunter, M. (1981): Pain behaviour in headache sufferers. *Behav. Anal. Mod.*, 4:257–266.
18. Philips, C., and Hunter, M. (1982): A laboratory technique for the assessment of pain behaviour. *J. Behav. Med.*, 5:288–294.
19. Rachman, S. J. (1978): *Fear and Courage.* W. H. Freeman, San Francisco.
20. Seligman, M. E. P. (1975): *Helplessness: On Depression, Development and Death.* W. H. Freeman, San Francisco.
21. Snaith, R. P., Ahmed, S. N., Melita, M. C., and Hamilton, M. (1971): Assessment of severity of primary depressive illness. *Psychol. Med.*, 1:143–149.
22. Sternbach, R. A. (1978): *The Psychology of Pain.* Raven Press, New York.
23. Turner, J. A., and Chapman, C. R. (1982): Psychological interventions for chronic pain: A critical review. I. Relaxation training and biofeedback. *Pain*, 12:1–21.
24. Turner, J. A., and Chapman, C. R. (1982): Psychological interventions for chronic pain: A critical review. II. Operant conditioning, hypnosis and cognitive-behavioral therapy. *Pain*, 12:23–46.
25. Wall, P. (1979): On the relation of injury to pain. *Pain*, 6:253–267.
26. Yen, S., and McIntire, J. W. (1971): Operant therapy for constant headache. *Psychol. Rep.*, 28:267–270.
27. Zarkowska, E. A. (1981): The relationship between subjective and behavioural aspects of pain in people suffering from low back pain. M. Phil. thesis. University of London, London, England.

Pain Measurement and Assessment,
edited by Ronald Melzack,
Raven Press, New York © 1983.

Assessment of Pain Behavior: Factors That Distort Self-Report

*Edwin F. Kremer, **Andrew Block,
and *J. Hampton Atkinson, Jr.

*Department of Psychiatry, University of California at San Diego School of Medicine,
La Jolla, California 92037; and **Department of Psychology, Indiana University—
Purdue University Indianapolis, Indianapolis, Indiana 46205

Following the seminal work of Fordyce (8,9), chronic benign pain is concep-
tualized as a constellation of acquired behaviors. Within this conceptualization,
pain itself has ceased to have any relevance for medical diagnosis or treatment.
But through a learning process, the patient develops a behavioral repertoire characterized by verbal report of discomfort, a level of function disparate from the
objective physical disability, excessive use of narcotic analgesics, and excessive
use of the health delivery system.

Consistent with this behavioral model, treatment for chronic benign pain has
focused largely on effecting behavioral change. According to Hendler (12), there
are now approximately 22 inpatient behaviorally oriented pain treatment centers in
the United States, and outcome studies generally indicate a high degree of success
(e.g., 1,9,15,24,28). Success typically involves some but usually not all of the
following behavioral changes: decreased pain-oriented speech; increased activity or
physical capability; decreased use of narcotic analgesics; and fewer hospitalizations
and visits to physicians.

Investigators commonly agree on the necessary and sufficient conditions for valid
and reliable documentation of behavioral change following treatment. Indeed, there
is a well-developed technology for the assessment of behavior (see 7). Unfortunately, the exigencies of clinical service rarely allow for the ideal. Thus, outcome
studies usually report some range of approximations to the ideal. Morgan et al.
(24), Painter et al. (26), and Chapman et al. (6) relied on mailed questionnaire data
or a combination of mailed questionnaires and telephone interviews to assess the
efficacy of their respective programs. Somewhat more rigorously, Seres and Newman (28) interviewed patients during a 3-month postdischarge visit and obtained
range of motion measures with a goniometer. Similarly, Wooley et al. (30) interviewed patients in their homes 1 year after discharge and used a modification of
the Gottschalk-Gleser verbal sample technique to assess the degree to which pain-
related talk had changed. These latter two studies, however, employed patient self-

report to assess medication use and reliance on the health delivery system. In weighing the contribution of each of these reports to our understanding of pain treatment, it is necessary to appreciate fully the reliability of self-report data. If such data are not reliable or valid, despite the convenience in acquisition, they only confound our attempts to understand pain.

This chapter reviews a growing literature that suggests that chronic pain patient self-report can be systematically distorted by several variables. Thus, outcome studies that fail to control for such variables are probably not interpretable. This chapter will not provide an exhaustive review of variables that confound self-report per se since comprehensive reviews are available in the literature (e.g., 25). Rather, the variables that are germane to assessment in a chronic pain population will be examined.

SELF-REPORT OF ACTIVITY AND DEPRESSION

Many workers use increased activity as an index of improvement in chronic pain patients. For example, Fordyce (8) asked patients to keep an hourly diary of activities during assessment, treatment, and follow-up. The patient recorded his major activities and whether he was sitting, standing, walking, or reclining. The major variable of interest was "up-time," the number of waking hours that a patient reports he is up and out of a reclining position. Brena and Koch (5), in their pain estimate model, required patients to indicate the time spent daily in designated activities (e.g., golf, washing windows, shaving, etc.). As with Fordyce, the major variable of interest was up-time activities.

Several investigators have attempted to determine the accuracy with which chronic pain patients record their own behaviors. Sanders (27), for example, has developed an "up-time clock" for objective measurement of patient activity levels. The clock is worn in a sealed pouch on the patient's waist and is activated whenever the patient is in a standing or walking position. At the end of the day, a technician records total up-time accumulated on the clock and resets the device. Patients are unaware of the real purposes of the clock, being told that it is devised to measure skin temperature. In addition, patients were asked to record up-time using the diary format developed by Fordyce (8). In order to provide a comparison of accuracy, the up-time clock was also worn by two other groups of subjects: psychiatric nonpain patients and staff members. Both of these comparison groups also self-monitored activity levels. Sanders found that all three groups underreported up-time relative to that measured by the clock. However, chronic pain patients engaged in significantly greater underreporting of activity than both staff and psychiatric patients. These last two groups did not differ in underreporting.

Kremer et al. (17) replicated part of Sanders' findings using a different methodology. Twenty chronic benign pain patients were required to record their major activity each hour for the waking hours of the day and to indicate the proportion of each hour spent standing, walking, sitting, or reclining. Concurrently, staff members unobtrusively observed patient behavior on a time-sample basis. Consistent with Sanders' work, patients significantly underestimated up-time. These patients, however, did not underreport social behavior (defined as being with at least one other person). In an attempt to understand the variables that influence underreporting, the up-time data were subjected to a multiple regression analysis. The results of this analysis demonstrated that depression and chronicity of the pain complaint were significantly related to underreporting. A subsequent path analysis indicated that these variables were orthogonal. Thus, underreporting did not occur simply because depression was more likely the longer the chronicity of the pain problem. Although each of these variables suggests explanations regarding the mechanism for underreporting, there has been no attempt to date to provide data to support one mechanism or another. Obviously, such data are urgently needed because rational treatment depends on definition of these mechanisms.

These data have important implications for pain behavior assessment. First, depression and chronic pain are highly correlated. Lindsay and Wyckoff (19) examined 300 consecutive referrals to two pain treatment centers and found that 85% had significant depressive symptomatology. Thus, the observation of depression-related underreporting of activity in a chronic pain population is quite understandable. Because many patients resolve their depressive symptomatology during hospitalization, it is unclear whether a concomitant increase in up-time represents a true improvement in physical function or simply a decrease in underreporting.

STIMULUS EFFECTS ON SELF-REPORTING

There is a well-developed literature describing the influence of target person characteristics on disclosure of health-related material (see 23). This literature suggests that disclosure of information is a function of the age, sex, and perceived professional stature of the target person. Ignelzi et al. (14) examined consistency of self-report of pain intensity to different health professionals. These workers found that in a single clinic visit, 46% of chronic pain patients reported significantly higher pain intensity to a neurosurgeon than to a psychiatrist or a psychologist. Pain reports to the psychiatrist and psychologist did not differ. Using responses to the McGill Pain Questionnaire as an anchor, this effect appeared to be an exaggeration of intensity to the neurosurgeon rather than a mitigation of intensity to the psychiatrist and psychologist. One implication of this observation is that pain patients use self-report to communicate information or requests in addition to their actual pain complaint. A possible motive for such embellishment of self-report is to manipulate treatment selection. Although this suggestion is in no way novel, it does emphasize the necessity of obtaining objective data.

Block et al. (4) examined the effect of perceived presence of spouse on pain intensity report. In this study, hospitalized chronic pain patients responded to a tape-recorded structured interview. During one-half of the interview, patients were informed that their spouse was observing the interview through a one-way mirror. In the balance of the interview, they were informed that the ward clerk (neutral observer) was observing, but in neither case was a stimulus person actually present.

An estimation of pain intensity was requested during each half of the interview. Patients whose spouses were solicitous toward pain complaints (as determined by a response to pain behavior questionnaire) reported significantly greater pain intensity under perceived spouse observation than under the neutral observer condition. For nonsolicitous spouses, the opposite effect was obtained.

One implication of these studies is that self-report of pain is under discriminative control. Thus, the level of infirmity presented by the pain patient might wax and wane with changes in stimulus conditions, which makes the task of assessment much more difficult. Not only must objective measures be sought for pain behavior assessment, but the potential impact of discriminative stimuli requires some consideration in methodology, such as matched stimulus conditions, random trials, etc.

COMPENSATION AND SELF-REPORT

As Fordyce (8) has noted, the influence of financial compensation on the chronic pain patient's presentation of illness behavior is probably much more complicated than has been appreciated in the literature to date. At the simplest level, the Law of Effect argues that if patients are compensated for illness behavior, the probability of occurrence of that behavior will increase. Thus, some behaviorally oriented pain treatment programs will not treat patients engaged in litigation (1,8). There is some empirical support for such an approach. For example, Block et al. (3) found that patients referred by Workman's Compensation to a pain treatment program improved significantly less than patients referred by medical subspecialists. Further, the compensation-seeking patients were significantly less compliant than other pain patients. Similarly, Kremer et al. (18) reported that compensation-seeking patients demonstrated as good an acquisition of communication skills as noncompensation-seeking patients but failed to show the same decreases in self-report of pain intensity. These investigators suggested that potential monetary reinforcement of high pain report outweighed any incentive to use other communication strategies as an alternative to pain complaint.

Many studies, however, have failed to find any relationship between compensation seeking and pain treatment outcome. Chapman et al. (6) compared patients with pending disability, patients currently receiving disability, and noncompensation-seeking patients in a number of outcome measures and failed to detect any influence of the compensation variable. Likewise, Swanson et al. (29) failed to find compensation seeking of much explanatory value in attempting to understand patients who were dissatisfied with their inpatient pain treatment. Finally, Painter et al. (26) compared patients who demonstrated continued improvement after pain treatment with patients who failed to maintain gains experienced while hospitalized. On admission, both groups were composed of exactly the same percentage of patients receiving compensation (72%). As with Swanson et al. (29), these researchers found personality variables more potent in accounting for differences in treatment outcome.

It is clear that the influence of compensation on outcome is not a simple one and that our understanding in this area is less than complete. Unfortunately, the same level of confusion applies to our understanding of the effect of compensation on self-report.

In a multiple case study report, Kremer et al. (17) found that compensation-seeking patients underreported level of activity whereas noncompensation-seeking patients tended to report activity levels consistent with staff observation. In a more extensive study, however, Kremer et al. (E. F. Kremer, A. Block, A. M. Kremer, M. Gaylor, *unpublished data*, 1982) failed to detect any effect of compensation seeking on report of activity. It is clear that an empirical understanding of the precise impact of compensation on the behavior of chronic pain patients is woefully lacking. Given the vast experimental literature demonstrating the potent influence of monetary reinforcers on a variety of behaviors (see 2), it is likely that the generalization of these latter findings to the chronic pain population has far exceeded the empirical work available.

EFFECT OF MEDICATION ON SELF-REPORT

Although no investigations directly assess the influence of medications on accuracy of self-report, there are sufficient data to argue that this is likely to be an important variable. First, the available literature suggests that central nervous system depressant medication and perhaps alcohol use are high among chronic pain patients. By some reports (12,13), 40 to 45% of patients admitted to an inpatient pain treatment center were taking benzodiazepines [diazepam (Valium®), oxazepam (Serax®), or others], and approximately 80% used narcotics. A similar study (22) examined hospitalized chronic pain patients and found that 24% had physical evidence of drug dependence, 41% could be characterized as drug abusers, and 18% had family histories of alcoholism. Second, medications commonly used by chronic pain patients have demonstrated effects on cognitive function. For example, Hendler et al. (13) studied 106 admissions to an inpatient pain unit and examined cognitive function by the performance and verbal scales of the Wechsler Adult Intelligence Scale (WAIS), the Bender-Gestalt test, and an electroencephalograph (EEG). Sixty percent of the patients in the study were taking benzodiazepines at the time of admission, and approximately 40% of the patients were taking both benzodiazepines and a narcotic. Patients on benzodiazepines alone or on benzodiazepines and a narcotic were significantly more likely to have objective evidence of cognitive impairment than those on narcotics alone.

Evidence from normal volunteers revealed that diazepam produced underestimation of time (11), inaccurate assessment of psychomotor function, and an inability to engage in self-assessment (16,20,21). One study (10) of the chronic effects of central nervous system depressants in a polydrug abuse treatment clinic examined a group of subjects using the Halstead-Reitan, WAIS, trail-making test, and EEG. In the initial evaluation, 46% of the patients showed deficits in abstract thinking and perceptual motor tasks. At testing 5 months later when the group was abstinent or on reduced dosage, 27% showed continued impairment. These data suggest that an important task for research is to delineate the precise effects of prolonged alcohol and medication use on self-assessment and self-report.

CONCLUSION

The work reviewed here indicates that patient self-report of pain intensity, activity, and social behavior is distorted by many variables, some of which are inherent to chronic benign pain, that is, depression, chronicity, and so on. Thus, in the assessment of pain behavior and pain behavior changes, these variables must be acknowledged and controlled. Clearly, unobtrusive observation of pain behaviors under neutral stimulus conditions must be the preferred method of assessment. But, given the demands of such endeavors, it is equally clear this will not always be possible. Sophisticated use of methodology can mitigate the confounding variables introduced by the variables identified in the work reviewed here. However, that work that does not control for the influence of these variables (such as simple outcome studies) fails to assess adequately pain behavior change, and therefore fails to contribute to our understanding of chronic pain.

REFERENCES

1. Anderson, T. P., Cole, T. M., Gullickson, G., Hudgens, A., and Roberts, A. (1977): Behavior modification of chronic pain: A treatment program by a multidisciplinary team. *Clin. Orthop.*, 129:96–100.
2. Bandura, A. (1969): *Principles of Behavior Modification*. Holt, Rinehart and Winston, New York.
3. Block, A., Kremer, E. F., and Gaylor, M. (1980): Behavioral treatment of chronic pain: Variables affecting treatment efficacy. *Pain*, 8:367–375.
4. Block, A. R., Kremer, E., and Gaylor, M. (1980): Behavioral treatment of chronic pain: The spouse as a discriminative cue for pain behavior. *Pain*, 9:243–252.
5. Brena, S. F., and Koch, D. L. (1975): "Pain estimate" model for quantification and classification of chronic pain states. *Anesth. Rev.*, 2:8–13.
6. Chapman, S. L., Brena, S. F., and Bradford, L. A. (1981): Treatment outcome in a chronic pain rehabilitation program. *Pain*, 11:255–268.
7. Cone, J. D., and Hawkins, R. P. (1977): *Behavioral Assessment: New Directions in Clinical Psychology*. Brunner/Mazel, New York.
8. Fordyce, W. E. (1976): *Behavioral Methods for Control of Chronic Pain and Illness*. C. V. Mosby, St. Louis.
9. Fordyce, W. E., Fowler, R., Lehmann, J., DeLateur, B., Sand, P., and Trieschmann, R. (1973): Operant conditioning in the treatment of chronic clinical pain. *Arch. Phys. Med. Rehabil.*, 54:399–408.
10. Grant, I., and Judd, L. L. (1976): Neuropsychological disturbances in polydrug users. *Am. J. Psychol.*, 133:1039–1042.
11. Healy, T. E. J., Lautch, H., Hall, N., Tomlin, P. J., and Vickers, M. D. (1970): Interdisciplinary study of diazepam sedation for outpatient dentistry. *Br. Med. J.*, 3:13–17.
12. Hendler, N. (1979): *Diagnosis and Nonsurgical Management of Chronic Pain*. Raven Press, New York.
13. Hendler, N., Cimi, C., Ma, T., and Long, D. (1980): A comparison of cognitive impairment due to benzodiazepines and to narcotics. *Am. J. Psychol.*, 137:828–830.
14. Ignelzi, R. J., Kremer, E. F., and Atkinson, J. H. (1980): Patient pain intensity report to different health professionals. Paper presented at Association for Advancement of Behavior Therapy, New York, New York, November 25–27.
15. Ignelzi, R. J., Sternbach, R. H., and Timmermans, G. (1977): The pain ward follow-up analyses. *Pain*, 3:277–280.
16. Kleinknecht, R. A., and Donaldson, D. (1975): A review of the effects of diazepam on psychomotor performance. *J. Nerv. Ment. Dis.*, 161:399–411.
17. Kremer, E. F., Block, A., and Gaylor, M. (1981): Behavioral approaches to treatment of chronic pain: The inaccuracy of patient self-report measures. *Arch. Phys. Med. Rehabil.*, 62:188–191.
18. Kremer, E. F., Block, A., Morgan, C., and Gaylor, M. (1979): Approaches to pain management:

Social communication skills and pain relief. Paper presented at First International Conference on Psychology and Medicine, Wales, U.K., July 8–11.

19. Lindsay, P. G., and Wyckoff, M. (1981): The depression-pain syndrome and its response to antidepressants. *Psychosomatics*, 22:571–577.

20. Linnolia, M., and Hakkinen, S. (1974): Effects of diazepam and codeine alone and in combination with alcohol on simulated driving. *Clin. Pharmacol. Ther.*, 15:368–373.

21. Linnolia, M., and Maki, M. (1974): Acute effects of alcohol, diazepam, thioridazine, flupenthixole and atropine on psychomotor performance profiles. *Arzneim. Forsch.*, 24:565–569.

22. Maruta, T., Swanson, D. W., and Finlayson, R. E. (1979): Drug abuse and dependency in patients with chronic pain. *Mayo Clin. Proc.*, 54:241–244.

23. Mechanic, D. (1968): *Medical Sociology: A Selective Perspective.* Free Press, New York.

24. Morgan, C. D., Kremer, E. F., and Gaylor, M. (1979): The behavioral medicine unit: A new facility. *Compr. Psychiatry*, 20:79–89.

25. Nelson, R. O. (1977): Methodological issues in assessment via self-monitoring. In: *Behavioral Assessment: New Directions in Clinical Psychology*, edited by J. D. Cone and R. P. Hawkins, pp. 217–240. Brunner/Mazel, New York.

26. Painter, J. R., Seres, J. L., and Newman, R. I. (1980): Assessing benefits of the pain center: Why some patients regress. *Pain*, 8:101–113.

27. Sanders, S. (1980): Assessment of uptime in chronic low back pain patients: Comparison between self-report and automation. Paper presented at Association for Advancement of Behavior Therapy, New York, New York.

28. Seres, J. L., and Newman, R. I. (1976): Results of treatment of chronic low-back pain at the Portland Pain Center. *J. Neurosurg.*, 45:32–36.

29. Swanson, D. W., Swenson, W. M., Maruta, T., and Floreen, A. C. (1978): The dissatisfied patient with chronic pain. *Pain*, 4:367–378.

30. Wooley, S. C., Blackwell, B., and Winget, C. (1978): A learning theory model of chronic illness behavior: Theory, treatment and research. *Psychosom. Med.*, 40:379–401.

Pain Measurement and Assessment,
edited by Ronald Melzack,
Raven Press, New York © 1983.

Nonverbal Measures of Pain

*Kenneth D. Craig and **Kenneth M. Prkachin

*Department of Psychology, The University of British Columbia,
Vancouver, British Columbia, Canada V6T IW5; and **Department of Health Studies,
University of Waterloo, Waterloo, Ontario, Canada N2L 3G1

People in pain convey their distress to others through a remarkably rich variety of expressive cues. Information about pain available to observers may include verbal report, paralinguistic vocalizations, escape and palliative behaviors, diffuse locomotor activity, and changes in facial expression (see Table 1). No single category is an exclusive or invariant index of the presence or severity of pain, nor are there direct linear relations between tissue insult and any observable manifestation of pain. In addition, all of the channels of expressive action are responsive to nonanalgesic influence; hence, observers are obliged to consider the sufferer's life history, current circumstances, and the context of the injury or disease when making judgments about pain.

Although there are numerous categories of expressive response to painful stimulation, verbal report has been relied on heavily for a variety of reasons. Self-report measures frequently are reliable, sensitive to variations in disease states and injuries, responsive to treatment, and allow reconstructions of experiences after they have occurred. On the other hand, verbal report has several serious limitations. Of

TABLE 1. *Potential expressions of painful distress[a]*

Vocal behavior
   Language: complaint, appeals, qualitative description, ratings, demands, exclamations
   Paralinguistic vocalizations: crying, screaming, moaning, sighing
Nonvocal expression
   Facial: distortion, grimacing, specific configurations described in the text
   Limbs: startle, withdrawal reflexes, clutching or rubbing painful area, locomotor activity
   Postural: guarded or unusual postures, inactivity
   Autonomic activity: blanching, flushing, panting, vomiting

[a]These categories of expression are not empirically derived. They represent a partial compilation of expressions of pain reported in the literature and observed in clinical settings. The emphasis is on immediate reactions to tissue insult rather than instrumental or coping activity.

173

particular concern is the fact that people tend to monitor their self-reports carefully and maintain high levels of control. Requests for self-report are highly obtrusive and sensitize people to situational demand. In consequence, verbal report may be distorted, both purposefully and unwittingly, and situational influences in the form of interviewer bias and experimenter demand are commonplace (5). A further limitation of self-report is that young children, and some disabled people, are unable to use language as a medium to convey their thoughts and feelings (4). Consequently, other components of the suffering person's expressive repertoire are used by observers to understand what is happening.

In natural and clinical environments, nonverbal expression is an important determinant of observers' judgments of others' distress. There is good reason to believe that verbal report comes into play late in the sequence of events during a pain episode (22), whereas other expressive channels may play a more immediate role in communicating the experience. The importance of nonverbal signs of subjective discomfort in adults was underscored in a study (15) in which nurses reported that physiological signs and nonverbal behaviors were more salient and easier to use in pain assessment than was verbal communication. The nurses' preference for nonverbal manifestations of pain was consistent with the more general findings that people attach greater credibility to nonverbal expression when it conflicts with self-report (7).

BRIEF HISTORY

Although nonverbal expressions play a crucial role during pain episodes, systematic study of these phenomena has been sparse, occasionally erroneous, and without substantial impact on the knowledge base in the field of pain. Charles Darwin (6) discussed pain expression briefly in his classic work on emotional expression. He emphasized the adaptive evolutionary role of expressive behavior and postulated the existence of universal components of pain expression that convey derivative meaning to others. From this perspective, expressive behavior may be a species-specific, prepotent reaction to pain, because it enables conspecifics to recognize dangerous events and may marshall aid for the individual in distress.

The value of naturalistic observation of pain expression was well illustrated by Zborowski (24). His descriptions of ethnocultural variations among residents of the City of New York were not restricted to accounts of verbal report, but included substantial observations on nonverbal expression. For example, "Old Americans" were described as unexpressive, attempting to control reflex responses of withdrawal, and avoiding screaming or crying. Jews engaged in more displays of crying and moaning and Italians appeared similarly disposed to cry, moan, and complain, but also expressed their distress through many gestures and body movements. Although ethnographic studies of pain expression have been subjected to considerable methodological criticism (23), the richness of the accounts has been invaluable.

Early observations in the experimental pain laboratory suggested an important role for nonverbal expression. Chapman and Jones (3) concluded that facial expressive behavior is insensitive to biasing influences unrelated to nociceptive processes. They asserted that subjects were unable to exert control over narrowing of the outer canthus of the eye in response to thermal pain, even when instructed to do so. Although this probably is not strictly the case, since remarkable control can be achieved over specific facial muscles with training, voluntary control requires effort and practice beyond what one would expect of most people.

OVERVIEW OF PRESENT STATUS

There is considerable reason to believe that observers, formally trained or otherwise, have success in using nonverbal cues about pain in others, although the precise nature of the cues and the manner in which they are perceived and interpreted are not understood.

Global Judgments

The extent to which facial displays encode information about the intensity of pain can be addressed by having judges make global ratings. Judges viewing videotaped facial expressions have success in identifying intensities of discrete electric shocks delivered to healthy, volunteer subjects (K. M. Prkachin, K. D. Craig, *unpublished data*, 1981), and in specifying the amount of distress or "pain" experienced by subjects exposed to electric shocks (16). The social context was found by Prkachin, Currie, and Craig (21) to have an impact on facial expressions, because judges had greater difficulty discriminating the current intensities that had been delivered if the subjects had accepted shocks conjointly with someone else who expressed greater tolerance for the shocks than the subjects.

These studies involved the administration of brief, discrete noxious stimuli to subjects. It may be that the graded intensities of expression described in the foregoing studies are limited to responses to brief, relatively novel stimuli. There is probably relatively rapid habituation of the facial response to repeated or prolonged noxious stimuli. The central role of psychological and social determinants in chronic pain would suggest that the relationship between tissue insult and extent of nonverbal expression would be less direct in such problems.

Discrete Signs of Pain

There have been attempts to identify the specific behavior patterns that signify pain to observers. Hjortsjo (12) described facial changes brought about by actions of the orbicularis oculi and masseter muscles that were believed to represent a specific pain expression. Leventhal and Sharp (19) developed a system for coding the morphology of facial changes induced by childbirth labor, and described reductions in comfort and increases in distress that correlated with the extent of cervical dilation. Izard et al. (13) recorded the facial expressions of 1- to 9-month-old infants during inoculations or the taking of blood samples. They identified a facial pattern that, they believed, was a discrete expression of pain relatively specific to infants. This was described as a lowering of the brows, broadening of the nasal root, an angular, squarish mouth, and tightly closed eyes.

Developmental changes have been observed in pain-related expression. Izard et al. (C. E. Izard, L. M. Dougherty, C. L. Coss, E. A. Hembree, *unpublished data*, 1981) recently reported that facial expressions of painful distress during inoculations decreased with age, whereas anger expressions increased with age. These reports provide some confidence that pain-relevant, possibly pain-specific, information is encoded in expressive behavior. This study also suggested that nonverbal expression offers prospects of studying facets of the pain experience other than its sensory properties. Several "basic" emotional states are encoded in discrete patterns of change in the facial musculature, and it should be possible to recognize their interplay with expressions of physical distress.

A broad range of behavioral differences in pain response associated with age in infants was observed by Craig et al. (K. D. Craig, R. H. McMahon, J. Morrison, C. Zaskow, *unpublished data*, 1982). Coders used a time-sampling behavioral observation system to distinguish among verbal expressive categories (language, crying, screaming, etc.) and nonverbal expressive categories (activity in the face, torso, and limbs) in expressive reactions to routine immunization injections in the first 2 years of life. The findings indicated that the reactions of children during the first year of life were more spontaneous, global, and linked to the tissue insult of the injection, whereas the children between 13 and 24 months displayed more anticipatory distress, used descriptive language during the session, and engaged in self-protective voluntary movements. Thus, expressions of pain change systematically during the first 2 years of life as the infant accumulates experiences and acquires motor skills and the capacity to recognize and influence others.

Skilled clinicians have also demonstrated considerable facility in identifying important patterns of nonverbal expression. Ambeau (*unpublished data*, 1982) suggested that pain disorders with greater contributions from psychological than organic determinants would be characterized by greater expressiveness in general, more verbal complaint and report, acute reactions when changing bodily position, groaning as opposed to sucking in the breath during pangs of distress, and tendencies to interrupt activities by stopping talking and averting the eyes when particularly hurting. Validity studies of clinicians' impressions and the checklists developed by nurse researchers for observing signs of pain (e.g., 2) would be of considerable value.

Individual Differences in Sensitivity to Pain Expressions

As in all forms of social judgment, decisions about another's painful experience are subject to recognition errors and systematic biases. The observer is at risk of failing to recognize painful distress, or attributing greater or lesser distress than is appropriate.

Propensities to be sensitive to minimal cues when making judgments about the amount of stress other people are experiencing appear to be characteristic of many people in natural settings. For example, parents of children suffering recurring abdominal pain without known organic origins have been characterized as overanxious, overprotective, and tending to have fears that the pain was a manifestation of some dangerous illness such as cancer (see 4). The parents' concerns appear to make them unduly sensitive and perhaps overreactive to minimal signs of physical distress.

Analogous conservative decision processes appear to be readily induced during laboratory studies of observers' judgments of others' nonverbal responses to noxious stimuli (21). Judges led to believe that subjects were hypersensitive to pain provided higher ratings of their pain displays than judges who were not misled. Thus, people appeared predisposed to conservative judgments when assessing others' painful distress. Self-protective and altruistic dispositions are well served by early recognition that others are experiencing painful distress.

Control of Nonverbal Expressive Behavior

The various modes of nonverbal expression of pain are familiar to most people and subject to voluntary control. Physical distress is expressed in various degrees with ease by children playing games and actors on the stage, and occasionally by children and adults seeking the privileges attached to being ill.

The process whereby emotional expression comes under voluntary control has been subjected to investigation. Ekman and Friesen (9) observed that through socialization, expression comes under the control of "display rules." People rapidly learn the occasions at which displays of specific affective states are appropriate, and act accordingly by expressing, suppressing, or masking feeling states. However, the display rules do not yield patterns of expression that are isomorphic to spontaneous or nondeliberate displays. There is evidence that facial behavior may provide sensitive information that it is being influenced by display rules. Ekman (8), for example, described a study in which subjects watched a stressful film while alone or in the presence of the research investigator. Slow-motion films of the subjects in the latter condition revealed the presence of initial facial movements indicative of distress that were rapidly suppressed and replaced by neutral or positive expressions, such as smiles.

The study of genuine and deliberate nonverbal expressions of pain may provide progress in understanding neurophysiological integration of pain. Nonverbal measures lend themselves to the possibility of distinguishing between spontaneous and deliberate social displays of pain. The independence of the physiological systems mediating these patterns of nonverbal expression has frequently been observed in studies of neurological disorders (15). For example, patients suffering from postencephalitic Parkinsonism have been observed to be capable of smiling on demand, whereas smiles in spontaneous social interaction are absent (20).

Behavioral evidence also supports the hypothesis of distinctive neural substrates for genuine and dissimulated displays. LaRusso (17) found that some observers could distinguish when videotaped subjects were anticipating electric shocks in contrast to others faking the anticipatory response. Unfortunately, the topographic features of genuine or faked facial displays were not identified. Others have focused on the possibility of facial asymmetries and more vivid expressions on one side of the face during posed and natural emotional expressions, but the findings have not been consistent (1,12). It would be of great value to isolate and describe the facial topographies associated with genuine and simulated pain states.

SPECIAL PROBLEMS THAT NEED SOLUTION

Major emphasis must be placed on the development of methodologies for decoding behavioral repertoires expressive of pain. Many empirical studies of emotional expression have suffered from the disadvantage of reliance on observational systems that require the acceptance of strong theoretical assumptions about the underlying meaning of expressive acts, and judges appear to impose them rapidly on nonverbal expression that is inherently subtle and ambiguous. Several observational coding systems appear promising. Behavioral time-sampling systems would appear to be useful because they require interobserver reliability and concrete operational definitions of the target behaviors being observed.

While real-time observational systems are likely to yield valuable information, the speed and complexity of changes in facial and other forms of nonverbal expression can exceed observers' capacities to decode them. Microanalytic studies of filmed material presented to judges in slow motion may be necessary to capture the complexity of visual displays. Ekman and Friesen (10) have developed a sophisticated system—the Facial Action Coding System (FACS)—that uses highly trained observers to recognize and identify discrete facial actions. The system is fine grained, in that it decomposes facial expressive behavior into 44 separate action units, and is relatively atheoretical, because the trained coders use explicit definitions of the action units that are based on the anatomy of the facial muscles. FACS has been used extensively in the study of emotional states, but it has not been applied to the study of pain, with one exception. LeResche (*unpublished data*, 1981) employed a modified version of FACS to characterize a limited sample of candid photographs of facial expressions of individuals apparently experiencing acute pain. Commonalities in these expressions led to the proposition that there is at least one prototypic pain expression characterized as "...brow lowering with skin drawn tightly around closed eyes, accompanied by a horizontally-stretched open mouth...."

In conclusion, it is expected that an expanded multidimensional formulation of pain assessment would contribute substantially to our knowledge of such diverse aspects of pain as its neurophysiological integration and the social sequelae it triggers, as well as suggesting new targets for therapeutic intervention. Expanding the range of dependent variables employed in evaluations of putative analgetic procedures, by incorporating indices of nonverbal expression, is a practice to be recommended.

ACKNOWLEDGMENT

Preparation of this manuscript was assisted by a grant from the Social Sciences and Humanities Research Council of Canada.

REFERENCES

1. Cacioppo, G. T., and Petty, R. E. (1981): Lateral asymmetry in the expression of cognition and emotion. *J. Exp. Psychol.*, 7:333–341.
2. Chambers, W. G., and Price, G. (1967): Influence of nurse upon effect of analgesic administered. *Nurs. Res.*, 16:228–233.
3. Chapman, W. P., and Jones, C. M. (1944): Variations in outcomes and visceral pain sensitivity in normal subjects. *J. Clin. Invest.*, 23:81–91.
4. Craig, K. D. (1980): Ontogenetic and cultural determinants of the expression of pain in man. In: *Pain and Society*, edited by H. W. Kosterlitz and L. Y. Terenius, pp. 37–52. Verlag Chemie, Weinheim.
5. Craig, K. D., and Prkachin, K. M. (1980): Social influences on public and private components of pain. In: *Stress and Anxiety, Vol. 7*, edited by I. G. Sarason and C. D. Spielberger, pp. 57–72. Hemisphere, New York.
6. Darwin, C. (1872): *The Expression of the Emotions in Man and Animals*. Philosophical Library, New York, 1955.
7. DePaulo, B. M., Rosenthal, R., Eisenstat, R. A., Rogers, P. L., and Finkelstein, S. (1978): Decoding discrepant nonverbal cues. *J. Pers. Soc. Psychol.*, 36:313–323.
8. Ekman, P. (1977): Biological and cultural contributions to body and facial movement. In: *Anthropology of the Body*, edited by J. Blacking, pp. 39–84. Academic Press, London.
9. Ekman, P., and Friesen, W. V. (1969): Nonverbal leakage and clues to deception. *Psychiatry*, 32:88–106.
10. Ekman, P., and Friesen, W. V. (1978): *Manual for the Facial Action Coding System*. Consulting Psychologists Press, Palo Alto.
11. Ekman, P., Hager, J. C., and Friesen, W. V. (1981): The symmetry of emotional and deliberate facial actions. *Psychophysiology*, 18:101–106.
12. Hjortsjo, C. H. (1970): *Man's Face and Mimic Language*. Nordens Boktryckeri, Malmo.
13. Izard, C. E., Huebner, R. R., Resser, D., McGinness, G. C., and Dougherty, L. M. (1980): The infant's ability to produce discrete emotion expressions. *Dev. Psychol.*, 16:132–140.
14. Jacox, A. K. (1980): The assessment of pain. In: *Pain—Meaning and Management*, edited by W. L. Smith, H. Merskey, and S. C. Gross, pp. 75–88. Spectrum Publications, New York.
15. Kahn, E. A. (1966): On facial expression. *Clin. Neurosurg.*, 12:9–22.
16. Kleck, R. E., Vaughn, R. C., Cartwright-Smith, J., Vaughn, K. B., Colby, C. F., and Lanzetta, J. T. (1976): Effects of being observed on expressive, subjective and physiological responses to painful stimuli. *J. Pers. Soc. Psychol.*, 34:1211–1218.
17. LaRusso, L. (1978): Sensitivity of paranoid patients to nonverbal cues. *J. Abnorm. Psychol.*, 87:463–471.
18. LeResche, L. (1982): Facial expression in pain: A study of candid photographs. *J. Nonverbal Behavior*, 7:46–56.
19. Leventhal, H., and Sharp, E. (1965): Facial expressions as indicators of distress. In: *Affect Cognition and Personality*, edited by S. S. Tomkins and C. E. Izard. Springer, New York.
20. Monrad-Krohn, G. H. (1924): On the dissociation of voluntary and emotional innervation in facial paresia of central origin. *Brain*, 47:22–35.
21. Prkachin, K. M., Currie, N. A., and Craig, K. D. (1983): Judging nonverbal expressions of pain. *Canad. J. Behav. Sci. (in press)*.
22. Wall, P. D. (1979): On the relation of injury to pain. The John J. Bonica lecture. *Pain*, 6:253–264.
23. Wolff, B. B., and Langley, S. (1968): Cultural factors and the response to pain: A review. *Am. Anthropol.*, 70:494–501.
24. Zborowski, M. (1969): *People in Pain*. Jossey-Bass, San Francisco.

V. PAIN ASSESSMENT IN THE CLINIC

Pain Measurement and Assessment,
edited by Ronald Melzack,
Raven Press, New York © 1983.

The Measurement of Pain in Children

Mary Ellen Jeans

School of Nursing, McGill University, Montreal, Quebec, Canada H3A 2A7

Although there has been great progress in pain research and management over the last 15 years, the problem of pain in children has remained relatively neglected. From 1970 to 1975, 1,330 papers were published on the topic of pain. Only 33 referred to pain in children, and of these, 32 focused on pain as a symptom of pathology (5). There was little research related to children's perception of pain or their responses to pain. Since 1975 there has been an increase in the number of publications addressing these issues, but compared with the growth of literature related to pain in adults, the increase is minimal. One reason for the lack of study of pain in children is the problem of pain measurement.

If the measurement of pain in adults is a challenge, pain measurement in children is further complicated by their lower verbal fluency and by continually changing developmental stages. Despite the added problems, recent research in the field has been devoted to the development of tools to assess pediatric pain. Because of the diversity of approaches, samples, and research designs involved, the organizing theme for reviewing these studies will be a developmental one. Attempts to measure pain in children at different stages of development from infancy to adolescence reveal a variety of problems unique to each age group.

INFANCY

The precise age at which pain is first perceived is a matter of contention. Some health professionals believe that infants are relatively insensitive to pain. Peiper (19) is critical of surgeons who continue to perform lengthy operations without anesthesia on neonates and infants whom they believe are completely insensitive to pain. Poznanski (20) states, "Many anesthesiologists do not use general anesthesia until about three months of age, though there are no firm data on which to base this practice." Such practices are probably based on the notion that pain perception is dependent on the degree of cortical development and myelination of the nervous system. Although cortical development may be necessary for memory of pain, most evidence suggests that some degree of pain awareness is present at birth (10). Myelination is only partially completed at birth, but proceeds at a rapid rate and

183

at different rates among infants (16). This does not lend support to the assumption that neonates do not perceive pain.

The only route to knowledge of pain in infants is the study of their behavior. Motor responses and crying are the major indices of pain in infants and young children. Fisichelli et al. (6,7) studied crying as a response to a rubber-band snap on the sole of the foot. They found a period of relative depression of crying at 5 hr of age, increased reactivity between 2 days and 12 weeks, followed by declining reactivity until the age of 1 year. They also described a significantly high number of no responses between 8 and 16 weeks. It is difficult to determine if these changes are directly related to changes in pain perception, to the development of the crying response, or to other changes in psychological and physical development. Crying can be a response to a variety of stimuli, not just to pain.

Wasz-Höckert et al. (25), using a spectrographic and auditory analysis of infant cries, found distinct differences between cries of pain, hunger, and birth. To date, these findings have not been replicated. The technique is somewhat complicated and costly, and its potential as an objective, indirect measure of pain in infants requires further exploration.

Motor responses to painful stimuli, such as pinprick or injection, have also been studied as indicators of pain in infants and young children. These responses develop from being an immediate, generalized body reaction with occasional reflex withdrawal to a localized, defensive response by 12 months of age (15). Anticipatory fear responses to a painful stimulus begin to appear at approximately 6 months of age (13). Although some progress has been made in categorizing the normal neonatal response to pinprick (21), whether these motor responses differ in any specific way from the neonate's responses to other sensory stimuli still must be determined.

PREOPERATIONAL CHILD (1½ TO 7 YEARS OF AGE)

There has been virtually no systematic study of pain in toddlers. Some may argue that there is very little that is systematic about toddlers. This is a stage of rapidly developing physical and psychosocial skills. Responses to pain are likely to be much more complex than infants' responses and are influenced by many more factors. That the repertoire of nonverbal responses to pain has increased dramatically by this age is apparent. Gildea and Quirk (8) report that toddlers may respond nonverbally to pain by clenching their lips, rocking, rubbing, opening their eyes wide, and showing agitated or aggressive behaviors such as kicking, hitting, or biting. The hospitalized toddler is likely to be found hiding under the bed or running down the hall at the sight of a nurse carrying a syringe (1). Fear appears to be a powerful component associated with painful situations in this age group. The development of methods to assess pain in toddlers may have to arise from more standardized naturalistic observations of the behavior of these children in response to common noxious stimuli.

Toward the latter years of the preoperational stage (4 to 7 years), the child begins to use language to express pain. Although vocabulary may be limited and verbal reports of pain encounter validity and reliability problems, the child can now understand simple instructions. Eland (3), however, found that 13 of 25 children aged 4 to 8 years did not know the meaning of the word pain. She advised that the word "hurt" would be more appropriate to this age group. Jeans and Gordon (12), on the other hand, found that children as young as 5 years of age understood the word pain and were able to describe a few sensory and evaluative qualities of pain. They frequently used intensifiers to express their pain: "It burns an awful, awful lot."

Some attempts have been made to develop nonverbal techniques for the assessment of pain in children. Color scales comprise one approach to the assessment of pain intensity (14,22). In most cases, the colors red and black are most commonly chosen by children to represent intense pain. Less vivid shades such as orange and yellow are chosen to represent less intense pain (9). It is difficult to know if children preferentially choose red to depict the color of pain or they respond to the brightness of the color. Certainly a brightness-matching technique may provide more precise estimates of pain intensity.

Hester (11) studied 44 children aged 4 to 7 years who were receiving immunization injections. She used a behavioral observation tool and a creative technique called the Poker Chip Tool to assess the pain of injection. The behavioral rating method revealed that 54% of the children remained quiet during the procedure. In fact, 63.6% made no sound at all. Sixty-one percent remained still, but 86.4% were rated as being tense. These data suggest that gross motor activity and spontaneous vocalization are probably not reliable indicators of pain for children in this age group. The Poker Chip Tool, in which poker chips are equated with "pieces of hurt" (one chip being a little hurt and four chips being the most hurt), was highly correlated with the child's verbal and behavioral response to the injection. Hester concluded that the poker chip method was a fairly reliable measure of the intensity of pain in children. Also, children found the method easy to use. Such nonverbal techniques as color scales and poker chips may be particularly appropriate for children at this stage of development, for whom cross-modal thinking is common (18).

CONCRETE OPERATIONAL STAGE (7 TO 12 YEARS OF AGE)

The concrete operational stage of cognitive development begins at approximately 7 years of age and lasts to approximately age 12. These children have more sophisticated verbal skills, observe relationships between objects, and understand cause and effect. In a study of 74 10- and 11-year-old school children, Shultz (23) attempted to determine how these children viewed pain. A written questionnaire was used to elicit responses. Some of the questions were open-ended and some were multiple choice. In response to the question "What does pain mean to you?", fear of bodily harm and death were frequent answers. To a sentence completion item, "pain is ———", a number of responses reflected fear and anxiety. The 11-year-olds often described pain in psychological terms, such as being scolded, failing at school, or having their feelings hurt. The 10-year-olds, on the other hand, described pain only in physical terms. Sex differences were evident in the answers given to a question about responses to pain. Boys reported being brave more often than girls, who admitted to being nervous or afraid.

Asking children to write responses to questions about pain has a number of limitations. Certainly this technique would not be feasible for most children who have moderate-to-severe pain at the time of assessment. Also, if children have to think about and carry out the task of writing, it is likely that they will provide fewer thoughts or ideas about the subject of study. Face-to-face interviews may provide an alternative approach. Jeans and Gordon (12) interviewed 54 healthy children aged 5 to 13 years about the subject of pain. One aspect of the study elicited words used by the children to describe various types of pain. Although the 5-year-olds had the most difficulty describing pain in words, the majority of the children used adjectives and adjective phrases. The pain vocabulary grew from 5 adjectives cited by the 5-year-olds to 26 adjectives used by the 13-year-olds. When compared with the McGill Pain Questionnaire (MPQ), the adjectives used by the children represented all but five subgroups of those listed in the questionnaire.

In a study of joint pain in child hemophiliacs, using the MPQ as one measurement tool, it was found that children under the age of 12 years had great difficulty in responding (17). The children 12 years of age and over, however, were able to describe their pain in response to the questionnaire. In addition to the adjectives included in the MPQ, children tended to use several additional miscellaneous words to describe pain. Further documentation of these words is needed and would contribute to the development of a pain questionnaire appropriate for children between the ages of 9 and 12.

Although more knowledge of the pain vocabulary of children is needed, DiLeo (2) reports that children communicate more clearly and openly through their drawings than they are willing or able to do verbally. Recently, researchers have begun to use drawings as a means of assessing pain in children. Unruh (24) has used this technique for evaluating migraine headaches in children. The majority of these children drew pictures of heads being pounded with hammers or other objects. The pictures provide information about the meaning of the pain and the child's fantasies about the cause of pain. The data are rich in ideas for cognitive control techniques of pain management.

Jeans and Gordon (12) have also used drawings in an attempt to understand the developmental characteristics of the concept of pain. Fifty-four healthy children aged 5 to 13 were asked to draw a picture that showed pain, and when it was completed, they were asked to describe what was happening in the picture. All of the children completed the task easily in a short period of time. The pictures and stories produced a wealth of descriptive data, which were subsequently analyzed along numerous dimensions. Overall, children drew pictures that represented pain they had experienced in everyday activities, such as falls, scrapes, sports accidents, and so forth. None of the children drew pain in relation to injections, contrary to the findings of Eland (4), who observed that 62% of 200 hospitalized children, aged 4 to 10 years, reported a shot or a needle to be the worst pain they had experienced. Certainly all of the healthy children had been subjected to immunization injections at some time in their lives. It is possible that the most recent experience of pain governs the child's immediate concept of pain. Further study may help to clarify the impact of pain in childhood on the overall development of pain perception and responses, as well as provide more information related to memory of pain.

Jeans and Gordon (12) also found that children's concepts of pain, as depicted in their pictures, followed a definite developmental trend. At approximately age 11, the concept broadened to include pain of a psychological nature, such as grieving. Prior to that age, all of the children drew accidental, physical pain usually localized in the limbs. There were no drawings of abdominal or internal pain by any of the children. Again at approximately age 11, the children began to draw pain that was purposefully inflicted either by another person (fighting, throwing rocks, etc.) or by themselves (endurance themes such as ballet or racing). Abstract representations of pain appeared exclusively in the pictures of the 13-year-olds. The use of drawing as a means of learning more about pain in children appears to have considerable potential for both research and clinical practice. Continued study may provide more systematic techniques for analyzing the content of the pictures in order to make meaningful comparisons among different groups of children.

CONCLUSION

Research on the topic of pain in children encounters many methodological problems. It is evident that one cannot ask for volunteer infants to be exposed to a noxious stimulus. Yet, in order to study pain perception and response, control of the parameters of the noxious stimulus is necessary. In lieu of laboratory-controlled studies, researchers have utilized noxious stimuli such as injections carried out in pediatric health centers. Unfortunately, control over the stimuli is difficult in these situations, and numerous other variables are introduced. The investigator has little control over such factors as the parental response to the child, the strange and potentially frightening environment, and so on.

In addition to the problem of finding appropriate independent variables, the choice of dependent variables for pain measurement also presents a challenge. A variety of dependent measures has been used, including crying, motor responses, verbal reports, matching techniques, and drawing. None of these measures has been evaluated to determine its reliability and validity. The interpretation of data based on different stimuli and varying response measures continues to impede the development of knowledge about pain in children.

In the absence of this knowledge, clinicians are prone to base their assessment and treatment of pain in children on vague notions and myths (such as infants are less sensitive to pain) or on knowledge of adult responses to pain. This may lead to faulty assessment and inadequate treatment. Our need for knowledge about the development of pain throughout childhood is pressing, not only for clinical practice but also for the continued refinement of theories of pain. It is frequently stated that past experience and early learning have an important influence on pain perception and response in adults. Little is known about the nature of past experience or the type of learning that may have a critical impact on the development of pain perception.

In order to continue to study the nature of pain in children, a concerted effort is needed to develop new tools to assess pain. Some standard methods are required to assess pain across age groups in order to make comparisons. Yet it is evident that pain responses vary from one age to another and become more sophisticated as the child develops. Comprehensive pain assessment will require methods appropriate to each stage of development. The research to date is just a beginning. Much more is needed to establish normative data related to the development of pain and methods of pain measurement. At this beginning level of knowledge, descriptive research methods will form the basis for formulating more objective instruments to assess pain in children.

REFERENCES

1. Brandt, P. A., Smith, M. E., Ashburn, S. S., and Graves, J. (1972): I. M. injections in children. *Am. J. Nurs.*, 8:1402–1406.
2. DiLeo, J. H. (1977): *Child Development: Analysis and Synthesis*, p. 82. Bruner/Mazel, New York.
3. Eland, J. M. (1974): Children's communication of pain. Master's thesis. University of Iowa, Iowa.
4. Eland, J. M. (1976): *The experience of pain in children.* Paper presented to the Mid-American Sigma Theta Tau Research Conference, Kansas City, Kansas.
5. Eland, J. M., and Anderson, J. E. (1977): The experience of pain in children. In: *Pain: A Sourcebook for Nurses and Other Health Professionals*, edited by A. K. Jacox, pp. 453–473. Little, Brown, Boston.
6. Fisichelli, V. R., Karelitz, R. M., Fisichelli, R. M., and Cooper, J. (1974): The course of induced crying activity in the first year of life. *Pediatr. Res.*, 8:921.
7. Fisichelli, V. R., Karelitz, S., and Haber, A. (1969): The course of induced crying activity in the neonate. *J. Psychol.*, 73:183.
8. Gildea, J. H., and Quirk, T. R. (1977): Assessing the pain experience in children. *Nurs. Clin. North Am.*, 4:631–637.
9. Gordon, D. J. (1981): The developmental characteristics of the concept of pain. Master's thesis. McGill University, Montreal.
10. Gross, S. C., and Gardener, G. G. (1980): Child pain: Treatment approaches. In: *Pain: Meaning and Management*, edited by W. L. Smith, H. Merskey, and S. C. Gross, pp. 127–142. Spectrum Publications, New York.
11. Hester, N. K. (1979): The preoperational child's reaction to immunization. *Nurs. Res.*, 28:250–255.
12. Jeans, M. E., and Gordon, D. J. (1981): Developmental characteristics of the concept of pain. Paper presented at the 3rd World Congress on Pain, Edinburgh, Scotland.
13. Levy, D. M. (1960): The infant's earliest memory of inoculation: A contribution to public health procedures. *J. Genet. Psychol.*, 96:3–46.
14. Loebach, S. (1979): The use of color to facilitate communication of pain in children. Master's thesis. The University of Washington, Seattle, Washington.
15. McGraw, M. B. (1941): Neural maturation as exemplified in the changing reaction of the infant to pinprick. *Child Dev.*, 9:31.
16. Mennie, A. T. (1974): The child in pain. In: *Care of the Child Facing Death*, edited by L. Burton, pp. 49–59. Routledge and Kegan Paul, London.
17. Monk, M. (1980): The nature of pain and responses to pain in adolescent hemophilics. Master's thesis. McGill University, Montreal.
18. Mussen, P. H., Conger, J. J., and Kagan, J. (1974): *Child Development and Personality*, 4th ed., pp. 271–325. Harper and Row, New York.

19. Peiper, A. (1963): *Cerebral Function in Infancy and Childhood*, 3rd ed., pp. 29–33. Consultants Bureau, New York.
20. Poznanski, E. O. (1976): Children's reactions to pain: A psychiatrist's perspective. *Clin. Pediatr.*, 15:1114–1119.
21. Rich, E. C., Marshall, R. E., and Volpe, J. J. (1974): The normal neonatal response to pin-prick. *Dev. Med. Child Neurol.*, 16:432–434.
22. Schroeder, P. (1979): Use of Eland's color method in pain assessment of burned children. Master's thesis. The University of Cincinnati, Cincinnati, Ohio.
23. Shultz, N. (1971): How children perceive pain. *Nurs. Outlook*, 19:670–693.
24. Unruh, A. (1982): Children's drawings of their headaches. Poster presented at the Second Pediatric Behavioral Medicine Conference, Ottawa, Canada.
25. Wasz-Höckert, O., Lind, J., Vuorenkoski, V., Partanen, T., and Valanne, E. (1968): The infant cry: A spectrographic and auditory analysis. *Clin. Dev. Med.*, 29:9–42.

Pain Measurement and Assessment,
edited by Ronald Melzack,
Raven Press, New York © 1983.

Pain Assessment in Rehabilitation Medicine

Etta Rybstein-Blinchik

*Department of Rehabilitation Medicine, New York University Medical Center,
Goldwater Memorial Hospital, Roosevelt Island, New York 10017*

In a rehabilitation medicine service, pain is sometimes associated with the primary diagnosis and related disability, and sometimes is a symptom of another health problem unrelated to the primary problem. In traumatic disability, acute pain is often related to the initial injury, and has usually been treated successfully prior to the patient's arrival at the rehabilitation unit. The list of disabilities that have pain as a primary or secondary symptom is lengthy. In stroke, pain is often found in relation to shoulder–hand syndrome and muscular contraction or spasticity. Patients with spinal cord injury frequently experience pain below the level of the cord lesion. In addition, the degenerative joint diseases, certain neuromuscular disorders, and the neuropathies are painful. Phantom limb pain, thalamic syndrome, various neuralgias, low back pain, and chronic headaches are also found with some frequency in a rehabilitation medicine service. The critical issue in the clinical assessment of pain in such patients often concerns their thoughts and beliefs about their capacity to exert control over pain and many other aspects of their lives.

Many of the characteristics of the disabled person relate to his potential to benefit from treatment. The attitude toward one's self and one's disability is a crucial determinant in general adjustment and productivity. Also critical is the willingness of the patient's family and friends to give up the commonly held position that the disabled person is different from physically normal people. These issues, while separate from the pain problem of the patient, feed into the whole experience. Thus, assessment of the disabled pain patient must take into account the potential existence of the view, often held by both the disabled person and his social environment, that the handicapping nature of the disability has affected the total personality and influences characteristics of the individual apart from his physical disability. These attitudes toward disability must be adequately studied.

The development of the Attitudes Toward Disabled Persons (ATDP) test has been one such attempt (8). The ATDP is a Likert-type scale in which the subject responds to 20 statements by expressing his degree of agreement or disagreement on a 6-point scale. Each statement suggests that disabled persons are either the same as physically normal persons or that they are somewhat different. The statements cover two aspects of this problem. Approximately one-half is worded to point out similarities or differences in "personality" characteristics, whereas the other suggests the need or lack of need for special treatment for the disabled. Thus, an attempt is made to measure attitudes of disabled persons toward themselves (self-acceptance versus self-rejection) and to measure the attitudes of nondisabled persons toward the disabled (acceptance versus prejudice).

Yospe et al. (10) have recently emphasized that family attitudes and responses toward sick behaviors frequently play a significant role both in the etiology and treatment of chronic pain syndromes. They note that the literature reveals few objective studies designed to test this general assumption. The authors use the Sickness Orientation Scale to evaluate orientation toward illness of patients and their spouses. Based on their scores, they were identified, as individuals and pairs, as belonging to specific illness orientation groups. At the time of discharge, treatment outcome for each patient was obtained by means of a Treatment Outcome Scale, which was administered to the treatment staff. Results of this study indicate that there is a relationship of patient–spouse illness orientation to treatment outcome.

In an attempt to examine the importance of cognitive factors in the experience and treatment of chronic pain within a physical rehabilitation hospital setting, Rybstein-Blinchik (7) included an expectancy of change measure in a pain assessment battery consisting of subjective and behavioral indices of pain. The results indicated that patients' attitudes about their own potential in relation to the treatment procedures and requirements could significantly determine the effectiveness of a given pain program. The implications for assessment with disabled pain patients are that instruments for the measurement of attitudes toward disability and treatment and the consideration of the interaction of these factors might be important predictors of response to treatment and thus valuable in pain assessment batteries used in rehabilitation medicine.

PAIN AS A VARIABLE IN REHABILITATION

The relationship of pain to progress in physical rehabilitation and the interaction of these two variables with certain affective and attitudinal states require examination in the pain assessment of disabled patients. Anxiety, hostility, and depression, as well as states sharing affective characteristics but reflecting more wide-ranging attitudes, such as motivation for recovery and the level of morale and hopeful expectations, require evaluation within the setting of a physical rehabilitation center.

Rosillo and Fogel (4) reported that in males rehabilitation improvement rated as high was associated more often with low levels of reported pain. In females a significant bipolar trend was found in which both high and low improvement were associated with low levels of reported pain. Females who showed moderate improvement tended to report high pain levels. In interpreting these data, the authors note that for both sexes, pain generally acts in an overall fashion as a drive mobilizer or may be considered as a drive state in itself. However, the effects of pain as a drive were different in the two sexes in the patient groups of this study. Certain female patients with generally low drive levels may not have had sufficiently high arousal from sources other than pain to be mobilized toward more adequate therapeutic efforts. For these patients, low pain level was one component of a characteristic pattern of deficiency in drives. A persistent lack of drive may well result eventually in a poor therapeutic outcome, particularly if a patient's overall motivation for recovery is significantly reduced. On the other hand, for some female patients, pain appeared to be a hindering or disintegrative stimulus. In these patients, absence or low levels of pain appeared to free them to direct their energies more efficiently toward therapeutic goals, unhampered by interferences owing to pain. Thus, for those female patients for whom pain acted most predominantly as a drive stimulator, there was an overall therapeutic benefit from pain; those female patients for whom the predominant results of pain were disruptive or debilitating were hindered therapeutically by its presence. The overall data suggested that beneficial results from pain occurred somewhat more often than did counterproductive results.

In a later study, Rosillo and Fogel (5) administered the Multiple Affect Adjective Checklist to physically disabled patients in a rehabilitation center. Patients were asked how they felt "today." The checklist assessed anxiety, hostility, and depression levels. The degree of physical improvement in patients was rated by a team of physiatrists who used a 7-point scale, ranging from "worse" to "markedly improved," to assess the global overall physical improvement shown by each patient from admission to discharge, irrespective of initial severity of disability. Because of the acknowledged difficulties in achieving interrater agreement in the evaluation of physical rehabilitation improvement, independent assessments made by each physiatrist on the team were pooled in order to arrive at an average judgment so as to increase rating reliability. A third, independent set of evaluations was provided by a rehabilitation psychiatrist who interviewed and rated each patient as soon as possible after admission. His ratings, on a 7-point scale ranging from "not at all" to "extremely," consisted of judgments concerning the degree to which the disability caused discomfort and pain, overall state of morale, and motivation for recovery. The results indicated that for females, the higher the pain level, the higher the checklist report of dysphoric affects. In males the higher the pain, the lower were the dysphoric affect levels. Also, females manifested lower levels of morale in association with high levels of pain than did males. Both pain and motivation for recovery were found to be significantly associated with rehabilitation progress when each was separately related to progress. High pain in males was associated with low improvement and low pain with high improvement. High pain in females was associated with high improvement and low pain with low improvement.

Motivation for recovery was positively related to improvement in both sexes. Improvement was positively related to morale-hopefulness, anxiety, hostility, and to a lesser degree depression. High levels of these affects were associated with higher improvement levels. It appears that the effects of pain and of motivation for recovery on improvement levels may be relatively independent. Thus, although pain may operate as a drive state by itself, it does not consistently or directly alter motivation for recovery. To elucidate further the relationship of pain to motivation, one needs to evaluate each patient's idiosyncratic interpretation of his painful experiences. Since pain appeared generally to reduce dysphoric affects that may have served as drive mobilizers, the attendant reduction in drive in male subjects could have operated as a mild overall deterrent toward improvement. In female patients, pain more often acted to heighten dysphoric affects, and in this way appeared to promote higher drive states. The higher drive level, in turn, could tend to promote higher improvement outcomes.

These findings are in marked contrast to earlier notions that viewed pain as a deterrent to rehabilitation progress. For example, Rusk (6) outlined some of the ways in which pain interfered with rehabilitation. Pain could: prevent the physical activities necessary for progress; lead to insomnia with resulting fatigue, impeding progress; result in surgical or pharmacological intervention that either slowed or stopped rehabilitation; lead to interpersonal problems with staff and fellow patients; lead to somatic preoccupation and withdrawal from rehabilitation program participation; and bring sources of secondary gain. In reference to the last, the pain complaint is viewed as an attempt to avoid participation, not because of physical limitations but because pain allows a rationale or legitimate excuse for uninvolvement, both in rehabilitation and in life. The patient experiencing pain over an extended period of time is expected to be less likely to avail himself in the rehabilitation effort.

INNOVATIVE PAIN ASSESSMENT APPROACHES FOR THE DISABLED PATIENT

Psychological assessment methods have not directly addressed the issue of how a patient's particular interpretation and consequent utilization of pain may be a critical factor with respect to the effect of pain on progress in physical rehabilitation. A consideration of several innovative pain assessment procedures discussed in papers presented at the Third World Congress on Pain of the International Association for the Study of Pain in Edinburgh, Scotland, Sept. 4–11, 1981, provides a means of developing a more comprehensive framework for measuring the dynamic process of pain in disabled patients. In an attempt to examine the characteristics of the concept of pain at different stages of normal growth and development, Jeans (1) asked 50 nonhospitalized normal children from ages 5 to 13, on an individual basis, to draw a picture that represents pain. The child was given five magic markers of different colors (red, yellow, blue, black, and green) and an 8 × 11-in sheet of heavy white blank paper. Upon completion, the child described the picture and told a story related to it. The interviews were taped and the interview techniques were similar to those used in projective testing.

Rogers (3) employed verbal and visual analogue methods in a study assessing pain and pain relief in children between the ages of 2 and 18 years with cancer. Verbal scales consisted of a 4-point categorical pain scale ("none," "slight," "moderate," and "severe") and a 5-point categorical pain relief scale ("none," "slight," "moderate," "a lot," and "complete"). In children 8 years and older, visual analogue scales for pain and pain relief, consisting of a 100-mm horizontal line that contained no markings, were used as well as a random display of seven pain descriptors. In children under 8 years, a series of five (happy–sad) drawings were employed. Preliminary observations suggested that children responded the same way as adults in reporting their pain and pain relief. Villamira et al. (9) used a battery of psychological tests consisting of the Minnesota Multiphasic Personality Inventory, Draw-a-Person Test, and Draw-a-Tree Test in diagnosing chronic pain syndromes. On occasion, a substantial discrepancy between structural and dynamic patterns of personality profiles was found. The projective tests balanced and biased the structural data, providing a more comprehensive frame of the dynamic process of chronic pain.

Reading and Newton (2) have described a card sort method of pain assessment, which is simpler than existing approaches. On each card are two words describing pain, one above the other, in balanced order to remove the effects of position set. The patient's task is to sort the cards according to whether the top or bottom word on each card most closely resembles the pain he is experiencing. At any one time, it requires patients to choose between two different words clearly presented on white cards, with the entire task taking about 5 min to complete. Zakrzewski (11) tested a different kind of technique at the Pain Centre of the Warsaw Medical School. One thousand pain patients completed a "Draw Your Pain" task on blank sheets of paper using colored crayons. More than 400 of them had also been administered several known psychometric tests. Computations were performed to reveal whether or not the characteristics of pain drawings reflected those of patients' personalities.

The development of such innovative procedures relates to a critical dilemma in the pain assessment of disabled individuals—that a broad evaluation of the perception of the pain experience may not always be obtainable, even in a comprehensive assessment procedure utilizing self-report questionnaires, observations by significant others, or the health care provider. The disabled chronic pain patient experiences a dual hurt, of the body and of the human being as a whole. The symbolic and the cognitive impact resulting from the experience of organic illness is a powerful one. This cannot always be expressed through verbal means by the disabled. Sometimes this is due to the very nature of the handicap, which precludes such expression, as in the case of expressive aphasia. Although gesturing may offer an alternate mode of response, other disabilities, such as impaired vision as from postcerebrovascular accident hemianopsia, auditory losses, perceptual deficits, language disorders such as receptive aphasia or brain damage, preclude satisfactory performance on assessment tasks. Moreover, interpretation of results is difficult. However, a more basic issue concerns the limitations of current verbal pain measurement methods for the disabled owing to the ambiguous nature of the very phenomenon involved. As the impact of bodily suffering on the wholeness of the self-image is influenced by many internal and external factors, no straight ratio between the medical severity of a handicap on the one hand and the varying degrees of anxiety and insecurity that spring from it exists. Symbolic representation of self-image, in various modes allowing for the creative–projective expression of balance and color, could provide an alternate means of assessing the emotional and cognitive processes involved in communicating one's body experience.

CONCLUSION

The literature on pain assessment in disabled patients testifies to the fact that the state of the art concerning the development of assessment procedures is in a rather primitive state. Pain assessment in rehabilitation medicine requires a holistic endeavor that attends to the total biopsychosocial constellation of factors making up any given individual. Psychological knowledge should not be limited to psychologists and psychological assessment techniques, but disseminated to all health care and educational professionals, thus utilizing a broad spectrum of procedures and involving a number of different patient modalities. Only in this manner can a truly comprehensive approach to the assessment of pain in disabled patients be achieved. Diagnosis in rehabilitation medicine has been synonomous with loss. The researcher must be sensitive to this relationship and explore what is meaningful to the patient within the total context of that particular individual's life. As psychological tests were neither designed nor standardized for use with the physically disabled, the examining psychologist must be cognizant of both limitations in the test and in the person taking the test. With knowledge of test and patient limitations, the psychologist can interpret findings with appropriate qualifications and attempt new alternatives so that the final report accurately reflects the patient's assets and liabilities. The superimposition of the disabled patient's personality on pain experience is the diagnostic issue central to pain assessment in rehabilitation medicine.

REFERENCES

1. Jeans, M. E. (1981): An investigation of the developmental characteristics of the concept of pain. *Pain*, 11:S11.
2. Reading, A. E., and Newton, J. R. (1978): A card sort method of pain assessment. *J. Psychosom. Res.*, 22:503–512.
3. Rogers, A. G. (1981): The assessment of pain and pain relief in children with cancer. *Pain*, 11:S11.
4. Rosillo, R. H., and Fogel, M. L. (1970): Progress in physical rehabilitation and psychological variables: I. Degree of disability and denial of illness. *Arch. Phys. Med. Rehabil.*, 51:227–229.
5. Rosillo, R. H., and Fogel, M. L. (1973): Pain, affects and progress in physical rehabilitation. *J. Psychosom. Res.*, 17:21–28.
6. Rusk, H. A. (1958): *Rehabilitation Medicine*, pp. 9–16. C. V. Mosby Co., St. Louis.
7. Rybstein-Blinchik, E. D. (1979): Effects of different cognitive strategies on chronic pain experience. *J. Behav. Med.*, 2:93–101.
8. Smith, N. J. (1978): "Attitude Towards Disabled Persons" Scale (A.T.D.P. Form O) on social work and non-social work students. *Int. J. Rehab. Res.*, 1:187–197.
9. Villamira, M. A., Buzzi, G. P., DeBenedittis, G., Nobili, R. M., and Villani, R. (1981): A psychological tests battery in chronic pain: Preliminary results. *Pain*, 11:S153.
10. Yospe, L. P., Seres, J. L., Newman, R. I., and Painter, J. R. (1981): Family orientations toward illness as a predictor of treatment outcome in chronic pain patients. *Pain*, 11:S172.
11. Zakrzewski, K. (1981): Pain drawing: Some personality correlates. *Pain*, 11:S153.

Pain Measurement and Assessment,
edited by Ronald Melzack,
Raven Press, New York © 1983.

Pain Classification and Vocational Evaluation in Chronic Pain States

*William Hammonds and **Steven F. Brena

*Department of Anesthesiology, Emory University Clinic,
and **Emory University Pain Control Center, Atlanta, Georgia 30322

Present cultural patterns in Western society depict pain as a symptom of disease. To the general public, pain is a problem to be solved by removing the alleged "cause of pain." If the "cause" cannot be found or—if found—cannot be removed, the cultural and legal systems in the United States view pain as a good reason for disability compensation, on the grounds that an individual with chronic pain is impaired and therefore cannot be gainfully employed. Fifty-one percent of all patients with chronic pain examined at the Emory University Pain Control Center have pending compensation cases, and 18% have pending litigation for car accidents. The average time interval between onset of the injury-related pain problem and the time they are examined at the Pain Control Center is 2½ years. Similar data are reported by many other Pain Control Centers in the United States; for instance, Seres et al. (13) report that 76% of the chronic pain patients interviewed at the Northwest Pain Center are covered by worker's compensation. Despite the overwhelming evidence presented in the work by Fordyce (9) and Sternbach (14) that conditioning factors, such as inactivity, drug misuse, and learned helplessness (12), play major roles in chronic pain states, there is little awareness among physicians or the general population that pathological conditions and illness behaviors are not invariably linked.

The cultural expectation that removal of pathological factors should naturally be followed by disappearance of pain, along with the idea that the persistence of chronic pain should be rewarded by disability compensation, is costly to the individual and to society. Data collected at the Emory Pain Control Center show that each pain-disabled individual costs society in excess of $21,000 per year. If only 2% of the U.S. population were pain-disabled every year, the total cost of chronic pain to the American taxpayer would be in excess of one hundred billion dollars per year (3). These and similar figures quoted by others (11) point clearly to the need to reach a consensus and an acceptance of clinical criteria for quantification and classification of chronic pain states, with related vocational disability evaluation.

A MODEL FOR QUANTIFICATION AND CLASSIFICATION OF PAIN

A model for quantification and classification of pain was presented in 1975 by Brena and Koch (5). The model is an operational definition of chronic pain patients, and is based on the analysis of three quantifiable sets of data: measures of organic pathology; measures of pain behavior; and relationships between pathological behavior correlates expressed in four different classes of chronic pain states.

Physician-Based Pathological Assessment

On the basis of all available medical data, the observed pathology is rated on a horizontal continuous scale of 0 to 10. Up to 2.5 points is assigned on the scale for evidence of pathology on each of the following sets of data: physical examination, neurological examination, radiological studies, and other studies.

Patient-Based Behavioral Assessment

Each patient routinely is given a paper-and-pencil testing packet that includes: measures of subjective pain intensity, including a visual analogue scale of 0 to 100 and the McGill Pain Questionnaire; activities of daily living, measured as the amount of time spent in activities requiring the use of muscles to stand and walk; drug use scale; and the Minnesota Multiphasic Personality Inventory.

Pathology Behavior Correlates

From the assessment of pathology and pain behavior, patients can be divided into four classes of chronic pain states. The characteristics of patients who fall into the four classes of the model were described by Brena and Koch (5). Class I describes patients with high levels of conditioned pain behaviors that are in excess of pathology scores, whereas Class III patients show high scores on both pathology and pain behaviors. Class II patients score low on both variables, whereas Class IV patients demonstrate low levels of pain behavior despite high pathology scores.

RELIABILITY OF THE PAIN ESTIMATE MODEL

Assignment of 15 case histories to classes by five physicians yielded a Pearson correlation of 0.85, indicating high interrater reliability of the model (6). Three validity studies have shown the ability of the model to predict empirical data (1).

THE PAIN ESTIMATE MODEL IN DISABILITY PATIENTS

An analysis of 252 cases was performed at the Emory Pain Control Center; 207 histories of back pain and 45 histories of headache were examined. Class I pain patients were found predominantly in the back-pain population, and 66.7% were patients with pending disability. Of the headache population, 83% were found to be Class II patients; only 4 headache patients were pending disability cases and 3 of them were assigned to Class I (1). The large number of Class I patients in the back-pain population demonstrates the impact of conditioning factors in chronic back pain. The conditioned process also influences responses to treatment. Brena et al. (2) have studied responses to sympathetic nerve blocks in 144 patients with chronic back pain; 70 subjects had no pending disability claims and 74 were worker's compensation cases; no significant differences in rating of physical pathology were found between the two groups, according to the Emory Pain Estimate model. Responses to sympathetic nerve blocks performed with a local analgesic agent (bupivacaine, 0.25%) and with a placebo normal saline solution were recorded. Statistical testing using the chi-square method indicated significantly different responses by worker's compensation patients and patients with no disability claim ($\chi^2 = 4.38$, $p < 0.05$). Only 17.6% of the worker's compensation patients displayed a placebo effect following the saline injections as compared with 35.7% patients in no-disability claim groups. Among the patients with no disability claim, 67% reported decreased subjective pain intensity from either the bupivacaine or saline injections or both. Only 50% of the worker's compensation group reported similar results.

THE VOCATIONAL DISABILITY EVALUATION

Because chronic pain is so often associated with disability claims, a vocational disability evaluation should be made a routine part of the process of pain evaluation in patients with such claims. In this field, health professionals, insurance companies, industry, government, legal professionals, and the patients themselves are faced with a system that is chaotic. A patient may find differences from physician to physician, state to state, company to company, and agency to agency. There are few, if any, institutions that provide a systematic approach to disability evaluation that assesses the medical status, provides an impairment rating, establishes a disability rating, matches potential for work to possible vocations, and classifies pain in a consistent way. All parties involved are currently forced to make judgements on an inadequate information base and often end up deciding who has chosen the best attorney rather than who has the most substantial claim. Although often used interchangeably, impairment and disability refer to different concepts. Impairment is defined as an anatomical or functional abnormality that is rehabilitated and nonprogressive; disability is determined by a combination of medical, social, and psychological factors, and is defined as task-specific limitation of performance.

Impairment Rating

The rating of bodily impairment can be made by a careful review of all available medical records for each patient, measurements of ranges of joint motion, and muscle strength. The rating is based on the American Medical Association (AMA) guidelines for physical impairment (8). While the AMA guidelines are imperfect, they are a widely used standard. Since 1961, the American Academy of Orthopaedic Surgeons has standardized a method for measuring and recording joint motion, which has become part of the AMA guidelines. Similarly, a standard method for recording muscle strength has also been approved by the American Congress of Rehabilitation Medicine and has also become part of the AMA guidelines.

Disability Rating

The disability rating is an interpretation of the effects of the individual's impairment on his ability to function, according to the requirements of his last job. This rating requires both an impairment rating and a vocational evaluation to assess the patient's vocational abilities. Among the numerous vocational evaluation systems, the Valpar and Hester systems have emerged as the most reliable. The Hester system, which presently is used at the Emory Pain Control Center, is composed of a battery of 22 vocational tests, which measures 26 basic work traits and covers motor, perceptual, and intellectual skills. After testing, the raw scores are fed into a computer and analyzed to determine how patients' abilities relate to those jobs contained in the U.S. Dictionary of Occupational Titles.

RELATIONSHIP OF CHRONIC PAIN, IMPAIRMENT, AND DISABILITY

Significant relationships among chronic pain states (as determined by the Emory Pain Estimate model), impairment, and disability have been found. Brena et al. (4) have studied the relationships among these three variables in 101 consecutive referrals for vocational evaluation at the Emory Pain Control Center. One-way analyses of variance were calculated to assess the effects of pain estimate class on both impairment rating and disability rating. Both analyses showed statistically significant effects ($p < 0.01$). A Newman-Keuls test revealed that Class III patients showed significantly higher ratings of impairment and disability than Class I patients, whereas Class I patients showed significantly higher ratings of impairment and disability than Class II patients (all p's < 0.01). The difference between Class I patients, with low physical pathology, high illness behavior, and higher impairment and disability ratings, and Class II patients, who have low pathology and low behavior scores, can most likely be attributed to learning rather than to pathological factors.

It can be concluded from these results that modification of illness behavior may be necessary to alter impairment and disability ratings in Class I patients. Even in Class III patients, reversal of pathology may not provide changes in these ratings unless illness behavior is also modified.

BEHAVIOR MODIFICATION IN CHRONIC PAIN PATIENTS

Basic goals of behavior modification in chronic pain patients can be summarized as follows: to detoxify patients in case of drug misuse; to change patients' perceptions of sensory inputs; to correct postural and gait abnormalities; to increase activities of daily living; to educate patients and their spouses in the roles that emotions, behaviors, and attitudes, as well as physical impairment, play in chronic pain and to teach them to cope with problems of daily living; and to remove rewards for illness behavior while encouraging and training patients in health behavior.

CHRONIC PAIN IN THE DISABLED PATIENT

In summary, one of the massive health problems facing our nation is the individual with chronic pain associated with temporary or permanent, partial or total disability. To find answers to this mammoth problem is not easy. No system of evaluation will avoid controversy, but the better the information on which decisions are made, the fairer the decisions will be. Workers lost from productivity may be restored to old or new occupations, a result that will benefit both the individual and the nation at large. The effects of treatment programs on disability levels may also be better defined. Treatment now given often has no proven record of efficacy, because of lack of systematic data collection and retrieval methods. The Emory Pain Estimate model is a simple, quantified and multidimensional clinical judgment. Because of its simplicity, it is easy to understand and apply in clinical practice. Its wide use would significantly enhance communication among professionals and improve management of chronic pain patients by allowing the health professional to target treatment toward the problems manifested by the patient.

For example, conventional medical procedures such as surgeries and nerve blocks can be expected to have little therapeutic effect for Class I patients; however, such modalities may be highly effective in Class IV patients and may also be helpful for many Class III patients if paired with counseling and rehabilitation to ensure return to healthy behavior. When pain classification is matched with impairment and disability evaluation, it enhances the outcome of rehabilitation programs and facilitates patients' return to gainful employment. Some results from the Emory Pain Control Center document the importance of such step-by-step processes in pain and disability evaluations. Out of a matched sample population of 61 patients with chronic pain and similar degrees of tissue pathology, 35 were receiving compensation for work-related accidents, and 26 were receiving no compensation for their illness behavior. In the noncompensation group, 69% of the patients successfully increased their activities of daily living and completed the pain rehabilitation program; in the compensation group, a large proportion of patients dropped out of the rehabilitation program, and only 43% demonstrated a similar increase in activities of daily living (10). This study was published in 1978 and refers to patients examined and treated at the Emory Pain Control Center between 1974 and 1976. During that period of time, no disability evaluation system was yet in operation at the Emory Center. A disability clinic for such services was started in November, 1976.

In 1980, a second study was performed, trying to assess treatment outcome in the Emory pain rehabilitation program (7). One hundred patients who completed structured pain control programs at the Emory Pain Control Center in 1977–78 were selected at random, and long-term follow-up data were obtained from mailings and telephone interviews in 80 of these 100 patients. Follow-up ranged from 15 to 33 months, with a mean of 21 months post-treatment. For the purpose of this study, the patients' responses at long-term follow-up were divided into a worker's compensation group and a no-worker's compensation group. Dependent measures to assess results from treatment were: subjective pain intensity rating; activities of daily living (ADL); and changes in drug intake. The results of the study showed no significant differences between the two groups for ADL, changes in pain intensity, and changes in drug intake. Nine patients of 100 were working for a wage at the beginning of treatment; 24 of 80 had returned to gainful employment at follow-up (11 of these 24 had been worker's compensation patients). Although the basic principles of the behavior modification and rehabilitation program were the same for both patients in the first and second studies, only the patients of the second study underwent disability evaluation, vocational evaluation, and vocational counseling.

In a pain rehabilitation program without systematic methods to evaluate disability in order to help patients to settle a disability claim and counsel them vocationally to return to gainful employment, patients with pending disability claims are likely to resist rehabilitation approaches for fear of losing the disability benefits and being unable to return to gainful employment. With disability evaluation and vocational counseling, such fears can be removed in a humane and efficient way, and the patient can be programmed efficiently for return to gainful employment, while being fairly helped in settling his disability claim.

CONCLUSION

The World Health Organization (WHO) has defined health as "a state of complete physical, emotional, and social well-being." In our Western culture, normal social roles include productivity and gainful employment to earn a living. We firmly believe that such goals as stated in the definition of health by the WHO cannot be achieved unless all the issues involved in a complex chronic pain problem—pathological, emotional, social, and vocational—are properly assessed and solved to the satisfaction and understanding of all parties involved.

REFERENCES

1. Brena, S. F., and Chapman, S. L. (1982): Validity of the Emory "pain estimate" model. Anesth. Rev., 9:42–45.
2. Brena, S. F., Chapman, S. L., and Bradford, L. A. (1979): Conditioned responses to treatment in chronic pain patients: Effects of compensation for work-related accidents. Neurol. Soc., 44:48–52.
3. Brena, S. F., Chapman, S. L., and Decker, R. (1981): Chronic pain as a learned experience. Emory University Pain Control Center. Natl. Inst. Drug Abuse Res., 36:76–83.
4. Brena, S. F., Chapman, S. L., Stegall, P. G., and Chyatte, S. B. (1979): Chronic pain states: Their relationship to impairment and disability. Arch. Phys. Med. Rehabil., 60:378–389.
5. Brena, S. F., and Koch, D. L. (1975): A "pain estimate" model for quantification and classification of chronic pain states. Anesth. Rev., 2:8–13.
6. Brena, S. F., Koch, D. L., and Moss, R. M. (1976): Reliability of the "pain estimate" model. Anesth. Rev., 3:28–29.
7. Chapman, S. L., Brena, S. F., and Bradford, L. A. (1981): Treatment outcome in a chronic pain rehabilitation program. Pain, 2:255–268.

8. Committee on Medical Rating of Physical Impairment (1958): Guides to the evaluation of permanent impairment: The extremities and back. *JAMA* (special edition).

9. Fordyce, W. E. (1975): *Behavioral Methods for Chronic Pain and Illness.* C. V. Mosby, St. Louis.

10. Hammonds, W., Brena, S. F., and Unikel, I. P. (1978): Compensation for work related injuries and rehabilitation of patients with chronic pain. *South. Med. J.*, 71:664–666.

11. Hirsch, T. (1977): Billion dollar backache. *Natl. Saf. News*, 116:51–54.

12. Seligman, M. E. P. (1975): *Helplessness.* W. H. Freeman, San Francisco.

13. Seres, J. L., Painter, J. R., and Newman, R. I. (1981): Multidisciplinary treatment of chronic pain at the Northwest Pain Center. *Natl. Inst. Drug Abuse Res.*, 36:41–65.

14. Sternbach, R. A. (1974): *Pain Patients: Traits and Treatments.* Academic Press, New York.

Pain Measurement and Assessment,
edited by Ronald Melzack,
Raven Press, New York © 1983.

The Temporal Aspects of Pain: The Pain Chart

Kenneth D. Keele

Leacroft House, Leacroft, Staines, Middlesex TW18 4NN, England

The pain chart records the timing and intensity of pain and the circumstances associated with it (10). Certain considerations must be included in a description of the chart. Its clinical context and criteria of intensity of pain must be defined. Almost all clinical charts described here are based on patients making a verbal complaint of pain. This, in the great majority of cases, brings the patient to the doctor. In all cases pain had been accepted as an unpleasant sensation leading to "complaint." However, a few patients with gross lesions did not complain of pain.

THE PAIN COMPLAINT

In normal circumstances the most sensitive quantitative evaluation of pain is expressed through the complaint of pain, that is, through the spoken word. The first step in evaluation, therefore, was to establish patients' vocabulary in this field. It should be noted here that all the subjects and patients were seen in London, England, since 1935. At that time, qualitative descriptions of pain were found to be composed of such a wide variety of adjectives and phrases that it was felt they defied analysis. In more recent decades, Melzack and Torgerson's use of a computer is making such "qualitative" analysis fruitful.

With regard to the intensity of pain, the vocabulary used was much more limited. Patients' observations were nearly always couched in the words "slight," "moderate," "severe," "agonizing," or "unbearable." These words constituting the y-axis were composed from the patients' own chosen vocabulary expressing intensity. Slight pain is defined as awareness of an unpleasant sensation that does not interfere with the normal activities of daily life. Moderate pain distracts attention from such activities so that they are modified—steps are taken to obtain relief, particularly if it is prolonged. Severe pain fills the field of consciousness to the exclusion of normal activities and demands relief. Agonizing or unbearable pain is manifested by disorganized movements that, unlike bodily movement with slighter degrees, may obscure its location.

THE VERTICAL *y*-AXIS

The above four grades of pain are suitable for charting visually on the vertical *y*-axis of the graph, whereas the horizontal *x*-axis represents units of time (Fig. 1). On it, events associated with pain or its relief are charted. The question that arises in making such a chart is how to relate the degrees of pain intensity. What, if any, is the mathematical relationship among these verbal degrees of pain intensity? This question has been answered in various ways, none of which is entirely satisfactory: by keeping the words on the vertical *y*-axis unaltered; by entering these words as grades 1, 2, 3, and 4, and treating them as numerals on an ordinal scale; by dividing pain tolerance or "ceiling pain" into "dols" by "just noticeable differences" (JND) [1 dol being equal to 2 JNDs; Hardy et al. (5) claim that the pain expressed as dols can be treated as mathematically related]; and by using statistical techniques of assessment, thereby reducing these grades of intensity to mathematical entities of various degrees from 4 to 100 (6). Aitken (1) has pointed out that the same word need not convey the same experience in different persons; neither does comparable positioning on a line. But by using observer judgment and a combination of statistical techniques, he has found that such psychological states as depression can be represented linearly on a visual analogue scale. This, he claims, bears mathematical significance. Huskisson deals with this method in this volume; he has used it in assessing relief of pain in patients with rheumatoid arthritis (7).

CALIBRATION

The method adopted for grading intensity in the pain charts shown here has combined one or more of these features with direct experimental calibration. The

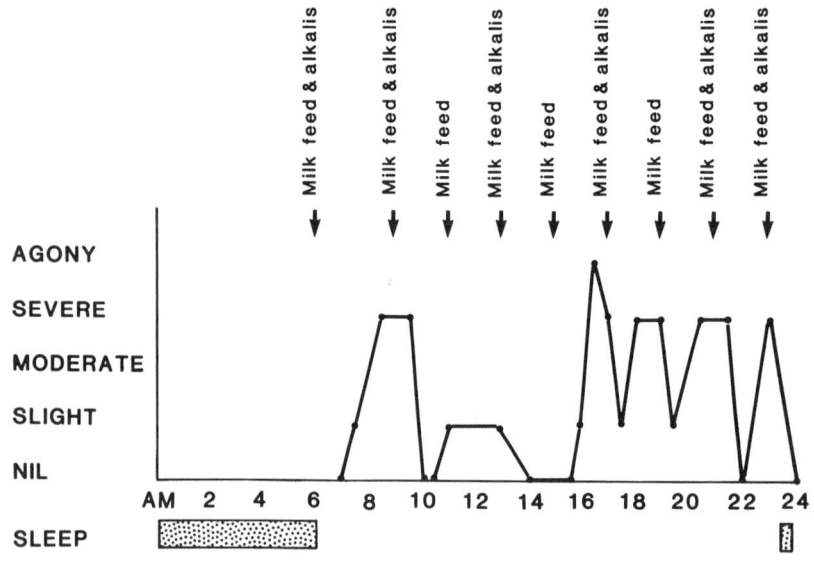

FIG. 1. Pain chart of a patient with a gastric ulcer showing the relief of pain with food and alkalis.

patients' vocabulary has been tested against the pain produced by the application of the pressure algometer to the forehead under standardized conditions at a standard rate of increase; that used has always been 1 kg/sec. Variation of this rate gives very different thresholds of sensitivity and tolerance. The pressure reading and the patients' vocabulary of intensity have been correlated. In performing these tests, careful appreciation of the background has to be given. Details of the technique were described in 1954 (11).

It is most important in algometric testing to minimize the psychological effects of anxious expectation. This is often high, particularly if the patient is confronted with formidable "scientific" apparatus and informed that he is about to have a "pain test." On the contrary, clinically calculated casualness should be practiced similar to that in using the stethoscope or sphygmomanometer. The application of the pressure algometer is accompanied by a brief standardized word pattern to minimize anxious expectation but to facilitate pain complaint. The principle of the calibration method described above—minimizing the element of the threat of pain—also applies to the recording of the pain chart. In both cases the investigation itself must avoid enhancing the phenomenon being investigated.

SELECTION OF PATIENTS

In view of the multifactorial elements involving pain complaint, that is, those sensory, cognitive, and affective factors that build up into the complex edifice of chronic pain, the most suitable patients for charting are those suffering from acute pain of visceral origin, often for the first time. In many cases, such patients have little or no suspicion of the cause of the pain. There is, therefore, a minimal cognitive element present. Large groups of the patients studied suffered from cardiac infarction and gastrointestinal pain. The pain experienced by many such patients between 1935 and 1965 was accepted by them as simple pain experience. Interpretation was minimal; even substernal chest pains were often thought of by the patient as "merely indigestion." In more recent years, patients have shown an increasing tendency to diagnose such chest pain as of cardiac origin. Increasing education, for good or ill, has added to this expectant cognitive element of a patient's reading of chest pains. The same applies elsewhere in the body to other forms of acute pain arising from organic disease.

VARIATION IN PRESSURE-PAIN SENSITIVITY IN RELATION TO THE PAIN CHART

The pressure-pain thresholds of individual persons vary significantly (Fig. 2). This finding is clearly relevant to the pattern of the pain chart. It is not uncommon to find patients who experience no pain at a pressure that to this writer is "unbearable." The range of pressure-pain thresholds by this technique was from 0.25 to 6.0 kg in 363 subjects. The writer's threshold (like that of many others) is 1.5 to 2.0 kg with a ceiling pain of unbearable degree at 4.0 to 5.0 kg. Subjects with a pain threshold above 4.0 kg have been called hyposensitive. Pressures greater

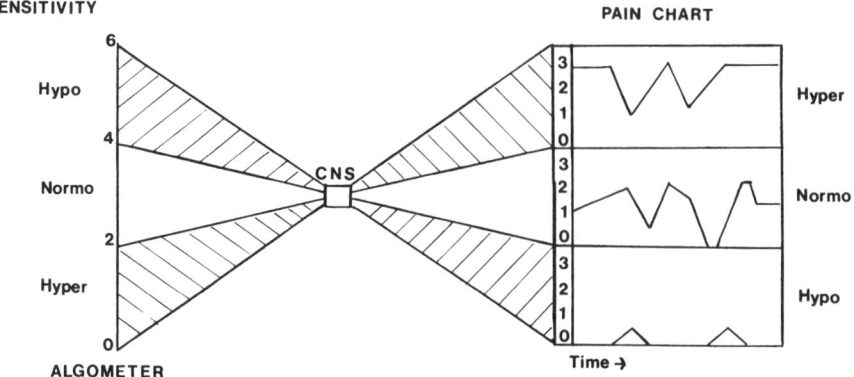

FIG. 2. Diagram illustrating the relation between pain sensitivity to pressure pain from an algometer measured in kilograms and the pattern of pain chart. Sensitivity is designated as hyposensitive, normosensitive, and hypersensitive.

than 6.0 are rarely used, because trauma is produced. However, even at this pressure a few patients do not experience pain. These constituted some 2 to 3% of the population tested. Such hyposensitive patients have been found to be the subjects of painless cardiac infarction (12), painless arthritis (8), and painless duodenal ulcers. They produce pain-free charts (which are described below).

All of the above suggested modes of measurement of pain intensity fail to include the time dimension. This is revealed by the pain chart, which combines intensity with the time factor.

THE x-AXIS TIME DIMENSION

The Hourly Clinical Pain Chart

In most cases of pain of organic origin, time intervals of 1 hr are most useful. Smaller intervals concentrate the attention of the patient too closely, or are likely to be omitted. Longer intervals give scope for errors of omission that express the remarkably short memory for even severe pain to which a patient attaches little or no significance, such as "cramp." Although recording is best done by the patient himself, a doctor's or nurse's tactful enquiry avoiding the use of the word "pain"— for example, "Are you comfortable?"—is invaluable in supplying objective judgment as well as revealing forgotten episodes. For example, one patient with pleurisy replied, "I had quite a severe pain last night but it did not last long and I did not bother the nurse about it." Relatively short charts, such as 24-hr charts, repeated at intervals of a few relevant days can be more informative than the continuation of charts over several consecutive days.

Long-Term Pain Charts over Weeks, Months, or Years

Daily records in diaries over weeks, months, or years clearly associated with particular physiological or psychological events reveal long periods of relief or exacerbation of pain. This may be observed in peptic ulcer, angina pectoris, biliary colic, and so on. The time scales of the chart are selected to be related to events that the clinical progress of the patient reveals as most significant with regard to both exacerbation and relief of pain.

The response to analgesics may well be revealed in the hourly recording of events. This also reveals the occurrences of exacerbation or relief related to significant physiological events, such as meals, exertion, bowel movement, etc., including the administration of drugs with specific physiological action such as alkalis. With regard to analgesic drugs, it reveals their duration and at the same time offers an opportunity to record side-effects. Moreover, comparison of the results of a potent analgesic like morphine with the effects of a placebo can be revealed, thereby helping to resolve one of the difficulties in assessment of analgesic potency.

The probability of the analgesic potency in a defined dose may be estimated by the mean duration of recorded relief on a composite chart obtained by repeating doses of the same drug on the same patient. In this way important information on the most suitable analgesic for that patient may be obtained. Charts may also be composed from the mean number of units and duration of relief from a fixed dose of analgesic given to different patients. This may give valuable information on the potency of the analgesic in general and therefore valuable information as to priority of choice.

The maintenance of continuous analgesia by spacing the dosage on the basis of the duration of relief obtained by the use of a particular analgesic can be determined from the pain chart (Fig. 3). In this way the optimum frequency and dosage of a potent analgesic may be assessed. Underdosage with recurrence of pain or overdosage with or without side-effects will be avoided. Such adjustments are of first

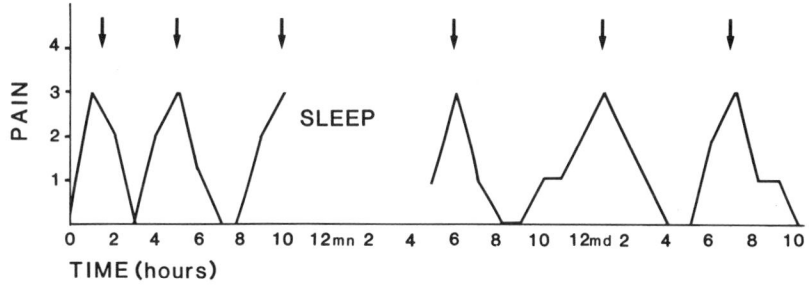

FIG. 3. A pain chart showing inadequate dosage of methadone hydrochloride of 7.5 mg by mouth *(arrows)* given to a patient with carcinoma of the cervix.

importance in the terminal care of patients with carcinomatous metastases and persistent bone pain.

THE PAIN CHART IN CLINICAL RESEARCH

Serum Lipid Changes and the Pain Chart

In 1959 Dodds and Mills (2) reported a fall in serum lipids during the days following myocardial infarction, rising to a peak some 3 weeks later. The possibility that this fall was closely associated with the pain of cardiac infarction was not considered. This has now been investigated (14). With the aid of a pain chart, a series of patients with cardiac infarction was studied for serum beta-lipoprotein and cholesterol changes during and after charted pain. A typical chart (Fig. 4) is shown with the beta-lipoprotein and cholesterol changes expressed on the y-axis in percentage of normal for that patient. The measurement was found to return to normal 7 days after the event. In a few cases, longitudinal follow-up was possible so that lipid values were known before the patient experienced further pain as well as during and after pain. The dramatic fall of serum beta-lipoprotein to below 50% of normal during pain revealed its close association with the pain. In a patient with

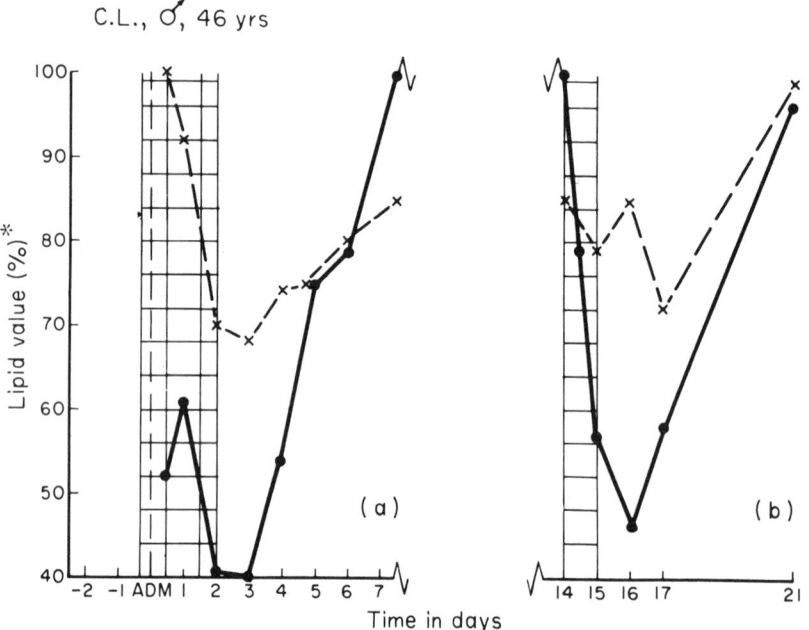

FIG. 4. The pain chart with cardiac infarction on two occasions (**a** and **b**). Duration of pain in days is shown by the hatched area. Beta-lipoprotein values in terms of a percentage of normal *(bold line)* and cholesterol values *(broken line)* are shown. This patient's second infarction occurred while in hospital so that the normal beta-lipoprotein level before his second infarction was known, and the rapid fall with pain was detected.

bouts of biliary colic, similar low beta-lipoprotein levels were found, rising to 100% after each of three episodes of pain. In this case the fall after cholecystectomy with postoperative pain was also charted. A similar fall of beta-lipoproteins in association with severe pain of cardiac, biliary, and renal origin strongly suggests that the finding of Dodds and Mills in 1959 was indeed associated with the pain rather than other pathological changes of cardiac infarction. This raises the probability that the serum beta-lipoproteins may provide a biochemical index of pain—a hypothesis that needs confirmation or refutation.

The Pain-free Chart with Noxious Stimulation

A phenomenon of particular interest is the occurrence of gross tissue damage in patients without the experience of pain and therefore with a negative, pain-free chart (12). The existence of subjects "indifferent" to pain was described by Ford and Wilkins (3) in 1938 and Jewesbury (9) in 1951. Another patient, admitted with painless fracture of the metatarsus, was seen by the author (13) in 1971. The etiology of such cases remains controversial. Insensitivity can be verified by such tests as Libman's test (15), pinching the Achilles tendon, pulling out locks of hair, stimulating the cornea—all painlessly. Stimulation of the cornea produces "tickle"; extraction of the hair "tug." According to the distribution curve of pressure-pain sensitivity, 15% of subjects is hyposensitive (11), whereas some 3% is insensitive as confirmed by the tests mentioned above. Of a series of 74 cases of cardiac infarction (12), 2 were painless and not accompanied by shock or arrhythmia. They presented as dyspnea, one being at first diagnosed as "hysterical dyspnea." His pain chart was flat on both the first and second occurrences of anteroseptal infarctions confirmed at post-mortem. Another patient presenting with repeated bouts of painless vomiting was found at operation to have two duodenal ulcers. These observations prompt the suggestion that pain sensitivity, like many other biological entities, may follow a normal distribution curve.

THE PAIN CHART IN EXPERIMENTAL RESEARCH

The use of the pain chart as an experimental procedure is exemplified by the results of the application of potassium chloride to blister bases in concentrations established as painful in a number of volunteers, for example, 64 mEq/liter. This noxious stimulus is found to be painless in subjects hyposensitive to pressure pain. Application of potassium chloride in concentrations of 8, 32, and 48 mEq shows a graded response. Slight pain is experienced by the majority of volunteers at 32 mEq and is reproducible on the pain chart. However, if the stimulus of a painful concentration of 64 mEq/liter of potassium is reapplied at 2-min intervals, analgesia is produced (Fig. 5). This may be prolonged indefinitely by continuous reapplication of the potassium at 2-min intervals. However, if washed and left for 6 min, sensitivity returns. A comparable phenomenon occurs on application of the potassium ion to the spinal cord of animals; for example, early enhancement of flexor reflexes, while with higher concentrations, profound inhibition is produced (17). Both these

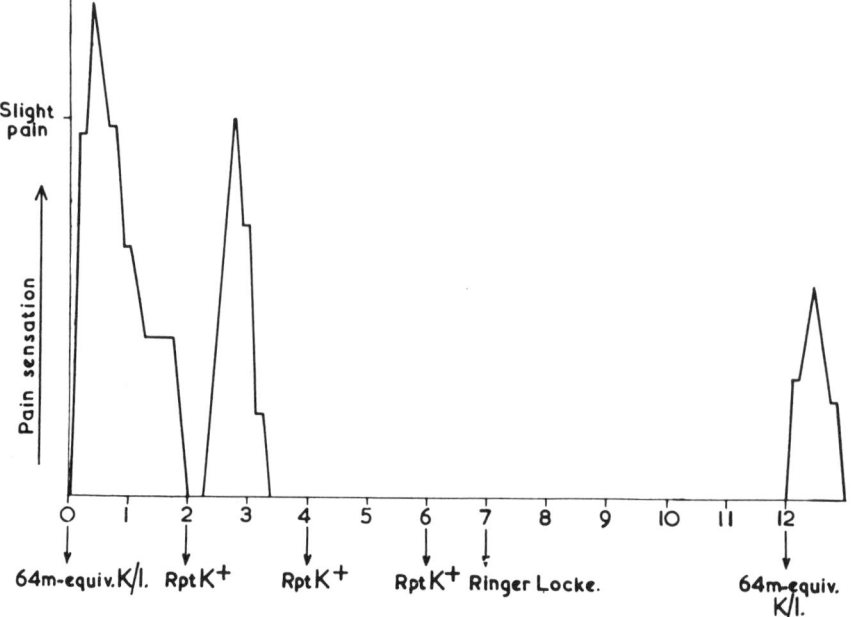

FIG. 5. Analgesia produced on a blister base by the repeated application of potassium chloride. The pain chart is calibrated at 2-min intervals, showing analgesia to the application of 4 and 6 min. After washing with Ringer-Locke solutions, sensitivity returned.

refractory phenomena may well represent depolarization of nerve endings by the potassium after stimulation.

CLINICAL PROBLEMS PRESENTED BY USE OF THE PAIN CHART

In the patient's history by hourly, daily, weekly, and even monthly charting, relationships of pain to any suspected, or sometimes unsuspected, physiological or psychological events can be revealed in the form of a visual record. One point, however, has to be insisted on and if possible monitored—the charting of pain must be as close to the time of its occurrence as possible. Even then errors will be made. A patient with cardiac infarction was admitted to hospital writhing in pain such that it was impossible to perform a physical examination. He responded well to morphine sulphate 16 mg. Next morning, that is within some 14 hr, on being asked about his pain, he replied, "What pain?" Such is the problem of amnesia for pain, particularly after adequate treatment with such drugs as morphine. This episode illustrates another important way of eliminating error. If possible, the patient should be observed while experiencing pain. This was clearly recognized by Mackenzie (16), a pioneer investigator of pain. Describing how the patient's recollection of pain was often so vague as to be misleading, he wrote, "I seized the opportunity...of observing the patient while in an attack of pain and then I carefully noted all the circumstances associated with the pain. . . . I had to train myself to observe accurately. . . . " Even today such self-training remains necessary. Mackenzie did not suggest keeping a pain chart. This omission of the time dimension left an obvious gap in his data on "all the circumstances associated with the pain"; hence the introduction of the pain chart as a clinical method.

Galen (4) divided the nervous system into three parts: motor, sensory, and nociceptive. He regarded pain as the "faculty of recognizing the experience of injury." Clinical experience brings appreciation of the individual physiological variation of the sensation of pain on the one hand, and its prominent psychological sources on the other. It emphasizes the fallibility of the experience of pain as a valid nociceptive index. It is commonly recognized that many organs of the body, such as liver and lung, undergo injury without pain. It is less commonly realized that there are patients who have gross nociceptive lesions in "sensitive" viscera—for example, a cardiac infarction—that fail to evoke this painful experience. However, important clues as to the relation between pain or its absence and injury can be obtained by calibrating the patient's pain sensitivity against his vocabulary on a pain chart.

Pain is an experience that may be dominated by emotional states and/or by peripheral noxious stimulation. In both spheres the pain chart carries with it the potential for revealing relevant data in the time dimension whether they be psychological or physical in nature. For this reason a pain chart is often more helpful than a temperature chart, but it remains far more rarely used in routine clinical practice. In many cases a pain chart may reveal guidelines for diagnosis and treatment unobtainable by any other means.

REFERENCES

1. Aitken, R. C. B. (1969): Measurement of feelings using visual analogue scales. *Proc. Rev. Soc. Med.*, 62:989–993.
2. Dodds, C., and Mills, G. I. (1959): The influence of myocardial infarction on plasma-lipoprotein concentration. *Lancet*, 1:1160–1163.
3. Ford, F. R., and Wilkins, L. (1938): Congenital universal insensitiveness to pain. *Bull. Hopkins Hosp.*, 62:448–466.
4. Galen, C. *De Usu Partium*. Book 5:9, quoted from Keele, K. D. (1957), p. 49. *Anatomies of Pain*. Blackwell, Oxford.
5. Hardy, J. D., Wolff, H. G., and Goodell, H. (1952): *Pain Sensations and Reactions*, p. 166. Williams & Wilkins, Baltimore.
6. Hewer, A. J. H., Keele, C. A., Keele, K. D., and Nathan, P. W. (1949): A clinical method of assessing analgesics. *Lancet*, 1:431–435.
7. Huskisson, E. C. (1974): Simple analgesics for arthritis. *Br. Med. J.*, 4:196–200.
8. Huskisson, E. C., and Hart, F. D. (1972): Pain threshold in arthritis. *Br. Med. J.*, 4:193–195.
9. Jewesbury, E. C. O. (1951): Insensitivity to pain. *Brain*, 74:336–353.
10. Keele, K. D. (1948): The pain chart. *Lancet*, 2:6–8.
11. Keele, K. D. (1954): Pain sensitivity tests: The pressure algometer. *Lancet*, 1:636–639.
12. Keele, K. D. (1968): Pain complaint threshold in relation to pain of cardiac infarction. *Br. Med. J.*, 1:670–673.
13. Keele, K. D. (1971): A physician looks at pain. *J. R. Coll. Surg. Edinb.*, 16:15–23.
14. Keele, K. D., and Stern, P. R. S. (1973): Serum lipid changes in relation to pain. *J. R. Coll. Physicians Lond.*, 7:319–329.
15. Libman, E. (1934): Observations on individual sensitiveness to pain. *JAMA*, 102:335–341.
16. Mackenzie, J. (1919): *The Future of Medicine*, pp. 66–67. Oxford University Press, London.
17. Vyklicky, L., and Sykova, E. (1981): May increased extracellular potassium be responsible for analgetic effects of electroacupuncture? *Pain [Suppl.]*, 1:S282.

Pain Measurement and Assessment,
edited by Ronald Melzack,
Raven Press, New York © 1983.

The Pain Chart: Spatial Properties of Pain

Michael S. Margoles

Orthopaedic Pain Center of San Jose, San Jose, California 95124

As an orthopedic surgeon, I was trained in diagnosis from a strictly anatomical perspective. Emphasis was placed on specific radicular components in suspected disc problems unless a specific joint was involved. Specific dermatomal patterns of sensory loss and deep tendon reflex deficits were always associated with specific nerve root dysfunction in the cervical and lumbar regions. Broadly speaking, low-back-pain problems were related to disc disease in the lumbar region, and neck-pain problems were related to cervical disc disease. The problems could be localized and were allowed to follow specific radicular pathways related to the cervical or lumbar regions involved. Generally speaking, any patients who deviated from the accepted standards became suspect of promoting secondary gain or were accused of having a purely psychological problem. Soon after entering the field of pain therapy, I saw the failures of conventional thinking: failed back and neck surgeries, the liberal diagnosing of "hysteria" and "conversion reaction," and the all too frequent use of "functional overlay." "Back strain" referred to irritation of the back anywhere from the upper thoracic to the sacral region.

I felt that too many patients from differing etiological backgrounds were too frequently given a psychological diagnosis for their pain problems, and that something had to be wrong with accepted concepts of radicular pain distribution. I designed the pain chart in Fig. 1 to see what my patients were feeling and where they were feeling it. After 5 years of studying 750 patients and thousands of pain charts, my observations include: (i) In chronic orthopedic pain patients, the paresthesias are frequently nonanatomical. (ii) The applied psychological diagnoses that have been given these patients have been deterrents to progress in the field of medicine and pain therapy. (iii) There is a need for new visualization techniques to aid pain therapists in understanding the complexities of the patients we treat.

DEFINITION

A pain chart is a two-dimensional graphic account, used by the patient, to report a number of the subjective components of the presenting pain problem. The contents of the sketch relate directly to the interest of the therapist and the honesty of the patient. There is a temporal component to the charting, and generally a number of the component symptoms will change slightly from visit to visit based soley on the

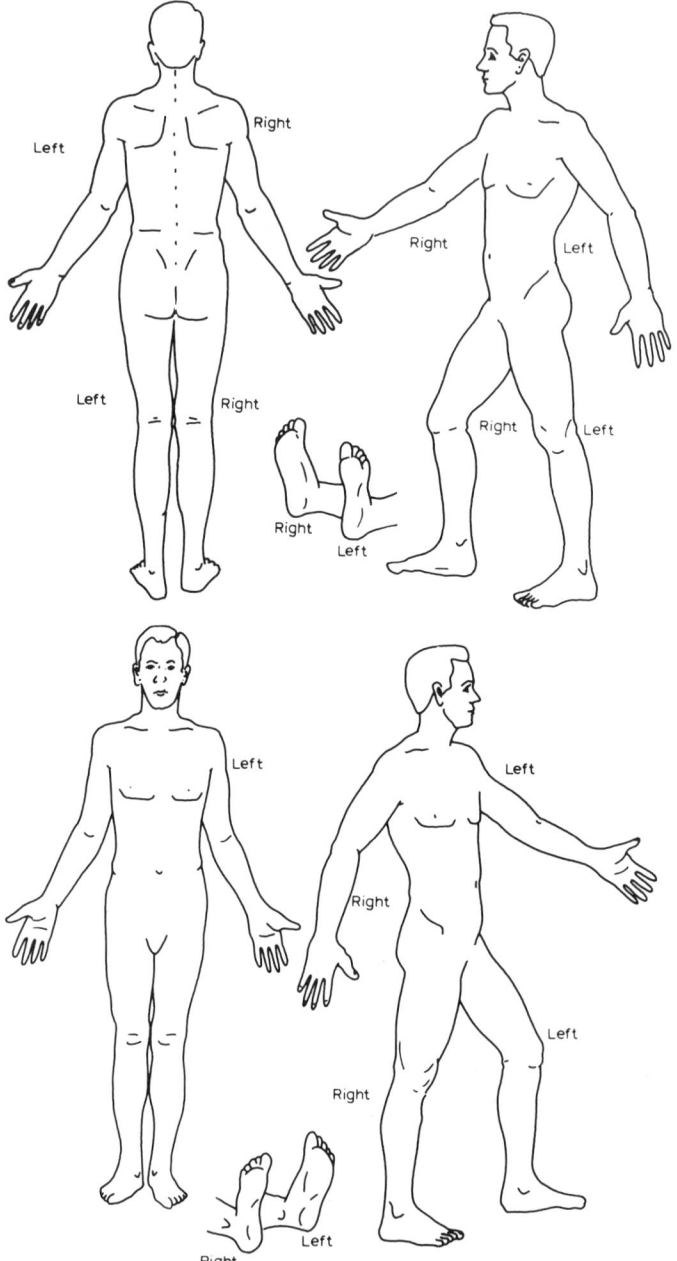

FIG. 1. The pain chart. Instructions to the patient are as follows. "Please use *all* of the figures to show me exactly where *all* your pains are, and where they radiate to. Shade or draw with *blue* pen. Only the patient is to fill out this sheet. Please be as precise and detailed as possible. Use *yellow marker* for numbness or tingling. Use *red marker* for burning or hot areas, and *green marker* for cramping. Please remember: *blue* = pain; *yellow* = numbness or tingling; *red* = burning or hot areas; *green* = cramping."

evanescent quality of some components of the sensations perceived as pain or discomfort. Word descriptors (3) may be added to enhance the communication value of the pain chart.

STRUCTURE

The pain chart concept can be adapted as a communication tool for any field of medicine or paramedical endeavor that requires the reporting of subjective somatic sensations. Dental charts show three facial projections, and headache charts employ four views of the head and neck. Rheumatologists, orthopedic surgeons, and neurosurgeons can readily use the general body charts shown in Fig. 1. I use an oblique angle of the lateral view because of interest in the latissimus dorsi in my current research.

COMPOSITION

Pain charts should be simple and easy to understand, and should address pertinent concerns. If pain is the only complaint, then a one-color chart will suffice. For the first 3 years I used blue for pain and yellow for numbness, tingling, and burning. Burning later became an area of separate interest because of work that began with B-vitamin research. Red was used to designate and follow the presence of burning on the pain charts. Because of an interest in using potassium to relieve cramping leg problems, the color green was added for the display and analysis of cramping as a component of chronic orthopedic pain problems.

Fast-drying felt-tipped markers that are not water soluble (water-soluble markers run and fade) are used by the patient. Thus, the color designation retains the individuality of the symptom that it was intended to report.

The resulting color display helps key the therapist's mind into a problem-solving approach, and aids in individualizing treatment for certain components of the depicted problem.

Many orthopedic pain patients have complained of tightness and stiffness in joints and nonarticulating areas. A suitable color will be chosen in the near future to represent and analyze that component of the presenting problem.

For simplicity and ease of printing, a totally black-and-white format has been utilized in this chapter. In the clinical setting I feel that a multicolor format gives the therapist a better sense of what the patient is trying to convey.

PURPOSE

Only the more salient aspects of the pain chart will be discussed. Therapists desiring commentary on other areas are encouraged to correspond with the author.

Communication

I believe that all pain is real. The pain chart lets the patient communicate its location and components. As long as the patient is told to put down all the components of the perceived discomfort, the pain chart often has the capability of demonstrating areas of involvement that are not always completely disclosed or understood in the verbal recording of the pain complaints.

Follow-Up

At present, there is a lack of objective parameters that can be used to assess some of the smaller gains made in pain treatment programs. The pain chart, when filled out in detail at each visit, presents an excellent subjective record of treatment response to any modality of treatment employed. When the pain charts are combined with follow-up physical examination and laboratory findings, the charts have been found to have potential objective value.

Multipurpose Format

The same chart format can be used by the therapist to document areas treated (such as injection sites), areas of palpable tenderness, and areas of neurological dysfunction (such as deficits in pinprick or temperature perception). The title and color of the chart can be changed appropriately, and the therapist can develop his own coding to designate areas of decreased or increased perception to pinprick, tenderness, trigger points, or other data being sought. This approach to data recording often provides a more accurate record than the verbal or written record.

For legal purposes, a good written or typed record should accompany the pictorial record. In my office charts, the pain chart is white, the tenderness chart is bright yellow, and the treatment chart is bright pink. The same four figures shown in Fig. 1 are used on the front and back of each type of charting. The color coding makes review of records easier because charts on chronic patients tend to become quite thick over relatively short periods of time.

Apportionment of Symptoms

There may be more than one injury incident in a patient being treated. Often industrially injured patients are reinjured weeks or months after returning to work. In many cases, the need for continuing medical care and the responsibility for the insurance payments are divided (apportionment) according to subjective complaints. If the patient has filled out a previous pain chart prior to his second or third injury, the previous pain chart can be utilized to assess what part the previous pain problem plays in his present pain complaints. The woman whose pain chart is shown in Fig. 2 was being evaluated for pain resulting from an auto accident that had occurred 3 months prior to her seeing me. Evaluation was completed (Fig. 2, top) and treatment started. One week later she was involved in a more severe car wreck, and subjective complaints are depicted in Fig. 2 (bottom). Review of these figures easily shows which parts of her most recent symptoms were residual from the first auto accident. All cases are not this easy to deduce!

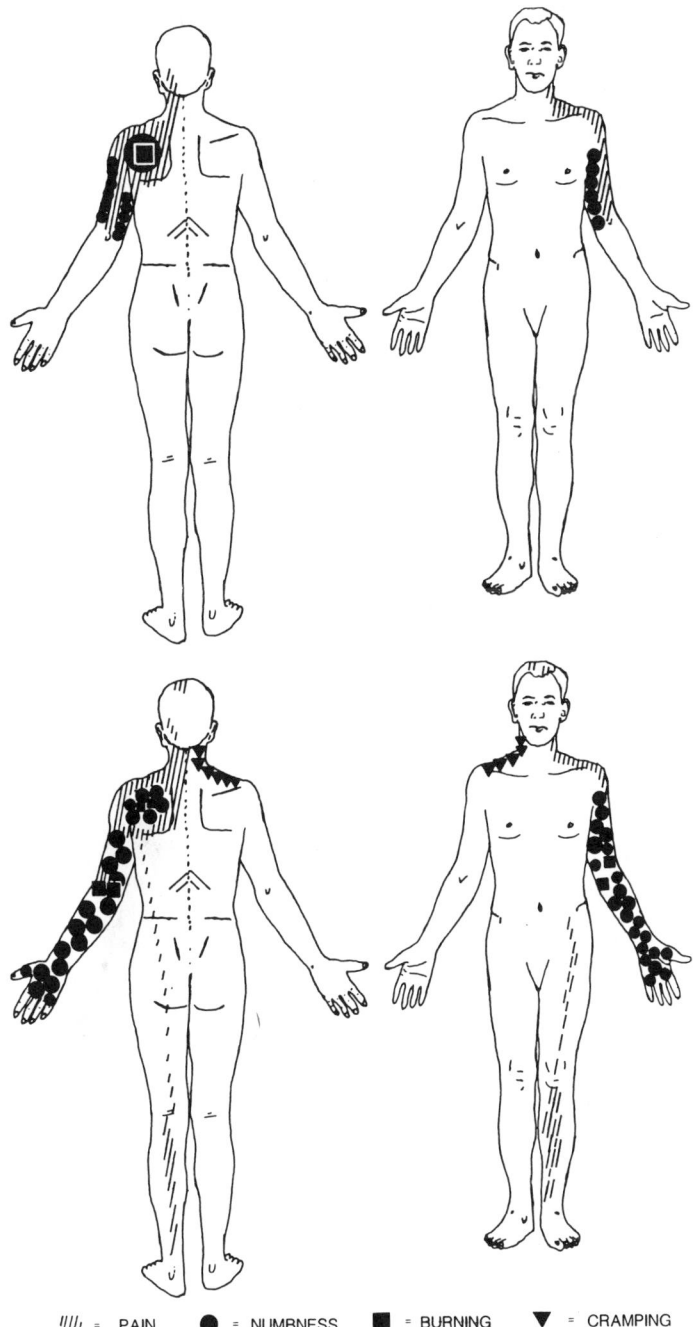

FIG. 2. Top: Patient 3 months after first automobile accident. **Bottom:** Patient 4 days after second automobile accident and 4 months after first automobile accident. Sensation symbols are shown at the bottom.

Surgical Decisions

Pain chart analysis may be of value in making a surgical decision. A patient drawing a pain chart as seen in Fig. 3 (left), having positive electromyogram (EMG) and appropriate physical findings would certainly be considered for appropriate lumbar disc removal. However, if the same patient depicts the extent of his pain as in Fig. 3 (right), having the same EMG and physical findings, lumbar disc removal will probably not be of value in eradicating the presenting pain problem.

Office Economy

The use of pain charts facilitates patient flow and cuts down on visit time. Once the clinician becomes proficient in assessing the pain charts, a quick review of it and pertinent neurological exam will be all that are usually necessary to assess the patient's progress and response to treatment.

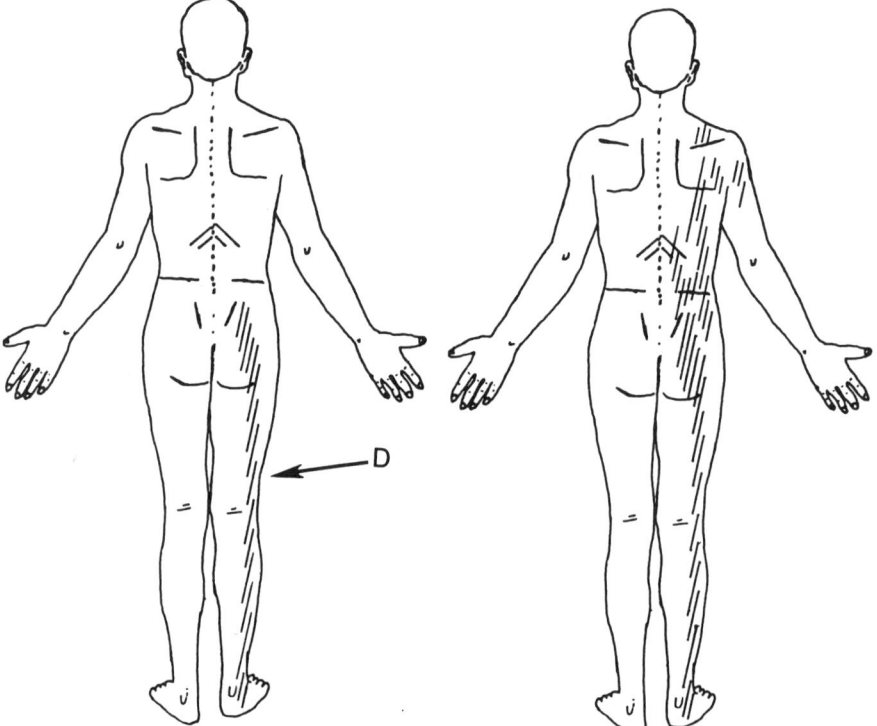

FIG. 3. Left: This chart is compatible with but not diagnostic of an L4,5 or L5,S1 disc rupture. **Right:** The more extensive involvement seen here should direct the therapist away from considering single-level disc pathology as the cause. Sensation symbols are as shown in Fig. 2.

Use in Research and Studies

Pain charts lend themselves well to blind, double-blind, and double-blind cross-over studies. They can be adapted to physical, pharmacological, and surgical studies in pain treatment.

The use of pain charts also allows regional classification of patients according to the regional area of the body involved. Thus, the therapist could review his records and study treatment response in all patients presenting shoulder pain with a radicular arm component. Once the regional groupings are made, then common laboratory, physical examination, historical and other data can be set up to subclassify the regional subgroups further.

A subgroup of back-pain problems that I defined (2), having grouped together 94 patients with similar pain chart findings, has been designated the Stress Neuromyelopathic Pain Syndrome. The pain chart characteristics consist of various degrees of vertical half-body involvement, usually one sided, with variable paresthesias and dysesthesias that in some cases involve one entire side of the body. The light form is depicted in Fig. 4A, moderate involvement in Fig. 4B, and severe involvement in Fig. 4C. Analysis of 27 of these patients revealed mild to moderate pyramidal tract involvement in 55%, posterior column involvement in 100%, nonanatomical pain and paresthesias in 90%, significant decrease of serum folic acid levels in 42%, with values suggestive of potential problems in 34%. Female:male ratio was 22:5. Average age at onset was 33 years; average duration of symptoms before coming to my office was 7.7 years, with a range of 2 months to 20 years. There was a history of weakness or "giving way" of the leg on the painful side in 78%. Also recorded was a 70% incidence of nonanatomical deficits to pinprick and cold perception testing. Forty-eight percent of patients offered complaints suggestive of a Lhermitte sign. Mild abnormalities of somatosensory evoked potential testing were found in 63% of these patients.

According to a similar case presented by Davison and Schick (1), there is suspected lateral spinothalamic tract degeneration in most of the SNPS patients. This could well explain the pain dysfunction and the vertical distribution. Patchy involvement of the lateral spinothalamic tract is postulated to explain the variable extent of vertical involvement. Also, in line with material from the same author (1), there is spillover or "mirror" involvement of the opposite side in the cases of severe involvement as shown in Fig. 4C. The severe cases also show the greatest degree of neurological dysfunction. SNPS has clinical similarities to subacute combined degeneration of the cord. No significant anemia has been found in these patients.

Recently, Pincus (4) has indicated that symptoms similar to subacute combined system disease are suspected in some cases of severe folic acid deficiency.

It was Dr. Janet Travell (*personal communication*, 1979) who first commented to me on this group of patients, indicating that they might have a problem of "spinal cord degeneration" or "postcordotomy syndrome."

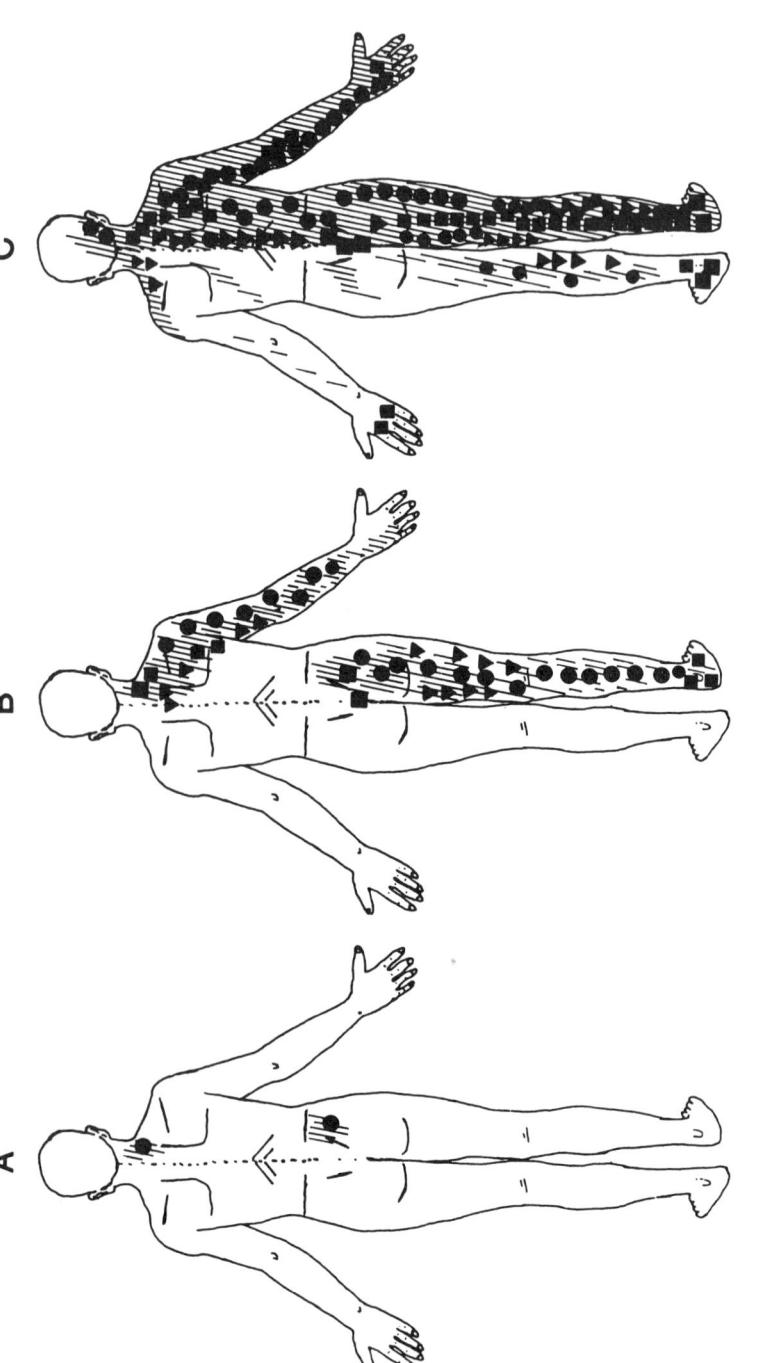

FIG. 4. A: Stress Neuromyelopathic Pain Syndrome—light involvement; may involve upper or lower area alone, both areas of involvement may present in the same patient, or upper and lower areas may present on opposite sides. **B:** Stress Neuromyelopathic Pain Syndrome—moderate involvement. **C:** Stress Neuromyelopathic Pain Syndrome—severe involvement; there is a spilling over or mirror involvement of a lesser magnitude on the opposite side. Sensation symbols are as shown in Fig. 2.

In the SNPS group, the only prognostic tool of value has proved to be the initial few pain charts. There has been no other consistent correlation with any other laboratory or physical finding.

Correlation with Physical Examination

The pain chart must correlate with the physical exam findings for the clinician to make a diagnosis of true organic pathology as a cause of the presenting problem.

WHO FILLS OUT THE PAIN CHARTS

Some therapists prefer to fill out the pain chart for the patient during the initial interview. However, when the therapist fills out the chart, he adds his personal bias to the interpretation, and may overlook other areas of related involvement.

In general, I believe the patients are more accurate at filling out the pain charts. Occasionally, the patient needs a bit of "practice" to understand what information is being sought by the therapist.

In order to maintain continuity of treatment and follow-up, the patient must be encouraged to fill in all areas of involvement at each visit. Having the patient fill out his own pain chart at each visit gets the patient actively involved in the problem and makes him responsible for communicating his complaints properly.

GRADING SYSTEMS

Pain charts are sometimes used to condemn patients based on an arbitrary point system used to "grade" what the patient puts on the pain chart. This is not fair to the patient, and may promote distrust, prejudice, and ill feeling between patient and therapist. Areas indicated as running outside of the designated figures usually represent proprioceptive dysfunction.

DEEP AND SUPERFICIAL PAIN

Although I have not done so on my charts, some centers ask the patient to designate whether the pain is superficial or deep by use of a specified letter such as the "D" in Fig. 3 (top). Use of this "D" tells the therapist that the patient perceives the pain as being deep or inside the leg.

ACUTE VERSUS CHRONIC PAIN

Acute pain often tends to be localized as depicted in the illustration on the left side of Fig. 5 (top). As the problem progresses to chronicity (see right side of Fig. 5 top), a recruitment phenomenon occurs, and pain begins to radiate further down the involved extremity. Other neurological dysfunctions accompany the radiating pain, such as the appearance of paresthesias and dysesthesias. I believe this represents progressive neurological deterioration in both the somatic and sympathetic

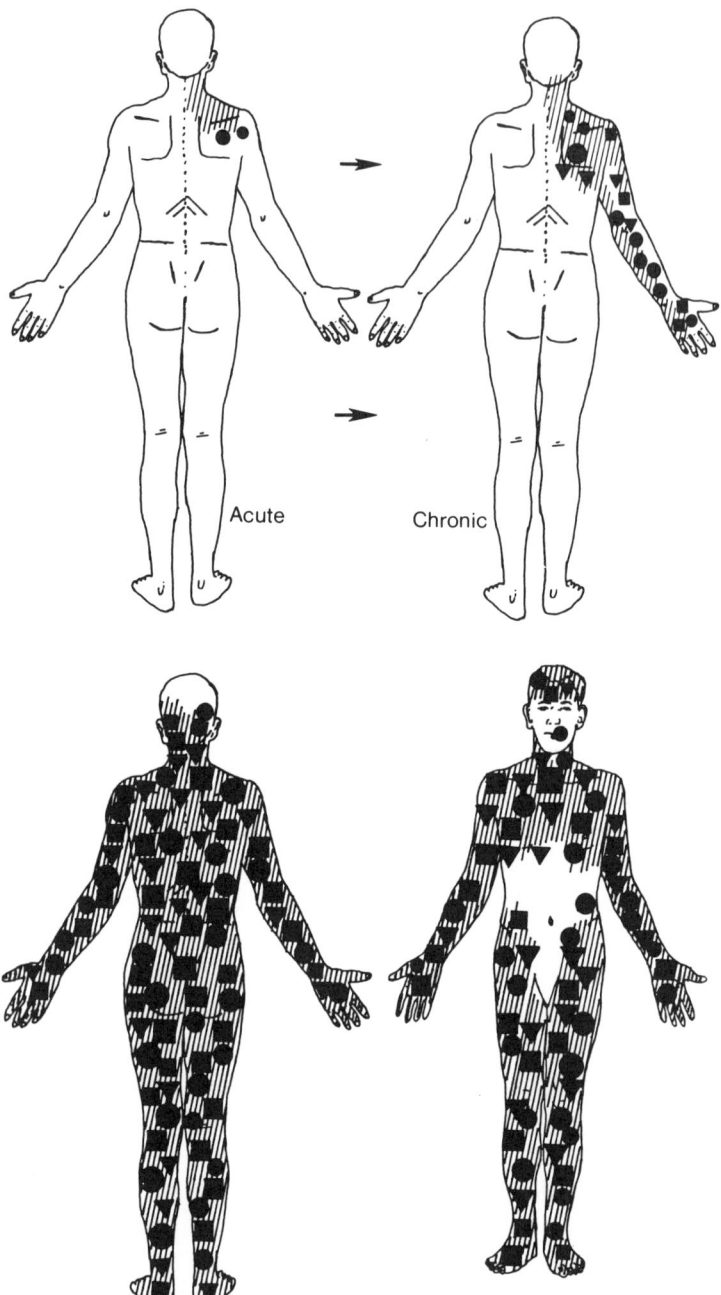

FIG. 5. Top: Neurological dysfunction occurs in a progressive fashion as chronicity replaces the acute phase. **Bottom:** This chart is compatible with but not diagnostic of a hysterical component to the pain problem. Sensation symbols are as shown in Fig. 2.

pathways, and that this phenomenon is accompanied or potentiated by chemical and metabolic derangements (5) in the patient.

PSYCHOPATHOLOGY

The most commonly encountered psychological problem in the 750 patients has been depression, usually stemming from situational and metabolic factors. I have seen no specific pain chart pattern characteristic of depression as such. A few patients have had a hysterical personality disorder concurrently with their pain problem, which usually presents as an exaggeration of perceived discomfort (Fig. 5, bottom). The pain chart can be used only as supporting evidence in asserting that there is a hysterical component to the clinical problem. The clinician is wise to have his pain chart-based psychological impressions corroborated by appropriate psychological consultation, preferably by a specialist familiar with chronic pain patients.

A pain chart that is solidly colored on the front and back does not imply psychopathology by itself. The general clinical impression of an experienced pain therapist, usually regardless of his basic specialty, is also important in deciding whether or not significant psychopathology exists in a chronic pain patient.

CONCLUSIONS

The observations described above indicate that at the present time the pain chart is a nonspecific, adjunctive diagnostic tool. It does not supplant the need for good clinical evaluation of the patient. If interpreted properly, however, pain charts can help the clinician appreciate the spatial extent of the patient's problem, and can aid in evaluation and treatment.

ACKNOWLEDGMENTS

I wish to express my sincerest appreciation to David Simons, M.D., for helping me with continued encouragement and instructions on chronic muscular pain problems.

REFERENCES

1. Davison, C., and Schick, W. (1935): Spontaneous pain and other subjective sensory disturbances: A clinicopathologic study. *Arch. Neurol. Psychiatry*, 34:1214–1215.
2. Margoles, M. (1984): The Stress Neuromyelopathic Syndrome. *J. Neurol. Orthop. Surg.*, *(in press)*.
3. Melzack, R., and Torgerson, W. S. (1971): On the language of pain. *Anesthesiology*, 34:50–59.
4. Pincus, J. (1979): Folic acid deficiency: A cause of subacute combined system degeneration. In: *Folic Acid in Neurology, Psychiatry, and Internal Medicine*, edited by M. I. Botez and E. H. Reynolds, pp. 427–432. Raven Press, New York.
5. Travell, J. (1976): Myofascial trigger points: Clinical view. In: *Advances in Pain Therapy and Research, Vol. 1*, edited by J. J. Bonica and D. G. Albe-Fessard, pp. 919–926. Raven Press, New York.

Pain Measurement and Assessment,
edited by Ronald Melzack,
Raven Press, New York © 1983.

Assessment of Body Image in Chronic Pain Patients: The Body Parts Problem Assessment Scale

Jon Kabat-Zinn

*Department of Medicine, University of Massachusetts Medical School,
Worcester, Massachusetts 01605*

One dimension of the chronic pain experience neglected by previous questionnaires is that of body image (3,6). Yet it is often important for clinicians and researchers to have reliable information on how the patient feels about his or her own body, particularly in terms of the degree of difficulty associated with problematic or malfunctioning regions. Body image is recognized to be a dynamic entity, continually being modified by new percepts and new experiences (3). For these reasons, a standardized instrument that can quantify the degree of difficulty associated with body parts and that permits an analysis of any change in body image as a function of treatment is potentially useful.

THE INSTRUMENT

The Body Parts Problem Assessment (BPPA) scale is a questionnaire specifically designed to provide information on body image to complement and augment information from other pain questionnaires such as the Pain Rating Index (PRI) (5), Dermatone Pain Maps (4), and assessments of the degree of interference of pain with normal activity (4). The BPPA assesses the extent to which different regions of a patient's body represent a problem to the patient. For chronic pain patients, it provides a rapid measure of the degree to which specific regions contribute to the overall pain complaint, and yields a useful summary score.

The questionnaire (Fig. 1) consists of a list of body regions (53 in the form currently in use) with a numerical scale from 0 to 5 listed next to each region. The patient is asked to circle the number that best describes the degree of problem or discomfort associated with each region, in a time frame of "the past week including today." Zero represents "no discomfort, no problem";[1] 5 represents "great discomfort, very problematic." The entire form can be completed by the patient in 5 min.

---

[1]The domain of positive body image is collapsed into the low end of the BPPA scale because for clinical use it is assumed that a low score reflects a positive body image.

forehead	0 1 2 3 4 5		l forearm	0 1 2 3 4 5
back of head	0 1 2 3 4 5		l wrist	0 1 2 3 4 5
scalp	0 1 2 3 4 5		l hand	0 1 2 3 4 5
temple, left	0 1 2 3 4 5		l fingers	0 1 2 3 4 5
temple, right	0 1 2 3 4 5		r upper arm	0 1 2 3 4 5
jaw	0 1 2 3 4 5		r elbow	0 1 2 3 4 5
face	0 1 2 3 4 5		r forearm	0 1 2 3 4 5
neck	0 1 2 3 4 5		r wrist	0 1 2 3 4 5
l shoulder	0 1 2 3 4 5		r hand	0 1 2 3 4 5
r shoulder	0 1 2 3 4 5		r fingers	0 1 2 3 4 5
l shoulder blade	0 1 2 3 4 5		l upper leg (back)	0 1 2 3 4 5
r shoulder blade	0 1 2 3 4 5		l upper leg (front)	0 1 2 3 4 5
upper back	0 1 2 3 4 5		left knee	0 1 2 3 4 5
middle back	0 1 2 3 4 5		left lower leg	0 1 2 3 4 5
low back	0 1 2 3 4 5		left ankle	0 1 2 3 4 5
chest	0 1 2 3 4 5		left heel	0 1 2 3 4 5
left hip	0 1 2 3 4 5		left foot (sole)	0 1 2 3 4 5
right hip	0 1 2 3 4 5		left toes	0 1 2 3 4 5
abdomen	0 1 2 3 4 5		r upper leg (back)	0 1 2 3 4 5
left side	0 1 2 3 4 5		r upper leg (front)	0 1 2 3 4 5
right side	0 1 2 3 4 5		right knee	0 1 2 3 4 5
buttock, left	0 1 2 3 4 5		right lower leg	0 1 2 3 4 5
buttock, right	0 1 2 3 4 5		right ankle	0 1 2 3 4 5
anus	0 1 2 3 4 5		right heel	0 1 2 3 4 5
genitals	0 1 2 3 4 5		right foot (sole)	0 1 2 3 4 5
l upper arm	0 1 2 3 4 5		right toes	0 1 2 3 4 5
l elbow	0 1 2 3 4 5			

FIG. 1. Body Parts Problem Assessment (BPPA) Scale. Patient is instructed to circle the number that best describes how he or she has felt for the past week about each region of the body. 0 means "no discomfort" and "no problem"; 5 means "great discomfort" and "very problematic."

SCORING

The BPPA is scored by summing the digits circled. The BPPA score can range from 0 to a theoretical maximum of 265. Scores above 25 usually reflect serious problems in the subject's relationship to his or her body. However, patients with chronic headache, facial pain, or pain in one extremity may have BPPA scores below 25 owing to the small number of body regions involved in their primary complaint. When the BPPA was given to 56 consecutive patients with a diagnosis of low back pain (with or without leg pain) seen in the Pain Clinic of our hospital, the mean BPPA score at initial assessment was 50.6 (SD = 38.0). The means for the men ($N = 32$) and women ($N = 23$) did not differ significantly (52.5 and 48.4, respectively). The highest BPPA score we have recorded was 218 for a male with a diagnosis of radicular low back pain.

MEANING OF THE BPPA SCORE

The BPPA scale probes the patient's feelings about his or her body. It does not mention the word pain. Strictly speaking, it is not a pain measure. It is more accurately described as an index of body image as it relates to somatic difficulty. For a cohort of 54 chronic pain patients referred to the Stress Reduction and Relaxation Program for a range of diagnoses, the BPPA score correlated positively with the McGill Pain Questionnaire PRI (5) ($r = 0.57$) as might be expected. It correlated highly with an index of somatization—the SOM dimension of the SCL-90-R (1) ($r = 0.79$)—and with the number of medical symptoms patients reported on a symptom checklist (4) ($r = 0.68$).

The BPPA supplies the clinician or researcher with an immediate picture of the patient's current problem and nonproblem areas from the patient's perspective. Specific body regions can be readily monitored and regional scores compared with clinical findings, body pain maps, and previously obtained BPPA data. The BPPA also provides important information when the PRI is atypical at the time of measurement, as is often the case for pain of an episodic nature such as headache or chest pain. These entities are less likely to be assessed by the PRI than by the BPPA because of the former's present-moment time frame.

USE AS AN OUTCOME MEASURE

The BPPA has proven sufficiently sensitive for use as an outcome measure with reliable results in a study of the effectiveness of training in meditation practices for the self-regulation of chronic pain (4; J. Kabat-Zinn, L. Lipworth, R. Burney, *unpublished data*, 1982). Twenty-one patients with a range of diagnoses were referred within our hospital from the Pain Clinic to the Stress Reduction and Relaxation Program, where they received training in mindfulness meditation. They began the 10-week program with a mean BPPA score of 47.8. Upon completion of the meditation training, the mean BPPA score for the 21 individuals was 30.1. This represents a reduction of the group mean of 37% ($p < 0.002$, df $= 20$; paired t-tests, two-tailed) and a mean percentage change as defined by Melzack (5) of 31%. Thus, a considerable statistically significant improvement in overall body image was measurable after meditation training. This improvement was maintained on follow-up for periods of up to 2 years (4; J. Kabat-Zinn, L. Lipworth, R. Burney, *unpublished data*, 1982).

A cohort of 21 comparable patients seen in the Pain Clinic for similar conditions but not trained in self-regulation showed no significant reduction in mean BPPA score over a 10-week period during which they received traditional medical treatment for their pain conditions (pre-treatment mean score: 44.4; posttreatment mean score: 43.4; mean percentage change: 4%). Neither repetition of the questionnaire at a 10-week interval nor conventional antipain therapy was sufficient to result in a net reduction in the mean BPPA score for this cohort of chronic pain patients (J. Kabat-Zinn, L. Lipworth, R. Burney, *unpublished data*, 1982).

CALIBRATION OF THE SCALE

Normative data for the BPPA were obtained for a population of first-year medical students at the University of Massachusetts Medical School on two occasions separated by 10 weeks. For 83 students reporting on both occasions, the mean BPPA scores were 14.9 and 11.4, respectively. These values are far below the range in which one finds the great majority of pain patients (25 and above). Of 119 consecutive patients seen in the Pain Clinic, 68% had initial BPPA scores above 25, whereas 17.5% of the students had initial scores above that level. The data, therefore, suggest good resolution between a nonpain population and a population of chronic pain patients. The 23% reduction in the group mean for the students during this time period was statistically significant in the paired t-test ($p < 0.01$, df $= 82$; paired t-test, two-tailed). However, the mean percentage change based on the net change for each individual was -8.3%, indicating an apparent deterioration in body image rather than the improvement suggested by the reduction in the group mean. This inconsistency is partially due to the fact that worsening among individuals with low initial scores tends to lead arithmetically to large negative percentage changes. The fact that the two methods of expressing the result of the two samplings of the normative population led to such different outcomes and the fact that the absolute difference between the two measurements of the group mean was small (3.5) imply that the difference observed on retesting the students, although statistically significant, did not reflect a major change in body image. It may reflect the sensitivity of the scale to fluctuations owing to the high stress levels characteristically found in medical students (2). In the case of the pain patients trained in meditation, the change in the group mean and the mean percentage change were both of comparable magnitude and in the same direction. The mean BPPA score in the comparison group was invariant at a high level on retesting, and the mean percentage change was near 0 and negative in spite of medical intervention (see above).

Discrimination between the student population and chronic pain patients was also obtained by counting the number of regions on the BPPA scored 4 or 5. The pain patients characteristically circled 4s and 5s with 10 times the frequency of the medical students.

USE AS A TOOL FOR FOCUSING AWARENESS

The BPPA obliges the subject to consider sequentially his or her whole body, region by region. It may be argued that such an exercise encourages exaggeration by triggering subliminal suggestions of discomfort in regions the patient might not have considered if not prompted. Even if this is sometimes the case for certain patients and certain body regions, the process serves the useful purpose of uncovering the entire body image of the patient. In the Stress Reduction and Relaxation Program, in addition to its function as a test measure, filling out the BPPA was seen as an initial therapeutic intervention, intended to elicit greater body awareness on the part of the patient and perhaps sensitizing him or her for subsequent meditation techniques that utilize intentional body scanning and awareness of proprioception as vehicles towards self-regulation of the pain experience (4; J. Kabat-Zinn, L. Lipworth, R. Burney, *unpublished data*, 1982).

WORK IN PROGRESS

The BPPA scale is currently being used in the Pain Control Unit of our hospital and in several other Boston area hospitals. Studies are in progress to separate the assessment of degree of *discomfort* from that of the degree of *problem* associated with the body regions.

ACKNOWLEDGMENTS

The author wishes to express his thanks to Deborah Hanna, R.N., for her support and help in collecting data in the Pain Clinic, to Dr. Robert Burney, Medical Director of the Pain Clinic, for his cooperation, and to Drs. Rob Goldberg and Leslie Lipworth for reading and criticizing the manuscript.

REFERENCES

1. Derogatis, L. R. (1977): *SCL-90-R Manual I*. Johns Hopkins University School of Medicine, Baltimore.
2. Huebner, L. A., Royer, J. A., and Moore, J. (1981): The assessment and remediation of dysfunctional stress in medical school. *J. Med. Ed.*, 54:547–558.
3. Gorman, W. (1969): *Body Image and the Image of the Brain*. Warren Green, St. Louis.
4. Kabat-Zinn, J. (1982): An outpatient program in behavioral medicine for chronic pain patients based on the practice of mindfulness meditation: Theoretical considerations and preliminary results. *Gen. Hosp. Psychiatry*, 4:33–47.
5. Melzack, R. (1975): The McGill Pain Questionnaire: Major properties and scoring methods. *Pain*, 1:277–299.
6. Secord, P. F., and Journard, S. M. (1953): The appraisal of body-cathexis: Body-cathexis and the self. *J. Consult. Psychol.*, 5:343–347.

Pain Measurement and Assessment,
edited by Ronald Melzack,
Raven Press, New York © 1983.

A Comprehensive Pain Questionnaire

*Richard Monks and **Paul Taenzer

*Pain Center, Montreal General Hospital, Montreal, Quebec H3G 1A4, Canada; and
**Pain Management Program, Tulsa Rehabilitation Center, Hillcrest Medical Center, Tulsa, Oklahoma 74104*

The pain problems suffered by patients seen in a pain clinic are typically intractable and appear to be maintained by interrelated biological, psychological, and social factors. This conceptualization of chronic pain states led to the establishment of multidisciplinary treatment programs. Although not yet supported by adequate controlled trials, therapeutic outcome studies of programs utilizing a multimodal approach have demonstrated impressive gains for patients refractory to more conventional medical regimens (2,6,8,19,20,21).

The complexity of the problems associated with chronic pain, the variety of treatment options now available, and the need for objective evaluation of the results of treatment all point to the necessity of using a comprehensive assessment strategy.

Assessment Goals

An adequate assessment would fulfill the following goals: identify biological (organic) pain generators and/or sources of impairment; identify significant psychosocial problem areas; delineate strengths and resources of the individual and his milieu; facilitate treatment planning; provide dependent variables for measurement of treatment outcome; and allow testing of research hypotheses.

Assessment Techniques

Many complementary techniques have been used to evaluate patients with pain. These include traditional medical and psychiatric examination (24), diagnostic anesthetic blocks (7), intravenous barbiturate interviews (24), psychophysiological response profiles (18), pain measurement methods (11,25), behavioral analysis (4,13), hypnotic susceptibility evaluation (12), psychological testing (23), and family or spouse interviewing (1,17,22). Appropriate assessment for the individual patient may include some or all of the above procedures.

PATIENT QUESTIONNAIRES

The comprehensive pain assessment questionnaire technique offers many advantages. The patient is encouraged to appreciate the complexity of his problem and

233

to become an active participant in the assessment process. A broad data base is obtained with a considerable saving in professional man-hours. This standardized method of obtaining information facilitates comparison of patients in treatment and research settings.

These instruments also have definite limitations. Difficulties in motivation or understanding may hamper patient responses. Inflexibility of format or content may inhibit patient and evaluator initiative and intuition. It is our impression that a combined patient questionnaire and interviewer review format minimizes these limitations.

A number of standardized patient questionnaires have been described. The original McGill Pain Assessment Questionnaire (MPAQ) devised by Melzack (16) is an interviewer guide that includes the McGill Pain Questionnaire (MPQ), as well as questions relating to pain description, history, treatment, and psychosocial consequences. Although the MPAQ addresses many relevant pain dimensions, some items are poorly defined and important areas are overlooked.

The Pain Profile of Duncan et al. (3) offers a computer-based chronic pain assessment method. Patient questionnaires are used to provide data regarding pain description, conditioned pain responses, health service and drug abuse, life events, patient psychopathology, functional impairment, and medical history. The information obtained is quantifiable, and a mathematical model has been suggested for research and clinical use. Unfortunately, like the MPAQ, the Pain Profile has not been subjected to formal reliability and validity testing. Additionally, the reductionistic methodology used and the absence of open-ended questions may, if improperly applied, discourage the exploration of further relevant factors.

The Psychosocial Pain Inventory (PSI) of Heaton et al. (9) is a recently reported assessment tool designed to quantify the impact of psychosocial factors in patients with chronic pain. A patient questionnaire is used to obtain details of pain treatment, pain behavior and social reinforcement, life changes, financial status and litigation, personal and family medical history, and the use of alcohol and medications. Preliminary results suggest good interrater reliability of PSI scores and some evidence for construct and predictive validity.

Several more specialized questionnaires have also been reported. Fordyce (5) described a structured interviewer guide to assess operant factors that maintain chronic pain behavior. Hendler et al. (10) devised a brief screening test based on an analysis of retrospective data differentiating successful and unsuccessful candidates for facet denervation. Leavitt and Garron (14) developed a modified version of the MPQ, the Low Back Pain Questionnaire, which differentiates patients with and without organic findings.

Many additional questionnaires and interview guides have been developed at individual Pain Centers and Clinics. At the present time, they remain unpublished and as a result have had little impact on the advancement of pain assessment methodology.

Each of the questionnaires and interviews reviewed above has obvious strengths and limitations regarding breadth of content, format, level of quantification, and demonstrated reliability and validity. The instrument reported here represents an attempt to develop a truly comprehensive pain assessment questionnaire, the McGill Comprehensive Pain Questionnaire (MCPQ). The MCPQ, medical history records, routine physical examination, and several psychological inventories comprise the initial assessment procedure at the Pain Center of the Montreal General Hospital.

The MCPQ is composed of two complementary parts, the Patient Questionnaire (Appendix A) and the Interviewer Guide (Appendix B).[1] The patient questionnaire is mailed to the patient prior to the first clinic appointment. A covering letter confirms the patient's referral and initial appointment. The multidisciplinary nature of the assessment and possible treatment approach are also outlined. The importance of the patient's active participation and observations regarding the pain condition is emphasized. The patient is requested to complete the questionnaire with care and bring it to the clinic for the first appointment.

The order of the content areas in the MCPQ is arranged to facilitate patient cooperation. The pain complaint is explored first. Emphasis on the complications of the pain then allows a transition to psychosocially oriented data in a fashion that is usually quite acceptable to the patient.

The content of the MCPQ has been derived empirically from clinical experience. Items reflect details of the illness, personality, milieu, and coping responses that have been useful in determining diagnosis and relevant treatment. Where feasible, items have been adapted from previously published instruments (3,5,15,16).

The McGill Comprehensive Pain Questionnaire

Each section of the MCPQ yields data designed to meet the previously stated assessment goals: (a) Organic factors may be suggested by details of the pain history, previous treatments, description, time pattern, accompanying symptoms and modifiers, medical history (past, present), and medications consumed; (b) Psychosocial problem areas may be inferred from all sections but are explicitly explored in those regarding the effects of pain, personal history, and items in the Interviewer Guide; (c) Resource recognition is aided by information on pain modifiers, effects, coping responses, and personal history; (d) Treatment planning is facilitated by the recognition of organic factors, previous responses to treatment, pain modifiers, effects of pain, and personal history; (e) Dependent variables are available for pain description, medications consumed, utilization of medical services, accompanying symptoms, and effects of pain.

The interviewer reviews the patient questionnaire, clarifies responses as necessary, and adds more complex or private inquiries such as those in the Interviewer Guide. While warm and respectful, the interviewer conveys a matter-of-fact expectation that the patient will be well motivated to deal with his problems. Evasions,

---

[1]The questionnaire and interviewer guide presented in the appendices have been shortened for inclusion in this publication. Although specific items have not been altered, space for recording responses has been abbreviated whenever possible. Full format copies of the MCPQ may be obtained for printing and postal costs from R. C. Monks, M. D., Dept. of Psychiatry, Montreal General Hospital, 1650 Cedar Ave., Montreal PQ H3G 1A4, Canada.

denial, and other forms of resistance are then subject to immediate clarification and exploration. Similarly, affective areas are highly valuable entry points for helping the patient to recognize internal states and to elaborate sensitive, relevant material.

Training personnel to administer the MCPQ is relatively straightforward. With increasing use, the interviewer can become more skilled in using the data base flexibly to explore areas that appear promising. Additionally, the MCPQ is useful as a teaching aid by introducing clinicians and students to the multidisciplinary approach to evaluation and treatment of chronic pain states.

We have found the MCPQ to be a valuable clinical assessment tool. If it is to be used for research purposes, further development will be required. We believe that the wide range of items available from the MCPQ will provide the basic material for constructing brief, reliable, and valid quantitative scales suitable for assessing specific pain-related hypotheses.

ACKNOWLEDGMENTS

The authors wish to thank Dr. M. E. Jeans, Dr. R. Melzack, Dr. J. Stratford, and Miss W. Lummis for their help in evolving the MCPQ and Miss I. Broitman for her technical assistance.

REFERENCES

1. Block, A. R., Kremer, E. F., and Gaylor, M. (1980): Behavioral treatment of chronic pain: The spouse as a discriminative cue for pain behavior. *Pain*, 9:243–252.
2. Chapman, S. L., Brena, S. F., and Bradford, L. A. (1981): Treatment outcome in a chronic pain rehabilitation program. *Pain*, 11:255–268.
3. Duncan, G. H., Gregg, J. M., and Ghia, J. N. (1978): The Pain Profile: A computerized system for the assessment of chronic pain. *Pain*, 5:275–284.
4. Fordyce, W. E. (1976): *Behavioural Methods in Chronic Pain and Illness*, pp. 12–19,86–90. C. V. Mosby, St. Louis.
5. Fordyce, W. E. (1976): Patient selection: Behavioural analyses of pain. In: *The Behavioural Management of Anxiety, Depression and Pain*, edited by P. O. Davidson, pp. 168–171. Brunner/Mazel, New York.
6. Fordyce, W. E., Fowler, R., Lehmann, J. R., DeLateur, B. J., Sand, P. L., and Trieschmann, R. (1973): Operant conditioning in the treatment of chronic clinical pain. *Arch. Phys. Med. Rehabil.*, 54:399–408.
7. Ghia, J. N., Toomey, T. L., Mao, W., Duncan, G., and Gregg, J. M. (1979): Towards an understanding of chronic pain mechanisms: The use of psychological tests and a refined differential spinal block. *Anesthesiology*, 50:20–25.
8. Gottlieb, H., Strite, L. C., Koller, R., Madorsky, A., Hockersmith, V., Kleeman, M., and Wagner, J. (1977): Comprehensive rehabilitation of patients having low back pain. *Arch. Phys. Med. Rehabil.*, 58:101–108.
9. Heaton, R. K., Getto, C. J., Lehman, R. A. W., Fordyce, W. E., Brauer, E., and Groban, S. E. (1981): A standardized evaluation of psychosocial factors in chronic pain. *Pain [suppl.]*, 1:154.
10. Hendler, N., Viernstein, M., Gucer, P., and Long, D. (1979): A preoperative screening test for chronic back pain patients. *Psychosomatics*, 20:801–808.
11. Huskisson, E. C. (1974): Measurement of pain. *Lancet*, 2:1127–1131.
12. Johnson, L. S., and Wiese, K. F. (1979): Live versus tape recorded assessment of hypnotic responsiveness in pain-control patients. *Int. J. Clin. Exp. Hypn.*, 27:74–84.
13. Klein, R. M., and Cherlton, J. E. (1980): Behavioral observation and analysis or pain behavior in critically burned patients. *Pain*, 9:27–40.

14. Leavitt, F., and Garron, D. C. (1980): Validity of back pain classification scale for detecting psychological disturbance as measured by the MMPI. *J. Clin. Psychol.*, 36:186–189.
15. Margoles, M. S. (1980): Letter to the editor. *Pain*, 8:115–117.
16. Melzack, R. (1975): The McGill Pain Questionnaire: Major properties and scoring methods. *Pain*, 1:277–299.
17. Mohamed, S., Wesiz, G., and Waring, E. M. (1978): Chronic pain, marital adjustment and family dynamics. *Pain*, 5:285–292.
18. Morgan, C. D., Kremer, E., and Gaylor, M. (1979): The behavioral medicine unit: A new facility. *Comp. Psychol.*, 20:79–80.
19. Newman, R. I., Seres, J. L., Yospe, L. P., and Gralington, B. (1978): Multidisciplinary treatment of chronic pain: Long term follow-up of low-back pain patients. *Pain*, 4:283–292.
20. Painter, J. R., Seres, J. L., and Newman, R. I. (1980): Assessing benefits of the pain center: Why some patients regress. *Pain*, 8:101–113.
21. Roberts, A. H., and Reinhardt, L. (1980): The behavioral management of chronic pain: Long term follow-up with comparison groups. *Pain*, 8:151–162.
22. Shanfield, S. B., Herman, E. M., Cope, D. N., and Jones, J. R. (1979): Pain and the marital relationship: Psychiatric distress. *Pain*, 7:343–351.
23. Sternbach, R. A. (1974): *Pain Patients: Traits and Treatments*, pp. 120–140. Academic Press, New York.
24. Walters, A. (1975): The psychogenic regional pain syndrome (hysterical pain). *Comp. Ther.*, 1:20–25.
25. Wolff, B. B. (1978): Behavioral measurement of human pain. In: *Psychology of Pain*, edited by R. A. Sternbach, pp. 129–168. Raven Press, New York.

VI. BRIDGING LABORATORY AND CLINICAL RESEARCH

Pain Measurement and Assessment,
edited by Ronald Melzack,
Raven Press, New York © 1983.

Interacting Approaches in Pain Research

Ronald Melzack

Department of Psychology, McGill University, Montreal, Quebec, Canada H3A 1B1

So far, this book has dealt with laboratory-produced pain and clinical pain examined from subjective and behavioral points of view. It is evident that none of these approaches excludes the others. Laboratory-produced pain, such as that evoked in the tourniquet test, has been used to evaluate clinical pain. The McGill Pain Questionnaire has also been used to study both laboratory-produced and clinical pain.

The subjective experiences of pain and "pain behaviors" are, presumably, reflections of the same underlying neural processes. However, the complexity of the human brain indicates that although experience and behavior are usually highly correlated, they are far from identical. One person may be stoic so that his calm behavior belies his true subjective feelings. Another patient may seek sympathy (or money, drugs, or some other desirable reward), and, again, behavior and subjective experience are poorly correlated. Generally, however, both features are good reflections of each other.

In Section V, we dealt with problems that urgently need to be solved: how to measure or assess pain in children or in severely handicapped patients; how to assess the temporal and spatial properties of pain in order to provide information that can be readily communicated and understood; how to carry out the assessment process so that it will reveal all the essential information about a patient that will allow the therapist to prevent further suffering and misery.

Finally, in the last section of the book, we deal largely with the future. Two authors (Chapman and Rollman) discuss the relationship between laboratory and clinical research. Important problems confront us here, and the judicious combination of the best of both approaches is certain to reveal important facets of pain mechanisms and the most effective procedures to control pain and suffering. Such research, however, may involve inflicting pain in order to understand it and find ways to relieve it. And this, clearly, brings us face to face with the question of ethics in pain research. Sternbach, in the concluding chapter, deals with this difficult issue, which each of us in this field must resolve to the satisfaction of his or her conscience. Sternbach presents the problem in a forthright manner and tells us that it is ethically unconscionable to relieve the suffering of one person at the cost of suffering by another. "Informed consent" is essential in the fullest and most real sense of that phrase. If the sensitivity of our measurement and assessment tools is an index of the degree of scientific development of the study of pain, then the adherence to ethical guidelines is a reflection of the degree of our humanity, of our genuine concern for the suffering and pain of our fellow humans.

Pain Measurement and Assessment,
edited by Ronald Melzack,
Raven Press, New York © 1983.

On the Relationship of Human Laboratory and Clinical Pain Research

C. Richard Chapman

*Departments of Anesthesiology, Psychiatry and Behavioral Sciences, and Psychology,
University of Washington Pain Center, University of Washington,
Seattle, Washington 98195*

For many decades, clinical and laboratory scientists have studied pain in human subjects, but the domains of their inquiries have been relatively independent. Although both groups write about pain, they have generated two separate literatures, and progress in one area has typically had little or no impact on the other. At the extremes, one finds clinicians who dismiss laboratory data as useless or irrelevant, and laboratory scientists who consider clinical data to be so poorly controlled and imprecise as to be of little value. This has led to problems in communication, enormous difficulty in the testing of new drugs for efficacy before marketing, and considerable confusion for practicing physicians who read the experimental literature.

The existence of a hiatus between clinical and laboratory research in humans is hardly a new observation. About 25 years ago, Beecher (1) attempted to relate research and clinical observation on postoperative pain control to the laboratory research of Hardy et al. (14), who studied the radiant heat pain threshold of human skin using laboratory volunteers. The well-known clinical effects of narcotic drugs and the difference in clinical response to placebo, aspirin-class agents, and narcotic analgesics could not be clearly or reliably shown with radiant heat dolorimetry in the laboratory. Beecher argued that such experimental pain investigations provided no information of clinical value, nd after an extensive review of the literature, he concluded that pain threshold change was simply not relevant to pain relief.

Nearly three decades have passed since this conflict first gained attention. New tools for scaling pain have been developed, and more importantly, today's researchers conceptualize the pain experience more comprehensively. The purpose of this chapter is to take another look at the relationship of laboratory and clinical pain in light of the progress in methodology and theory in recent years. General guidelines for integrating the information yielded by these two traditionally independent realms of research are provided.

243

WHAT IS MEASURED IN THE LABORATORY AND IN THE CLINIC?

The difference between laboratory and clinical research is seen more clearly if one considers the types of variables measured in each. Laboratory researchers have traditionally measured pain threshold, but in recent years reports of experienced sensations, various measures of performance accuracy in discrimination or detection tasks, response bias, and reaction time have been assessed. Fortunately, the use of threshold measures in pain research is now infrequent. A significant part of the problem with response reliability in the research of Hardy et al. (14) and others who followed their approach was probably attributable to the vagaries of threshold assessment. Such measures tend to confound sensory changes with response proclivity, so that they often reflect the incidental psychological variables in the testing situation rather than the expected treatment effects (4,21). Sensory decision theory (SDT) methodology (5,6,11), evoked potential studies (6,7), and magnitude estimation paradigms (13) now provide powerful alternatives that yield more reliable outcomes.

These procedures all have a common theme: they attempt to relate precisely controlled change in an external stimulus to subjective experience or to some indicator of performance that reflects the accuracy of information acquisition and transmission within the nervous system. In short, investigators using these methods have tacitly construed pain as a sensory modality that can be studied with the same tools one might use for vision, touch, or hearing. The literature produced in such investigations has shown sufficient reliability to support this assumption. Subjects can perceive and discriminate painful stimuli much as they process other information, and this perceptual ability is reduced by analgesic interventions. Of course, this assumption may be correct and yet still be insufficient to explain the natural experience of pain.

Clinical investigators have typically assessed pain intensity via a visual analogue scale or other simple device. In some cases they have quantified patient activity levels or measured amount of medication intake. Lacking precise control over the stimulus, the clinical researcher makes no effort to measure the accuracy of nociceptive information acquisition and transmission. Instead, he or she seeks to measure the ways in which the patient's expressed experience and behavior differ from normal. Beecher described the clinical acute pain problem as one of emotion, and argued that postoperative pain management was really a problem of sedation rather than analgesia (2). Another approach would argue that pain is a motivational state, or a "drive," since it organizes and directs the patient's perception and behavior (9). It determines what is relevant or irrelevant for the patient at any given moment and directs the patient to behave in a way that will reduce, stop, or minimize the pain.

One could argue that, intentionally or otherwise, clinical studies measure the aversive quality of pain. For example, the postoperative patient with pain suffers from the compelling and emotionally unpleasant nature of the experience rather than from the sheer "loudness" of the sensation. The emotionally neutral intensity dimension of pain is an abstract concept not really relevant to distressed patients marking visual analogue scales, and it is doubtful that such scales can yield pure measures of pain intensity.

In an attempt to help bridge the gap between laboratory and clinical pain from the side of the laboratory researcher, Wolff and associates (22) developed the "drug request point" measure for experimental pain studies. This has not been widely adopted, however, because a laboratory subject does not really suffer and can leave the experiment at any time he or she chooses. Thus, the subject's drug request point is really an "as if" measure that may provide an indicator of the subject's imagination and role-playing ability more than it measures pain sensibility.

Alternative approaches to assessing the aversive dimension of pain in the laboratory have been developed, largely in response to Beecher's attack (1) on the work of Hardy et al. (14). Smith and colleagues in Beecher's group, for example, attempted to measure the aversive dimension of pain in the laboratory by using a tourniquet tolerance test, termed the submaximum effort tourniquet technique (20). This proved more effective than radiant heat procedures in the evaluation of analgesics. In addition, the cold pressor test (ice water immersion) (15), esophageal inflation (10), colon inflation (19), and a tight headband (12) have been employed in laboratory studies, to name only a few of the many creative attempts. These procedures clearly elicit an emotional–motivational experience in subjects. Just how good an approximation of clinical pain they provide is uncertain, because the subject is free to quit the experiment at any point and never feels the desperation of the postoperative or traumatized patient. Because these approaches yield dependent measures with poor precision and large variances in data sets, such studies are a minority in the laboratory pain literature.

PAIN AS A MULTIDIMENSIONAL PHENOMENON

In the three decades since the conflict between Beecher (1) and Hardy et al. (14), a broader, more comprehensive concept of pain has evolved. No longer is pain thought of as simply a sensory modality, but rather as a complex multidimensional experience. A landmark article by Melzack and Casey (16) described pain in terms of sensory–discriminative and motivational–emotional dimensions in a model that extended the original concepts of gate control theory. Pain experience was construed as a process that included sensory information and motivational drive together with higher-level brain processes involved in the evaluation and integration of these factors with other perceptual experiences and memory. Both Melzack and Casey have further elaborated on this concept.

The McGill Pain Questionnaire, developed by Melzack and Torgerson (17), has had a great impact on clinical research on pain. It assesses the language patients use to describe pain in terms of sensory–discriminative, motivational–emotional, and evaluative dimensions by listing words that express these dimensions of subjective experience. This instrument provides a comprehensive basis for evaluating clinical pain, and it can be used in the laboratory as well.

Casey (3) has developed a neurophysiological model that specifies separate spinal and supraspinal pathways for the sensory–discriminative and motivational–emotional aspects of pain. The former utilizes the dorsal column medial–lemniscal system and the ventrobasal thalamus. The latter employs paleospinothalamic pathways that send collaterals to the reticular formation of the brainstem, medial thalamus, and hypothalamus from which they may influence the limbic system. Casey ascribes the aversive dimension of pain primarily to the activity of the reticular formation. This model has strong implications for the problem of relating laboratory and clinical studies.

Differences in the dependent variables used to measure pain in the laboratory and in the clinic suggest that laboratory investigators have been concerned primarily with the sensory–discriminative aspect of the pain experience, whereas clinical researchers have focused on the motivational–emotional side of pain. Casey's model (3) asserts that these two dimensions reflect different underlying physiological systems and perhaps even two separate classes of psychological experience. There seems to be little redundancy between these two putative systems from the viewpoint of the organism's perception and behavior, and consequently information coming to the brain via one system is unlikely to generalize to the other. Moreover, some pain experiences may involve one system heavily but use the other hardly at all. For example, cutaneous laboratory pain may have little or no motivational–emotional quality but be rich in sensory–discriminative input, whereas the visceral pain generated by the stretching of a hollow organ may be rich in aversive quality but poor in sensory–discriminative information.

Thus, clinical and laboratory investigators (excepting those using tolerance techniques) may have been studying nearly independent physiological and psychological phenomena. Each realm of inquiry has generated valuable scientific information, but attempts to force the two bodies of knowledge into a single line of evidence have been unsuccessful. It is entirely possible, however, to integrate information provided by these two areas of research into a multidimensional model such as that articulated by Melzack and Casey (16). Some approaches to achieving such integration are considered below.

TOWARD INTEGRATING CLINICAL AND LABORATORY RESEARCH

Past problems in the interchange between laboratory and clinical research are primarily due to the misapplication of findings from one area of investigation to the other rather than methodological shortcomings of either. Attempting to generalize the sensory effects of an analgesic treatment in the laboratory to the aversiveness of clinical pain is a bad bet at best, and drugs that alter clinical pain may not appear analgesic in the laboratory. The challenge for the future is to develop these two lines of research into complementary bases of knowledge that expand our understanding of a multidimensional model of pain. The following four approaches, which are not mutually exclusive, can help achieve this goal.

First, one can design laboratory studies that are multidimensional at the outset. That is, an investigator could endeavor to quantify both the sensory–discriminative and motivational–emotional aspects of pain in any given study. An example is provided by an investigation of the possible analgesic effects of diazepam by Chapman and Feather (8). We examined the effect of this tranquilizer as contrasted with placebo on pain tolerance using the submaximum effort tourniquet technique, and then carried out a second study to determine whether diazepam might alter sensory capability (d') in a SDT task using radiant heat stimulation. We found that the drug significantly increased tourniquet tolerance time over a placebo in a double-blind design, but it had no affect on d'. State anxiety scores obtained during the tourniquet testing session indicated that with diazepam, subjects showed less anxiety over time during tourniquet testing than with placebo. We concluded that diazepam altered the aversive or emotional aspect of pain but not the sensory–discriminative aspect. Certainly, experiments that provide assessment of both aspects of the pain experience can go further toward the achievement of a broad understanding than a unidimensional study.

Such an approach cannot completely solve the problem, however, because the investigator, no matter how clever he may be, is still restricted to a laboratory study. There are two reasons why laboratory investigations with human subjects can never accurately approximate clinical situations. One is that ethical issues become murky, and few precedents exist for studies in which subjects suffer emotionally and existentially significant pain. Even if the investigator could devise a method of generating intense, persisting pain that was totally harmless to the subject, ethics committees would still be reluctant to approve a project that would subject a volunteer to prolonged pain with extreme discomfort over time. In all such cases, subjects must have the right to quit the experiment whenever they choose. This factor alone makes it impossible for the experimenter effectively to model clinical pain, because in cases of traumatic injury or recovery from surgery, patients cannot escape their situations. The other reason is the problem of the time frame used in conventional laboratory studies. Most investigators do not keep subjects more than 2 or 3 hr in the laboratory, but pathological pain is rarely so kind. The pain investigator, like the sleep investigator, would need to study a subject 8 to 24 hr or even longer to evaluate the experience of pain comprehensively. Few laboratories for testing human subjects are equipped or prepared to do this. Thus, laboratory procedures seem irreconcilably limited.

Second, it is possible to undertake team research that involves parallel studies in the clinic and the laboratory. When carried out within a carefully developed and comprehensive conceptual framework, such a program of research could make major contributions to our understanding of pain and to the evaluation of analgesic treatments. For example, electrical tooth pulp stimulation studies could be carried out in the laboratory using evoked potential methodology and psychophysics, while at the same time conceptually parallel work could be done in a clinical context. Investigators could develop parallel lines of evidence about motivational–emotional and sensory–discriminative aspects of pain through such a paradigm.

Third, an investigator could bring patients into the laboratory for experimental testing. The research data gathered could be of value clinically or gathered in parallel with clinical pain measures. If patients perform differently from normals on laboratory tests, this may indicate abnormality in central levels of pain modulation or other nervous system dysfunction. Alternatively, from such testing the researcher could derive measures that might serve as valuable covariates in a clinical context. For example, one might conduct an experiment designed to evaluate the effects of a new analgesic in this way. By using an index of sensory–discriminative changes obtained in the laboratory as a covariate in analysis of clinical visual analogue scale data, the experimenter could obtain a clearer estimate of the effect of the treatment on the motivational–emotional aspect of pain.

Fourth, and finally, investigators can employ a more optimal decision strategy for the overall evaluation of the literature. Claims that laboratory findings are useless or uninformative reflect a narrow concept of pain, and such thinking effectively prevents useful integration of information about sensory and aversive aspects of pain. One problem is that there has been an inordinate emphasis on obtaining positive rather than negative outcomes in laboratory experiments. Sensory studies conducted in the laboratory that show that certain drugs do not alter sensory function have typically been dismissed as useless and in conflict with clinical data. In fact, the combined studies show that the drug acts on the motivational–emotional aspect of pain, as seen in the clinical context, and not on the sensory as seen in the laboratory. As Platt (18) has emphasized, one of the best indicators of progress in science is the negative finding. Given a well-conceived, logical framework, an investigator can make effective inferences from a series of negative outcomes by showing which hypotheses are not true. If a given treatment does not alter the sensory–discriminative aspect of pain but does, in turn, affect the motivational–emotional, then considerable understanding has been gained. It is very important to specify which treatments do or do not affect each of the two dimensions of pain and not only to show positive outcomes when a given analgesic is investigated. Relatively few investigators take the time to design experiments and select dependent variables so carefully that outcomes are unambiguous. In the past, casual experimentation has been combined with the attempted attribution of treatment effects to the two categories of pain, and the scientific inference prcess has become muddied. There is a need, therefore, to accompany multidimensional pain research with careful planning and experimental design that will yield clear outcomes.

REFERENCES

1. Beecher, H. K. (1959): *Measurement of Subjective Responses: Quantitative Effects of Drugs*, pp. 92–190. Oxford University Press, London.
2. Beecher, H. K. (1969): Anxiety and pain. *JAMA*, 209:1080.
3. Casey, K. L. (1980): Supraspinal mechanisms in pain: The reticular formation. In: *Pain and Society, Dahlem Konferenzen*, edited by H. W. Kosterlitz and L. Y. Terenius, pp. 183–199. Verlag Chemie, Weinheim.
4. Chapman, C. R. (1974): An alternative to threshold assessment in the study of human pain. In: *Advances in Neurology, Vol. 4*, edited by J. J. Bonica, pp. 115–121. Raven Press, New York.

5. Chapman, C. R. (1978): Pain: The perception of noxious events. In: *The Psychology of Pain*, edited by R. A. Sternbach, pp. 169–202. Raven Press, New York.
6. Chapman, C. R. (1980): Pain and perception: Comparison of sensory decision theory and evoked potential methods. In: *Pain*, edited by J. J. Bonica, pp. 111–142. Raven Press, New York.
7. Chapman, C. R. (1980): The measurement of pain in man. In: *Pain and Society, Dahlem Konferenzen*, edited by H. W. Kosterlitz and L. Y. Terenius, pp. 339–354. Verlag Chemie, Weinheim.
8. Chapman, C. R., and Feather, B. W. (1973): Effects of diazepam on human pain tolerance and pain sensitivity. *Psychosom. Med.*, 35:330–340.
9. Chapman, C. R., and Gagliardi, G. J. (1980): Clinical implications of Bolles and Fanselow's pain/fear model. *Behav. Brain Sci.*, 3:305–306.
10. Chapman, W. P., and Jones, C. M. (1944): Variations in cutaneous and visceral pain sensitivity in normal subjects. *J. Clin. Invest.*, 23:81–91.
11. Clark, W. C. (1974): Pain sensitivity and the report of pain: An introduction to sensory decision theory. *Anesthesiology*, 40:272–287.
12. Dudley, D. L., Holmes, T. H., and Ripley, H. S. (1967): Hypnotically induced and suggested facsimile of head pain. *J. Nerv. Ment. Dis.*, 144:258–265.
13. Gracely, R. H., McGrath, P., and Dubner, R. (1978): Ratio scales of sensory and affective verbal pain descriptors. *Pain*, 5:5–18.
14. Hardy, J. D., Wolff, H. G., and Goodell, H. (1943): The pain threshold in man. In: *Research Publications, Association for Research in Nervous and Mental Disease, Vol. 23*, pp. 1–15. Williams & Wilkins, Baltimore.
15. Hilgard, E. R., and Hilgard, J. R. (1975): *Hypnosis in the Relief of Pain*. William Kaufmann, Los Altos.
16. Melzack, R., and Casey, K. L. (1968): Sensory, motivational and central control determinants of pain: A new conceptual model. In: *The Skin Senses*, edited by D. Kenshalo, pp. 423–443. Charles C Thomas, Springfield.
17. Melzack, R., and Torgerson, W. S. (1971): On the language of pain. *Anesthesiology*, 34:50–59.
18. Platt, J. R. (1964): Strong inference. *Science*, 146:347–353.
19. Ritchie, J. (1973): Pain from distension of the pelvic colon by inflating a balloon in the irritable colon syndrome. *Gut*, 14:125–132.
20. Smith, G. M., Lowenstein, E., Hubbard, J. H., and Beecher, H. K. (1968): Experimental pain produced by the submaximum effort tourniquet technique: Further evidence of validity. *J. Pharmacol. Exp. Ther.*, 163:468–474.
21. Watson, C. W. (1973): Psychophysics. In: *Handbook of General Psychology*, edited by B. B. Wolman, pp. 275–306. Prentice-Hall, Englewood Cliff.
22. Wolff, B. B. (1980): Measurement of human pain. In: *Pain*, Publ. Assoc. Res. Nerv. Ment. Disease, *Vol. 58*, edited by J. J. Bonica, pp. 173–184. Raven Press, New York.

Pain Measurement and Assessment,
edited by Ronald Melzack,
Raven Press, New York © 1983.

Measurement of Experimental Pain in Chronic Pain Patients: Methodological and Individual Factors

Gary B. Rollman

*Department of Psychology, University of Western Ontario,
London, Ontario, Canada N6A 5C2*

A recent issue of the journal *Pain* includes five papers with the word "pain" in their titles. One (34) superbly reviews the literature on cognitive methods for pain control in humans and provides an overview of studies in which the discomfort arose due to muscle ischemia, ice water, electrical shock, heat, pressure, endoscopic examination, knee arthrogram, cast removal, cardiac catheterization, surgery, dental procedures, muscle contraction headache, childbirth, and duodenal ulcer, among others. The remaining four examine the pain due to electrical shock, chronic low back pain, diverse pain syndromes, and phantom limb pain.

Those interested in the measurement or treatment of pain wish to generalize across studies—to read reports emerging from one laboratory or clinic and apply the findings to their own specific needs. However, even a casual review of the pain literature reveals repeated instances of inconclusive outcomes and failures to replicate effects reported elsewhere. Given the enormous range of pain-inducing stimuli and syndromes described above, such discrepancies are not surprising.

An understanding of the sources of these differences, however, is crucial for an adequate theory of pain. In recent years, scientists have made considerable progress in isolating specific neural, biochemical, psychological, and social factors that influence the response to noxious stimulation. This chapter presents a selective examination of some of those elements that appear to be important in comprehending the existing literature and in planning future studies.

THE VARIETIES OF PAIN

Laboratory-produced pain and acute and chronic clinical pain differ in both the source of the discomfort and the motivational and cognitive reactions of the individual. Other chapters in this volume emphasize some of the dominant issues concerning the validity of generalizing from the laboratory to the clinic. A declared feature of experimental pain is the capacity to control precisely the spatiotemporal characteristics of the stimulus. This, however, is hardly advantageous if the results obtained in the laboratory are irrelevant to the demands of the clinic. Such a pessimistic stance is unwarranted; nonetheless it is imperative that laboratory procedures and measures be verified in a wide variety of clinical studies.

Pain Induction Methods

Stimuli that can be readily controlled, precisely calibrated, and easily applied, and that are nonhazardous are widely available (26). They fall into a number of broad physical categories, containing considerable choice within each: mechanical (pressure on skin, tourniquet), thermal (heat, cold), electrical (cutaneous or tooth pulp stimulation), and, less satisfactory, chemical (cutaneous, subcutaneous, intramuscular).

Are these interchangeable in pain investigations? Discrepancies in the literature may relate to either the source of the pain or the responses signalling its presence. In humans, these components can be isolated. If indices of responsiveness are obtained for several different stressors, will individuals show similar patterns of sensitivity to all?

Past results (5,9,10,36) have been equivocal, so Georgina Harris and I tested the convergent and discriminant validity (6) of three different pain induction procedures in a group of 40 subjects. Pain thresholds and tolerances were obtained, along with subjective ratings, for (a) a train of electrical impulses delivered to the forearm, (b) a cold pressor test, in which the forearm was immersed in a tank of circulating ice water, and (c) pressure applied through a plastic wedge against the first phalanx of the subject's forefinger (12).

The stimuli varied in locus, energy, and method for determining thresholds. For electrical shock, the stimuli were presented intermittently in ascending intensity, whereas for cold and pressure the physical intensity was constant, and the duration of the stressors was extended. Nonetheless, observers were relatively consistent in their behaviors. Correlations tended to be significant both within a given pain source and across stressors.

Despite the evidence for validity (6) of both traits (pain measures) and methods (stressors), there are a number of reasons for caution in concluding that these electrical, thermal, and mechanical stimuli are equally satisfactory in testing pain attenuation. First, the correlations, although statistically significant, were generally between 0.3 and 0.5. Second, some serious differences among stressors were revealed by the concurrent rating data. Subjects received instructions to report when the stimulus became painful and to tolerate the discomfort as long as possible. At both decision points, they also described their pain experience by marking a scale that included both words and numbers: slight pain (1 to 4), moderate pain (4 to 7), severe pain (7 to 10), and very severe pain (10).

For the three stressors, the following are the average ratings provided at pain threshold and tolerance points:

	Shock	*Cold*	*Pressure*
Threshold	1.77	3.80	3.72
Tolerance	5.92	7.92	7.12

It appears that for shock, subjects withdrew from the experiment while their pain was still fairly moderate; for cold and pressure it was described as somewhat severe. Clearly, threshold and tolerance do not mean the same thing for different stressors.

Which, then, is the preferred induction method? Shock was the only one of the three stressors that showed significant correlations with personality measures (17). Is shock unacceptable because it is subjectively the one that is most unlike clinical pain and the one for which the tolerance criterion may be the lowest, or is it desirable precisely because factors such as anxiety, which are responsible for this cautious behavior, are also the ones that provide the closest parallel to the affective and evaluative components prominent in the clinic?

The method of pain induction is not an issue that can be examined in isolation. Interactions between pain source and pain attenuation may occur, leading one laboratory to conclude that a putative analgesic is without effect while another laboratory, using a different source of pain, proclaims its striking antinociceptive properties. Often, the pain source is chosen on the basis of what apparatus is readily available rather than by an informed judgment regarding its capacity to mimic the sensory, affective, or evaluative properties of particular clinical disorders. Even a single form of energy, such as electrical shock, can produce vastly different effects as a function of both its pulse properties and experimental locus (27). Pain researchers should expand their arsenal and replicate their results with a variety of stressors, thereby establishing a meaningful comparative perspective on the interaction of different treatment modalities and different forms of pain.

Pain Measures

Just as there are a wide variety of pain induction methods, there is now a plethora of direct and derived pain measures: thresholds, tolerances, categorical judgments, magnitude estimations, signal detection theory (SDT) indices, visual analogue scales, multidimensional scaling, cross-modality matches, scaled verbal descriptors, functional measurement, the McGill Pain Questionnaire (MPQ) and other checklists, nonverbal pain expressions, cortical evoked potentials, autonomic indices, withdrawal reflexes, and, in the case of clinical pain, behavioral correlates such as activity levels or drug intakes.

It would be folly to assume that each of these reflects the same attribute, yet relatively few investigators (e.g., 1,2,4,13) utilize more than one nociceptive measure. As was the case with pain induction, a comparative perspective is required here, so that the full complexity of the human pain experience can be adequately expressed.

The emphasis of the gate control theory (23) on the sensory–discriminative, motivational–affective, and cognitive–evaluative components of pain has fostered attempts to develop scales which assess each of these dimensions. The MPQ (22) and the verbal descriptors and cross-modal matches utilized by Gracely and his colleagues (e.g., 14) represent important steps in quantifying the multidimensional nature of nociception.

However, since pain is a complex integration of these elements, it remains to be seen whether they can be measured independently. Melzack (22), for example, determined correlations between the rank values of each MPQ subscale: sensory, affective, evaluative, miscellaneous, as well as total. All correlations were significant at the 0.01 level.

Although Gracely has presented data that indicate that sensory and affective components can be dissociated (e.g., 14), both judgments were generally not obtained at the same time. More recent results (37) demonstrate that not all psychophysical attempts to assess these two components are equivalent; in a group of chronic low-back-pain patients, verbal scales of both sensory intensity and unpleasantness of noxious thermal stimuli were significantly reduced when compared with a placebo by administration of morphine, whereas handgrip measures of each were not reduced by the drug.

Pain measures utilizing verbal responses may include items not understood by sizeable numbers of patients or subject to multiple interpretations. Even simple words create difficulties: "Intense" and "miserable" are both included on the evaluative subclass of the MPQ; others (15) used the former as a sensory descriptor and the latter as an affective one.

In my own laboratory, SDT measures of discrimination of electrical shocks presented to the forearm were not reliably affected by instructions to rate the intensity, unpleasantness, or painfulness of the stimuli, although discriminability was improved when observers concentrated on distinguishing the stronger signal from the weaker (30). More recently, Elizabeth Nowicki and I compared the MPQ with concurrent visual analogue scales and direct magnitude estimations of the sensory intensity and unpleasantness experienced by a group of patients receiving spinal blocks. The correlations of the MPQ subscales were similar to those reported by Melzack (22). As well, for both visual analogue scales and ratio judgments, intensity and unpleasantness showed highly significant correlations with each other. The changes in pain, both within and across sessions, were not reflected equally by these measures (see also 19). Further attempts to refine multidimensional techniques and identify the limiting characteristics of verbal and performance scales (e.g., 14) are clearly in order.

Subject Characteristics

Research on pain generally involves either the endogenous discomfort of patients or induced stress in pain-free volunteers. Rarely do investigators study experimental pain with clinical subjects. Several years ago (29), I presented data that suggest that judgments of pain are based on comparisons with other pain levels and proposed an adaptation level model for such decisions. I suggested, as well, that whereas pain-free individuals refer to other stimuli in the pain-inducing set, chronic pain patients may utilize their internal discomfort as an anchor in describing an external signal's intensity or unpleasantness. Anecdotal reports reinforce this view. A newspaper columnist (32) related the story of an arthritic woman who failed to recognize an attack of acute appendicitis, adding "you must be in considerable pain when you can't recognize the addition of a new pain of that magnitude."

Recently, Naliboff et al. (24) tested the adaptation level concept, contrasting it with a hypervigilance model (see 8). The adaptation level model predicts that pain patients should have higher pain thresholds than controls—that is, the externally produced pain should not seem very severe when compared with the internal distress. The hypervigilance model assumes an exaggerated focus on painful sensations and predicts that pain patients will have lower pain thresholds than controls. In their study, Naliboff et al. compared radiant heat thresholds and ratings provided by low-back-pain patients, chronic respiratory patients, and nonpatient controls. The pain patients (as well as the respiratory disease ones, perhaps as a result of a history of painful diagnostic tests) had substantially higher pain thresholds than controls and showed poorer discrimination at lower intensity levels, thus supporting the adaptation level model. Related demonstrations that experimental pain thresholds or tolerance levels are reduced by successful treatment of painful conditions are available from the research of Nyquist and Eriksson (25) and Greenhoot and Sternbach (16).

Interestingly, in a study of patients with myofascial pain dysfunction (MPD) syndrome, a disorder attributed to muscle tension arising from emotional stress and anxiety, Malow et al. (20) found that they reported lower thresholds than nonpatients with the Forgione and Barber (12) pressure algometer and significantly lower discriminability in a signal detection task. A subsequent experiment by Malow and Olsen (21) found similar distinctions between unimproved and improved MPD patients. The threshold data suggest possibly important differences in the judgmental behavior of individuals suffering from psychogenic versus organic disorders; the signal detection results provide a challenge to those advocates of SDT (28) who argue that reductions in discriminability are the expected consequences of analgesic procedures, since the pain-free individuals exhibited increased discriminability indices.

These findings indicate that a synergistic relationship may be obtained from a convergence of traditional approaches. Experimental pain can be adjusted and quantified; clinical pain involves special affective and evaluative components. Testing chronic pain patients under laboratory conditions captures the benefits of both conceptual models.

Subject characteristics are not defined only by pain patient versus nonpatient distinctions. A massive body of literature has developed demonstrating the influence of other factors on the pain experience, and further research is needed to uncover their interactions with pain production, pain measurement, and pain state. Among these factors are age, sex, cultural and racial group, prior social experiences, psychiatric status, intelligence, expectation for pain relief, laterality, endorphin levels in cerebrospinal fluid, menstrual cycle, diurnal cycle, circannual cycle, and a host of personality variables including anxiety and coping style. As well, pain responses are affected by interactions between the subject's characteristics and those of the experimenter.

Cognitive strategies appear to be particularly promising in assessing the response to pain (17,33,35) and in planning appropriate treatments (34). Harris (17), for example, has shown that self-generated strategies (emphasizing "coping" rather than "catastrophizing") influence base-line responses to painful stimuli and interact with subsequent instructions in determining the success of brief cognitive therapies.

DOLORMETRICS

This chapter has emphasized the importance of methodological and individual factors in understanding pain experience. Pain cannot be studied in isolation. Judicious selection of induction techniques, response scales, and subject characteristics constitutes a critical part of the measurement process.

The problems identified here are not unique to the study of pain. Questions relating to individual differences and the relation between affect, evaluation, and behavior in both laboratory and natural situations have arisen in areas as diverse as social cognition (18), sexual behavior (11), aggression (3), intelligence testing (7), and the psychological factors underlying placebo effects (31). Psychometrics is a vibrant discipline that concerns itself with the measurement of mental traits and processes. Given the theoretical and empirical advances in pain research that have taken place in the recent past, dolormetrics, a science devoted to the measurement of pain, appears similarly promising. The task will not be easy. Pain source, measure, and subject characteristics each includes a multitude of categories, leading one to imagine a rather unwieldy Rubik's cube to describe the conceptual trinity presented here. Since even the conventional cube has the potential for 43 quadrillion configurations, considerable challenge and excitement lie ahead.

ACKNOWLEDGMENTS

Preparation of this chapter was supported by Grant A0392 from the Natural Sciences and Engineering Research Council of Canada. I am grateful to Eldon H. Bossin, Terence J. Coderre, Georgina Harris, Patricia McGrath, and Elizabeth A. Nowicki for many fruitful discussions.

REFERENCES

1. Adams, J., Brechner, V. L., and Brechner, J. (1979): The reliability of some techniques utilized in quantifying the intensity of clinical pain. *J. Pharmacol. Ther.*, 4:629–632.
2. Anderson, I., Thompson, W. R., Varkey, G. P., and Knill, R. L. (1981): Lumbar epidural morphine as an effective analgesic following cholecystectomy. *Can. Anaesth. Soc. J.*, 28:523–529.
3. Berkowitz, L., and Donnerstein, E. (1982): External validity is more than skin deep: Some answers to criticisms of laboratory experiments. *Am. Psychol.*, 37:245–257.
4. Bromm, B., and Seide, K. (1982): The influence of tilidine and prazepam on withdrawal reflex, skin resistance reaction and pain rating in man. *Pain*, 12:247–258.
5. Brown, R. A., Fader, K., and Barber, T. (1973): Responsiveness to pain: Stimulus specificity versus generality. *Psychol. Rec.*, 23:1–7.
6. Campbell, D. T., and Fiske, D. W. (1959): Convergent and discriminant validation by the multitrait-multimethod matrix. *Psychol. Bull.*, 56:81–105.
7. Carroll, J. B., and Horn, J. L. (1981): On the scientific basis of ability testing. *Am. Psychol.*, 36:1012–1020.

8. Chapman, C. R. (1978): Pain: The perception of noxious events. In: *The Psychology of Pain*, edited by R. A. Sternbach, pp. 169–203. Raven Press, New York.

9. Clark, J. W., and Bindra, D. (1956): Individual differences in pain thresholds. *Can. J. Psychol.*, 10:69–76.

10. Davidson, P. O., and McDougall, C. E. (1969): The generality of pain tolerance. *J. Psychosom. Res.*, 13:83–89.

11. Fisher, W. A., and Byrne, D. (1978): Individual differences in affective, evaluative, and behavioral responses to an erotic film. *J. Appl. Soc. Psychol.*, 8:355–365.

12. Forgione, A. G., and Barber, T. X. (1971): A strain-gauge pain stimulator. *Psychophysiology*, 8:102–106.

13. Francini, F., Maresca, M., Procacci, P., and Zoppi, M. (1981): The effects of non-painful transcutaneous electrical nerve stimulation on cutaneous pain threshold and muscular reflexes in normal men and in subjects with chronic pain. *Pain*, 11:49–63.

14. Gracely, R. H. (1980): Pain measurement in man. In: *Pain, Discomfort and Humanitarian Care*, edited by L. s2K. Y. Ng and J. J. Bonica, pp. 111–137. Elsevier/North-Holland, New York.

15. Gracely, R. H., McGrath, P., and Dubner, R. (1978): Ratio scales of sensory and affective verbal pain descriptors. *Pain*, 5:5–18.

16. Greenhoot, J. H., and Sternbach, R. A. (1974): Conjoint treatment of chronic pain. In: *Pain: Advances in Neurology, Vol. 4*, edited by J. J. Bonica, pp. 595–603. Raven Press, New York.

17. Harris, G. (1981): Pain and the individual. Unpublished doctoral dissertation. University of Western Ontario, London, Canada.

18. Higgins, E. T., Kuiper, N. A., and Olson, J. M. (1981): Social cognition: A need to get personal. In: *Social Cognition: The Ontario Symposium*, edited by E. T. Higgins, C. P. Herman, and M. P. Zanna, pp. 395–420. Laurence Erlbaum Associates, Hillsdale.

19. Kremer, E., Atkinson, J. H., and Ignelzi, R. J. (1981): Measurement of pain: Patient preference does not confound pain measurement. *Pain*, 10:241–248.

20. Malow, R. M., Grimm, L., and Olson, R. E. (1980): Differences in pain perception between myofascial pain dysfunction patients and normal subjects: A signal detection analysis. *J. Psychosom. Res.*, 24:303–309.

21. Malow, R. M., and Olson, R. E. (1981): Changes in pain perception after treatment for chronic pain. *Pain*, 11:65–72.

22. Melzack, R. (1975): The McGill Pain Questionnaire: Major properties and scoring methods. *Pain*, 1:277–299.

23. Melzack, R., and Wall, P. D. (1965): Pain mechanisms: A new theory. *Science*, 150:971–979.

24. Naliboff, B. D., Cohen, M. J., Schandler, S. L., and Heinrich, R. L. (1981): Signal detection and threshold measures for chronic back pain patients, chronic illness patients, and cohort controls to radiant heat stimuli. *J. Abnorm. Psychol.*, 90:271–274.

25. Nyquist, J. K., and Eriksson, M. B. E. (1981): Effect of pain treatment procedures on thermal sensibility in chronic pain patients. *Pain [Suppl.]*, 1:591.

26. Procacci, P., Zoppi, M., and Maresca, J. (1979): Experimental pain in man. *Pain*, 6:123–140.

27. Rollman, G. B. (1974): Electrocutaneous stimulation. In: *Cutaneous Communication Systems and Devices*, edited by F. A. Geldard, pp. 38–51. Psychomic Society, Austin.

28. Rollman, G. B. (1977): Signal detection theory measurement of pain: A review and critique. *Pain*, 3:187–211.

29. Rollman, G. B. (1979): Signal detection theory pain measures: Empirical validation studies and adaptation-level effects. *Pain*, 6:9–21.

30. Rollman, G. B. (1982): Multiple subjective representations of experimental pain. In: *Advances in Pain Research and Therapy, Vol. 5*, edited by J. J. Bonica, U. Lindblom, and A. Iggo. Raven Press, New York.

31. Ross, M., and Olson, J. M. (1981): An expectancy-attribution model of the effects of placebos. *Psychol. Rev.*, 88:408–437.

32. Slinger, A. (1982): The trouble with pain is that it hurts. *Toronto Star*, April 6:A2.

33. Spanos, N. P., Radtke-Bodorik, L., Ferguson, J. D., and Jones, B. (1979): The effects of hypnotic susceptibility, suggestions for analgesia and the utilization of cognitive strategies on the reduction of pain. *J. Abnorm. Psychol.*, 88:282–292.

34. Tan, S. Y. (1982): Cognitive and cognitive-behavioral methods for pain control: A selective review. *Pain*, 12:201–228.
35. Weisenberg, M. (1980): The regulation of pain. *Ann. N.Y. Acad. Sci.*, 340:102–114.
36. Wolff, B. B. (1971): Factor analysis of human pain response: Pain endurance as a specific pain factor. *J. Abnorm. Psychol.*, 78:292–298.
37. Wolskee, P. J., and Gracely, R. H. (1980): The effects of morphine on experimental pain response in chronic pain patients. *Soc. Neurosci. Abstr.*, 6:246.

Pain Measurement and Assessment,
edited by Ronald Melzack,
Raven Press, New York © 1983.

Ethical Considerations in Pain Research in Man

Richard A. Sternbach

*Pain Treatment Center, Scripps Clinic and Research Foundation,
La Jolla, California 92037*

In these nightmarish times, when unspeakable tortures are performed on human beings by their governments and by terrorist groups, when horrors are contemplated as instruments of governmental policy, it seems almost quaint and archaic to consider ethical problems in pain research. As compared with the monstrous cruelties regularly reported (13), of what significance is the transient and noninjurious pain we inflict in the laboratory or manipulate in the clinic?

The answer to this question is very simple and very important. We are ultimately responsible for our own actions as individuals. Unless each of us is scrupulously ethical in our own behaviors, particularly in those situations in which we have the possibility of committing an offense to human dignity, there is little hope of influencing others for the better and of shaping a more ethical world.

Those of us committed to the alleviation of pain must pause when contemplating pain research. To inflict pain deliberately, or to permit pain to continue when it can be abated, raises the serious ethical question of cruelty. The conditions under which it may be acceptable to do pain research, and the guidelines for doing so, represent the topics of this chapter. But such situations occur in social, interpersonal contexts in which the goals and aspirations of the researcher also are influential, and so must be taken into account.

MOTIVATIONS IN PAIN RESEARCH

We are well aware that injury signals seem to be a basic biological mechanism for survival. Those who do not normally appreciate pain usually seem to have greater difficulty in surviving than those who do (10). Despite this, the long-term experience of pain (the apparent subjective correlate of injury signals) seems frequently to be quite harmful in both a psychological as well as physical sense (6,11). The justification for pain research seems therefore to be quite obvious: It is necessary in order better to be able to control (alleviate) pain.

To achieve this goal, it is necessary to understand the mechanisms of pain and analgesia in humans. This, of course, requires studies in which pain is inflicted,

259

or manipulated, to determine the variables influencing these mechanisms, and what could be a loftier justification than the possibility of abolishing unnecessary pain?

But there is a very serious reason for hesitating even at this preliminary statement of goals. There is the empirical fact that every advance in scientific knowledge has been perverted to some harmful purpose. One can easily imagine that advances in pain research will also be so abused. It takes no science fiction author's imagination to predict that there will soon be deliberate manipulations of prisoners' brain amines and peptides to create yet more fiendish tortures. The results of one's lifetime of dedicated research to a noble cause is as likely to be used for evil as for good. This must be recognized. What researcher would wish to have this development on his or her conscience?

There is another problem with the assumption that the study of pain, like the study of all natural phenomena, is of primary importance. This is the emphasis on knowing, with its corollary of being able to manipulate the environment. Such an emphasis makes scientific research an activity that takes precedence over other conflicting values (12). In the Western world, for example, limited financial resources are weighted far more toward knowing than toward such other values as feeling or relating. Perhaps because it is assumed that knowledge (science) is power, those in power are more easily disposed to support scientific research than the arts or humanities. But it should be clear that there is no intrinsic superiority of knowing or learning over creating beauty, for example, or over being kind. Scientists tend to promote the precedence of science, and biomedical scientists find it all too easy to justify the infliction of pain to learn more about it. But as there is nothing inherently superior about scientific activity as compared with artistic or literary or social activity, the insistence by some scientists of their "need" or "right" or "obligation" to do research reflects only their arrogance.

This arrogance is manifested in the attitude that human subjects and patients similarly have an "obligation" to participate in such research. It is argued that such persons are already the beneficiaries of an improved medical science because of sacrifices made by previous subjects and patients. Although it is not possible now to repay those earlier subjects, the "system" of biomedical research can be repaid. This may, in turn, benefit the patient and his family in the future, as well as other patients yet to come. Even if there is no immediate benefit to the subject, he is obligated to participate in research to repay the debt he owes to subjects of the past (5).

This example of the attitude of some scientists obviously lacks an essential element. There is no provision for prior consultation with the subject, and he is given no possibility of negotiation. He is placed into a contractual arrangement without his consent, as one is at birth placed into a contractual arrangement with society and the state. Yet this is an arrangement made unilaterally by the biomedical research establishment, which is not part of the legal or political system, and no such obligation on the part of the subject actually exists.

No one has an obligation to participate in any research, as subject or patient. To argue otherwise would be to assume that subjects could be coerced into any sort of experiment that the investigator or the research establishment thought worthwhile. Here is the consequence of scientific arrogance, as scientists inform subjects and patients that they "should" submit to research protocols. The assumption is that what biomedical scientists do is good, and refusal to acquiesce to their requests is bad.

One might be tempted to consider noble scientific ends justifying such coercive means if only there were noble motives involved. Actually, as we are frequently reminded by news of falsified data and bogus research, the medical research scientist is a complex human being with mixed motives. Although an image of the disinterested scientist who dedicates his or her life to the welfare of humanity is still being propagated these days (2), it is received with somewhat less innocence than formerly. Increasingly, we are aware that practical matters replace the noble ideals of the young student. It soon becomes necessary to obtain grants, to impress one's superiors and colleagues, to publish or perish, to win promotions, to support a family, to win a prize, to obtain power.

The old phrases about benefiting humanity and human welfare have become merely propaganda, skillfully used to obtain compliant subjects who help to further one's career. There is, in fact, a record of abuse of subjects by medical researchers, who are quite callous and indifferent to suffering (8). It appears that biomedical scientists have the same lusts for power and recognition as any other group. They are not uniquely blessed with pure and noble motives, nor do they have a special claim on the cooperation of other persons.

Thus, the special arguments used to justify human pain research are: the need to learn about pain is more important than other needs or rights; the work is done by selfless scientists disinterested in any personal gain; the research is done solely for the future benefit of humankind.

None of these statements is the complete truth. The persistent use of these arguments is explained by the need of biomedical scientists for status and power. There are experimental studies that show clearly how easy it is for persons to inflict great pain and suffering on others, in the setting of "legitimate" pain research (7). Acts of apparent cruelty are easily rationalized and justified in the appropriate social settings.

AVOIDING EXPLOITATION OF HUMAN SUBJECTS

The pain researcher is under two conflicting obligations: to perform research that significantly improves our understanding of pain and analgesic mechanisms and therefore improves our ability to treat pain; and to avoid treating subjects in ways that have the potential for causing physical or mental harm or affronting their dignity. It should be quite clear that any research that involves inflicting or prolonging pain may be considered only for significant purposes, and not for such trivial reasons as to clear up a technical or procedural question.

The outcome of the proposed research should answer important questions, whether or not the hypotheses tested are confirmed. That is, even if negative findings are obtained in the study, this result should contribute significantly to the advancement of knowledge in the area.

Furthermore, it is necessary that alternative strategies be considered first. Before inflicting pain on humans, can mathematical or statistical modeling provide answers to the questions being considered? If not, can research on "lower" species do so?

If it is considered that the research is indeed necessary and justified, then some additional issues must be considered.

(a) The fewest possible number of subjects and the least intense and shortest duration of pain must be employed.

(b) The potential subject must be informed of all possible risks of physical or mental discomfort or harm, and must be assured that participation is purely voluntary, with no adverse consequences for refusal to participate. For example, patients must be informed that they will receive the best of care and pain relief possible whether or not they participate in the clinical trial. In short, subjects must be able to give fully informed (of the alternatives and consequences), voluntary consent to participate in the pain study, with no coercion nor any implied threat for refusal.

(c) Every possible precaution must be taken to minimize distress and danger. In the laboratory, measures of maximum pain tolerance should not be obtained if not necessary and if mere changes in estimations of suprathreshold noxious stimuli will suffice. In the clinic, pain relief should not be withheld; placebo conditions should not be used if adequate control for experimental treatments can be made by comparison with standard analgesics or procedures. No pain research design should be extended beyond the minimum duration necessary to obtain valid data.

(d) The participant in the research must gain something of value for participation. There must be some *quid pro quo* for having helped the researcher. "Knowledge that you have contributed to the welfare of humanity" is mere propaganda and cannot suffice. Voluntarily being subjected to pain must bring immediate benefit or reward to the person experiencing it. The laboratory subject must be given some monetary or other reward, which is stipulated in advance and to which the subject agrees. The clinic patient must be given legitimate pain relief for his participation.

These precautions for protecting pain subjects from our well-intentioned manipulations have been summarized in an ethical principle by the American Psychological Association (1). "Principle 7: The ethical investigator protects participants from physical and mental discomfort, harm and danger. If the risk of such consequences exists, the investigator is required to inform the participant of that fact, secure consent before proceeding, and take all possible measures to minimize distress. A research procedure may not be used if it is likely to cause serious and lasting harm to participants."

The Declaration of Helsinki, adopted by the 18th World Medical Assembly in Helsinki in 1964 (3) and revised by the 29th World Medical Assembly in Tokyo in 1975 (9), is even more emphatic: "I.5 . . . Concern for the interests of the subject must always prevail over the interests of science and society. 6. The right of the research subject to safeguard his or her integrity must always be respected. Every precaution should be taken to respect the privacy of the subject and to minimize the impact of the study on the subject's physical and mental integrity and on the personality of the subject.... III.4. In research on man, the interest of science and society should never take precedence over considerations related to the well-being of the subject (9)."

The ethical investigator cannot alone be the judge of the adequacy of his compliance with these precautions. It is obvious that his enthusiasm for his own ideas and his mixed motives for conducting the pain study may well blind him to alternative designs and to less harmful or painful procedures. It is necessary to have a "human subjects research committee" to evaluate the need for the research, the cost/benefit ratio, the possible alternatives, protection of subjects, the adequacy of informed consent, remuneration, etc.

Such a committee should not be composed entirely of colleagues of the researcher, who themselves rarely question the necessity for biomedical research. The committee should probably have only 50% of the membership drawn from the clinical and research sciences, and the others should be lay persons and members of the legal and religious professions. Only then can there be careful sensitivity to such issues as these: Will male subjects in a Veterans Hospital feel that their participation is a sign of their masculinity, and that refusal to participate will weaken their esteem among their fellows? Are excessive inducements being offered to subjects for participation, thus clouding their judgment? Will subjects really feel free to terminate participation at any time during the study, or will they feel coerced to continue?

Such questions as these are all too easily glossed over by the pain researcher, rather than faced squarely. It is therefore necessary to provide a social mechanism to protect the interests of the subjects and of society in general.

THE BASIC ETHICAL PRINCIPLE

The volunteer subject or patient in a pain study should immediately be benefited by participating. "The interests of the subject must always prevail (9)." Other considerations are irrelevant, and are usually used by researchers only to justify unethical behavior.

For example, it is clearly unethical to attempt to persuade a reluctant subject by referring to the importance of the study of science or to society or to humankind. It causes the subject to feel unworthy or morally inferior if he does not participate. Even if coerced into participating, he feels ashamed or guilty for having been reluctant in the first place.

Other considerations may also be used to weaken the basic ethical principle of human pain research. For example, what if inflicting pain may help to ensure the life or health of another? This situation is almost impossible to imagine, but it is approached indirectly in instances of organ transplantation. In organ transplantation, however, pain is an incidental effect of surgery, not a central issue; yet even so, clinicians must be extraordinarily cautious about coercing a relative into being a donor. The voluntary nature of the participation in a research study must never be compromised. It is assured by the use of a "contract," or mutual agreement, in which the subject or patient is compensated by an adequate consideration, either a fee or clinical benefit.

As pain researchers we may be tempted to use appeals about benefiting science or humanity. But we must be aware that there are social forces that would erode the individual's rights to dignity and nonparticipation by appeals to the need of the state or of the party. But "the interest of science and society should never take precedence over considerations related to the well-being of the subject (9)."

There is another way of conceptualizing this matter. It is that each individual must be dealt with as he or she wishes to be. This is a modification of the Golden Rule: "Do unto others as they wish done unto them." This requires a consultation prior to any action. It is a principle that does not assume that the other person has the same values as we (the researchers) do, but may hold different ones. The principle assumes that the individual is a free agent with the right of negotiation and is, thus, to be treated with respect to his dignity, and such a free agent cannot be forced or coerced into any relationship without compromise of this freedom (4). This is the basic principle of ethics that underlies all relationships in an ethical society and that applies particularly to pain research.

CONCLUSIONS

No researcher has an inherent "right" to inflict or prolong pain for research purposes. Subjects are not obligated to suffer such pain for the benefit of others. Society merely awards the research scientist the privilege of conducting pain research under quite specific and restricted conditions.

The individual subject or patient is a free agent with the right of negotiation without coercion regarding participation in the research. He (or she) must be capable of giving fully informed voluntary consent to participate. He must understand the purpose of the study, the procedures to be used, and the benefits and risks of participation. The patient, especially, must understand that alternative treatments are available and that he may withdraw from participation at any time without sacrificing rights to the best care available. The normal subject also must be aware of his right to terminate participation immediately at any time without penalty. Both subject and patient must receive some consideration or personal benefit from participating in the study. If a new pain-relieving technique or drug is studied in the clinic, a comparison with a standard method is preferable to a no-treatment (placebo) control group, as the latter prolongs unnecessary suffering. If there is any risk of serious or permanent harm, the study must not be done.

Each of these rules must be followed in pain research, and compliance must be assured by a committee that oversees human research. To ensure that the committee does not automatically rubber-stamp approval of a colleague's plans, at least half the members should be lay persons, with adequate representation of the legal and religious professions.

As pain researchers, we must temper our tendency to be overenthusiastic about our work. We must remind ourselves that it is intrinsically a cruel activity. The results of single studies are usually much less important and less far-reaching than we had hoped. Strict controls are necessary to protect the subjects from our tendency to be callous or indifferent from constant exposure to suffering. Each subject is a free agent whose dignity and integrity must always be respected.

REFERENCES

1. American Psychological Association (1973): *Ethical Principles in the Conduct of Research with Human Participants*, pp. 58–69. American Psychological Association, Washington, D.C.
2. Cournand, A. (1977): The code of the scientist and its relationship to ethics. *Science*, 198:699–705.
3. Declaration of Helsinki: Recommendations guiding doctors in clinical research (1972): *World Med. J.*, 19:28–29.
4. Engelhardt, Jr., H. T. (1980): Ethical issues in pain management. In: *Pain and Society*, edited by H. W. Kosterlitz and L. Y. Terenius, pp. 461–480. Verlag Chemie GmbH, Weinheim.
5. Gilbert, J. P., McPeek, B., and Mosteller, F. (1977): Statistics and ethics in surgery and anesthesia. *Science*, 198:684–689.
6. Merskey, H., and Spear, F. G. (1967): *Pain: Psychological and Psychiatric Aspects*, pp. 71–87. Bailliere, Tindall & Cassell, London.
7. Milgram, S. (1974): *Obedience to Authority: An Experimental View*. Harper & Row, New York.
8. Pappworth, M. H. (1968): *Human Guinea Pigs*. Beacon Press, Boston.
9. Refshauge, W. (1976): Research on humans: The place for international standards. I and II. *World Med. J.*, 23:60–63; 75–77.
10. Sternbach, R. A. (1968): *Pain: A Psychophysiological Analysis*, pp. 95–115. Academic Press, New York.
11. Sternbach, R. A. (1974): *Pain Patients: Traits and Treatment*, pp. 12–19, 40–51. Academic Press, New York.
12. Tukey, J. W. (1977): Some thoughts on clinical trials, especially problems of multiplicity. *Science*, 198:679–684.
13. (1981): Torture. *World Med. J.*, 28:17–32.

Appendix

APPENDIX A. McGILL COMPREHENSIVE PAIN QUESTIONNAIRE©

To be completed by the person with pain

1. PAIN HISTORY

    a) When did this pain begin? Year: _____ Month: _____

    b) Did this pain begin: gradually _____ suddenly _____

    c) How did this pain begin? *Please check (√)*, then give more specific details on the lines below.

        i) accident at work   ☐
        ii) accident at home   ☐
        iii) following an illness ☐
        iv) following surgery   ☐
        v) pain just began   ☐
        vi) other (e.g., car accident) _____

    d) Were there any changes in your life during the year before this pain began? (For example: job change, buying or selling a home, death or loss of a friend or family member, marital problems) _____

    e) Is the pain the same now as it was when it began? YES ☐ NO ☐

2. PAIN TREATMENTS

Please place a check (√) in the box before any of the professionals you have consulted for the pain problem.

☐ Acupuncturist	☐ Gynecologist/Obstet	☐ Physiatrist
☐ Allergist	☐ Hypnotist	☐ Physiotherapist
☐ Anesthesiologist	☐ Internist	☐ Plastic Surgeon
☐ Cardiologist	☐ Neurologist	☐ Proctologist
☐ Chiropractor	☐ Neurosurgeon	☐ Psychiatrist
☐ Clergyman	☐ Nurse	☐ Psychologist
☐ Dentist	☐ Oncologist	☐ Radiologist
☐ Dermatologist	☐ Ophthalmologist	☐ Rheumatologist
☐ Ear-Nose-Throat	☐ Orthopedist	☐ Social Worker
☐ Endocrinologist	☐ Osteopath	☐ Surgeon (General)
☐ Faith Healer	☐ Pain Clinic	
☐ General Practitioner	☐ Pediatrician	

Please list all the treatments you have had and are currently having for your pain. Include operations, hospitalizations, anesthetic procedures, physiotherapy and psychological treatments:

Name & type of specialist	Date started	Type of treatments and number of treatments (i.e. once a week/every day)	Effect	
			Helped	Did not help
≠	≠	≠		

3. PAST MEDICAL HISTORY

Please list any illnesses *other than your pain* problem that you have had *at any age.*
Also include: allergies, hospitalizations, operations, anesthetic procedures, physiotherapy,
and psychological illnesses and/or treatments. Please make an (×) beside any painful
condition.

Year	Problem	Treatment

4. PRESENT MEDICAL HISTORY

a) Please list any illnesses or health problems (other than the pain problem) you may
have *now,* (i.e. high blood pressure, ulcer, etc.)

Problem	Present treatment

b) Are you still menstruating? YES ☐ NO ☐   If YES, is there any effect on the
pain problem? YES ☐ NO ☐

5. MEDICATION

a) *Please read the following list of drugs below and on page 3A carefully. Place a (√)
in the box beside any drug you have used for any reason. If you have taken a drug
for pain:* please mark in the box a + if it increased pain; please mark a − if it
lessened the pain; please mark a 0 if it did not help; if you are ALLERGIC to ANY
of these drugs please mark it with an A.

i)
- ☐ acetaminophen
- ☐ Alka-Seltzer
- ☐ Anacin
- ☐ Ascriptin
- ☐ Aspirin
- ☐ Atasol
- ☐ Atasol with codeine
- ☐ Bufferin
- ☐ Darvon
- ☐ Darvon mixtures
- ☐ Entrophen
- ☐ Excedrin
- ☐ Equagesic
- ☐ Fiorinal
- ☐ Fiorinal with codeine
- ☐ Frosst "217"
- ☐ Frosst "222"
- ☐ Frosst "282"
- ☐ Frosst "292"
- ☐ Frosst "642"
- ☐ Frosst "692"
- ☐ Propoxyphene
- ☐ Tylenol
- ☐ Tylenol with codeine

ii)
- ☐ Demerol
- ☐ Dilaudid
- ☐ heroin
- ☐ Leritine
- ☐ Methadone
- ☐ morphine
- ☐ Paragoric
- ☐ Percodan
- ☐ Talwin

iii)
- ☐ Butazolidin
- ☐ Clinoril
- ☐ Cortisone
- ☐ Dexamethasone
- ☐ Feldene
- ☐ hydrocortisone
- ☐ Indocid
- ☐ Malgesic
- ☐ Motrin
- ☐ Nalfon
- ☐ Naprosyn
- ☐ Prednisolone
- ☐ Prednisone
- ☐ Tanderil
- ☐ Tolectin
- ☐ Zomax

iv)
- ☐ Arlidin
- ☐ Cafergot
- ☐ Ergotrate
- ☐ Gynergen
- ☐ Inderal
- ☐ Sandomigran
- ☐ Sansert
- ☐ Vasodilan

v)
- ☐ Dantrium
- ☐ Flexeril
- ☐ meprobamate
- ☐ Norgesic
- ☐ Robaxin
- ☐ Soma

vi)
- ☐ Ativan
- ☐ diazepam
- ☐ Equanil
- ☐ Librium
- ☐ Miltown
- ☐ Serax
- ☐ Tranxene
- ☐ Valium
- ☐ Vivol

vii) ☐ Amytal
☐ Butisol
☐ Nembutal
☐ phenobarbital
☐ Seconal

viii) ☐ Benadryl
☐ chloral hydrate
☐ Dalmane
☐ Doriden
☐ Halcion
☐ L-Tryptophan
☐ Methaqualone
☐ Noludar
☐ Paraldehyde
☐ Placidyl
☐ Periactin
☐ Quaalude

ix) ☐ amitriptyline
☐ Anafranil
☐ Aventyl
☐ doxepin
☐ Elavil
☐ Etrafon
☐ lithium
☐ Ludiomil

☐ Marplan
☐ Nardil
☐ Norpramin
☐ Parnate
☐ Pertofrane
☐ Sinequan
☐ Triavil
☐ Tofranil
☐ Vivactil

x) ☐ Atarax
☐ Haldol
☐ Largactil
☐ Mellaril
☐ Moditen
☐ Navane
☐ Parasan
☐ Phenergan
☐ Sparine
☐ Stelazine
☐ Trilafon

xi) ☐ amphetamines
☐ hashish
☐ LSD
☐ marijuana
☐ mescaline

☐ phencylidine (PCP)

xii) ☐ Bensedrine
☐ Dexedrine
☐ Ionamin
☐ Ritalin
☐ Tenuate
☐ Tenuate Dospan

xiii) ☐ Dilantin
☐ Tegretol

xiv) ☐ penicillins
☐ Erythromycin
☐ Keflex
☐ Tetracycline

xv) ☐ multivitamins
☐ vitamin "A"
☐ vitamin "B"
☐ vitamin "C"
☐ vitamin "D"
☐ vitamin "E"
☐ vitamin "K"

xvi) ☐ birth control pill

xvii) ☐ other _____

b) Please list *ALL* drugs you are *NOW* taking for any reason, including drugs which MAY NOT be on the list, whether prescribed by a doctor or not (include: home remedies; over the counter medications; birth control pills).

Name of drug	Dosage	How many times per day/ per week	Reason for taking
⨍	⨍	⨍	

6. ACCOMPANYING SYMPTOMS LIST

Please read the following list carefully. If you have *any* of these symptoms *with your pain*, mark it with *W.P.* If you have them at *other times,* mark it with *O.T.*

_____ blurred vision
_____ constipation
_____ cough
_____ diarrhea
_____ difficulty breathing
_____ difficulty urinating
_____ dizziness
_____ excessive sweating
_____ numbness at non-pain sites
_____ fainting
_____ fatigue
_____ headache
_____ other _____

_____ itching
_____ memory loss
_____ nasal stuffiness
_____ nausea
_____ rash
_____ ringing in the ear(s)
_____ swelling of tissues
_____ skin color change
_____ skin temperature change
_____ tearing of eyes
_____ vomiting
_____ weakness

7. PAIN DESCRIPTION

a) Using the body figures shown below, please mark in *with a pencil* the areas where you feel the pain.

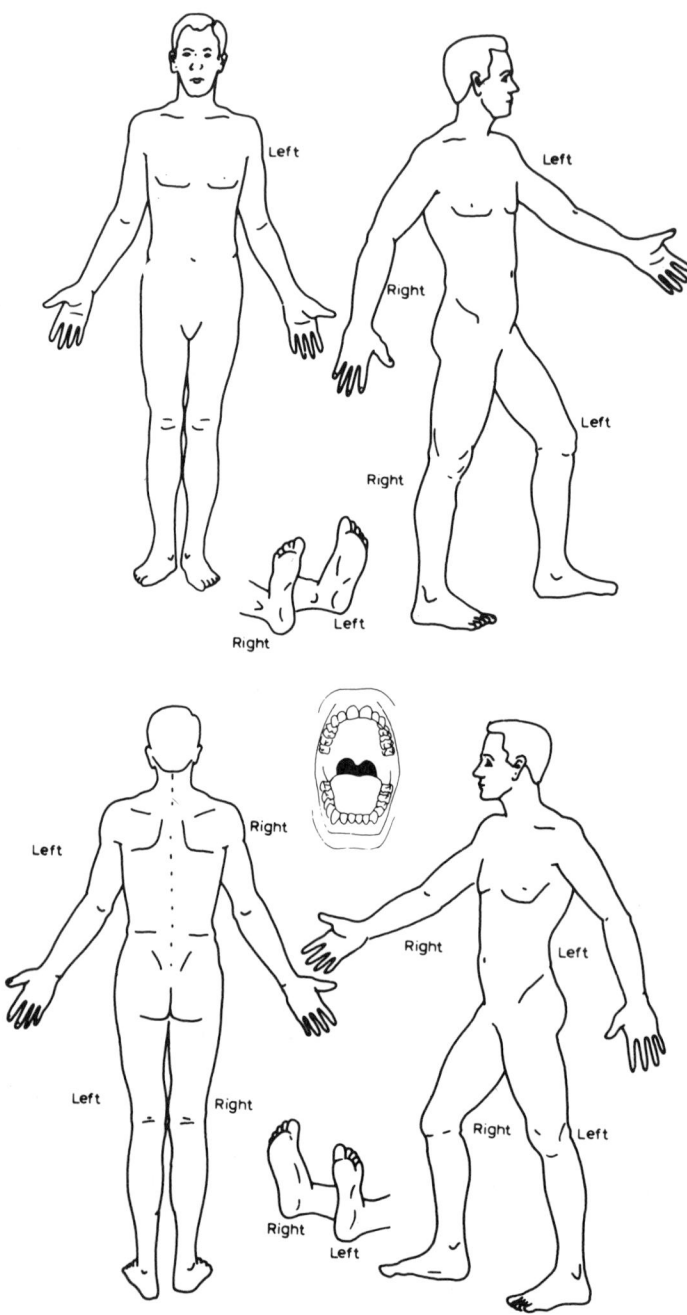

8. TIME PATTERN DURING THE DAY

   a) Do you have the pain immediately on waking? YES ☐ NO ☐   If NO, when does the pain begin? _____

   b) Does the pain change during the day? YES ☐ NO ☐
      If YES, what part of the day is the pain *worse?* _____
      What part of the day is the pain *better?* _____

   c) How many hours of the day are you *in pain?* _____

   d) How many hours of the day are you *pain free?* _____

9. PAIN MODIFIERS

   a) For each of the following: please mark with a + if it increases the pain; please mark with a − if it decreases the pain; please mark with a 0 if it has no effect on the pain.

☐ bright lights	☐ housework	☐ vigorous exercise
☐ casts	☐ loud noises	☐ walking
☐ cold	☐ lying	☐ weather
☐ collars	☐ massage	☐ work related
☐ corsets	☐ mild exercise	☐ others _____
☐ coughing, sneezing	☐ sitting	_____
☐ going to toilet	☐ standing	_____
☐ heat	☐ vibrator	_____

   b) Using the same signs (+, −, 0) as in the above question, please indicate how any of the following feelings and social situations affect your pain.

☐ anger	☐ frustration
☐ being with others	☐ happiness
☐ contentment	☐ sadness
☐ enjoying things	☐ talking with others
☐ fatigue	☐ when others are sympathetic

   c) If parts of your body (e.g., stomach or muscles) are tense or tight, does the pain get worse? YES ☐ NO ☐
      Which parts of your body get tense or tight? _____

   d) Have you found that pain changes when you are with certain people (e.g., relatives, boss, etc.)? YES ☐ NO ☐   If YES, please specify. _____

   e) Does rest decrease your pain? YES ☐ NO ☐   How many hours do you rest each day? _____ Where and how do you usually rest? _____

   f) Have you learned any *specific* ways to relax yourself when the pain is bad?
      YES ☐ NO ☐   If YES, what do you do? _____

   g) How do people around you know that you are in pain? _____

10. EFFECTS OF PAIN

   a) WORK
      i) At what age did you start working full time? _____
      ii) How many jobs have you had? _____
      iii) What is the longest length of time you have held a job? _____
      iv) What type of work do you do, or did you do last (include housewife)?

      _____

      For how long? _____ Number of hours per week _____

Duties (particularly physical activities, body postures, emotional stresses)

_____

v) Has the pain caused any change in your work? YES ☐ NO ☐
   If YES, do the changes include:
   change in number of hours worked? YES ☐ NO ☐
   from _____hours per week before to _____hours per week now
   change of type of work? YES ☐ NO ☐   from _____to _____
   satisfaction with work?   ☐ more   ☐ same   ☐ less
   efficiency at work?   ☐ more   ☐ same   ☐ less
   change in how you get/got along with co-workers, clients, etc? YES ☐ NO ☐
   If YES, please specify. _____
vi) Was/is your salary adequate for what you did/do? YES ☐ NO ☐
   In general, before the pain began, did your employer treat you fairly?
   YES ☐ NO ☐   Since the pain began? YES ☐ NO ☐
   If NO, please specify. _____
vii) *If you are not working presently:* If you did not have a pain problem, would
   you go back to work? YES ☐ NO ☐
viii) What job would you really like to have? _____

b) FINANCES
   i) Are you receiving any income for your disability? YES ☐ NO ☐
   If YES, from whom (i.e. Workman's Compensation, Pension, Insurance)

   _____

   When did this begin? _____
   When will it be stopped? _____
   Do you feel it is adequate? YES ☐ NO   ☐ Specify _____
   ii) Number of individuals on family income: _____   Who is the main
   contributor to this income? _____
   Do others contribute? YES ☐ NO ☐   Which others? _____
   Since when? _____
   iii) Do you have any debts? YES ☐ NO ☐
   Are you in financial need? YES ☐ NO ☐
   If YES, what steps have you taken to correct this? _____
   iv) Do you have health insurance? YES ☐ NO ☐ Details: _____

c) LEGAL PROCEEDINGS (LITIGATION)

   i) Are you involved in a lawsuit concerning the pain? (Specify: lawyer, against
   whom, what are you requesting) _____

   _____

   ii) Have you been involved in a legal suit in the past? YES ☐ NO ☐   Results: __

   _____

d) LEISURE
   i) Are there any hobbies, sports, recreational and social activities that you no
   longer do because of the pain? YES ☐ NO ☐
   If YES, what activities? _____
   ii) What hobbies, social activities etc. do you still do? _____
   iii) Do any of your present activities help take your mind off the pain?
   YES ☐ NO ☐   If YES, which ones? _____
   iv) Are there any new activities that you have begun since the pain began?
   YES ☐ NO ☐   If YES, what activities? _____

e) SLEEP
   i) When do you usually go to bed at night? _____
   ii) Approximately how long does it take to fall asleep? _____

iii) Do you have trouble falling asleep? YES ☐ NO ☐
iv) What body position do you use to sleep? _____
v) Do you awaken in the night? YES ☐ NO ☐   How many times? _____
What hours? _____Do you empty your bladder? YES ☐ NO ☐
Do you take medication? YES ☐ NO ☐
Do you awaken others? YES ☐ NO ☐
If YES, what do they do? _____
When do you finally awaken for the day? _____
vi) Do you feel refreshed or worse in the morning? _____
vii) Was your sleep pattern different before the pain? YES ☐ NO ☐
If YES, please specify _____

f) WEIGHT/DIET
i) How is your appetite?   ☐ too good   ☐ good   ☐ poor   ☐ very poor
ii) Has your weight changed since the pain began? YES ☐ NO ☐
If YES, from _____lbs. or _____kilos to _____lbs. or _____kilos
Have you dieted? YES ☐ NO ☐   Are you now? YES ☐ NO ☐
What is your weight now? _____   Your height? _____

g) HABITS

i) Do you smoke? YES ☐ NO ☐   If YES, what/how much? _____
ii) Please indicate the number of cups/bottles you drink of the following each day:
coffee _____   tea _____   cola _____
iii) Do you drink alcohol? YES ☐ NO ☐   If YES, what type of alcoholic beverage(s)?
_____
How much do you drink per day? _____
iv) Do you drink to: relieve the pain? YES ☐ NO ☐,   relax? YES ☐ NO ☐,
sleep? YES ☐ NO ☐,   socialize? YES ☐ NO ☐
v) Have you had any problems because of alcohol (i.e. physical, legal, psycho-logical, social)? YES ☐ NO ☐   If YES, please explain (i.e. loss or difficulty with friends, family, job, liver disease, blackouts, passing out, seizures, fits, hallucinations, etc.). _____
_____

11. PERSONAL HISTORY

a) PARENTS
i) Were you adopted? YES ☐ NO ☐   Your age at the time _____
ii) Has either of your parents died? YES ☐ NO ☐
If YES, please indicate: which parent, his/her age at the time, your age at the time and the cause of death _____
_____

iii) Please indicate with a check in the appropriate boxes if any of these words apply to your MOTHER or FATHER

MOTHER	FATHER	
☐	☐	sad
☐	☐	happy
☐	☐	loving
☐	☐	unloving
☐	☐	rejecting
☐	☐	accepting
☐	☐	rewarding
☐	☐	punishing
☐	☐	satisfying
☐	☐	frustrating

☐	☐	sickly
☐	☐	healthy
☐	☐	supportive
☐	☐	critical
☐	☐	selfish
☐	☐	giving
☐	☐	honest
☐	☐	dishonest
☐	☐	cooperative
☐	☐	competitive
☐	☐	encouraging independence
☐	☐	overprotective
☐	☐	intrusive
☐	☐	allows privacy
☐	☐	authoritarian
☐	☐	democratic
☐	☐	easygoing
☐	☐	strict

other words you feel apply to MOTHER or FATHER _____

b) SIBLINGS

Do/did you have any brothers or sisters? YES ☐ NO ☐
If YES, how many brothers and sisters do/did you have? _____
Where did you fit in the birth order (i.e., first, last, etc.)? _____
If any brothers or sisters have died please indicate: which ones, their age at the time, your age at the time and the cause of death _____

c) PERSONAL DETAILS

i) Check (√) any of the following which applied to you during your childhood.

☐ bed wetting	☐ fire setting	☐ stammering
☐ cruel to animals	☐ happy	☐ teeth grinding
☐ destructive	☐ hostile	☐ temper tantrums
☐ extremely shy	☐ like to play with others	☐ thumb sucking
☐ fears	☐ lying	☐ unhappy
☐ finicky with food	☐ night terrors	☐ others _____
☐ nail biting	☐ no friends	_____
☐ withdrawn	☐ overactive	_____

ii) Please check (√) any of the following describing your school experience.

☐ afraid to attend
☐ enjoyed school
☐ frequent absenteeism
☐ frequent discipline
☐ suspended
☐ picked on
☐ alone
☐ shy
☐ others _____

☐ joined group activities
☐ athletic
☐ leader
grades: ☐ superior
        ☐ very good
        ☐ fair
        ☐ poor
        ☐ very poor

iii) Which of the following describe your friendship patterns? Please check (√)

☐ anxiety with others
☐ avoid groups
☐ loner
☐ difficulty keeping friends
☐ no good friends
☐ sociable
☐ join groups
☐ other _____

☐ leader
☐ follower
☐ have good friends
☐ long friendships
☐ can share thoughts/feelings with others
☐ date(d) opposite sex
☐ enjoy(ed) dating opposite sex

iv) Do you daydream? YES ☐ NO ☐   Dream at night? YES ☐ NO ☐

d) MARRIAGE

i) Please check (√) and, if relevant indicate the length of time you have been:

☐ married _____
☐ remarried _____
☐ common law _____
☐ separated _____

☐ single _____
☐ living together _____
☐ divorced _____
☐ widowed _____

ii) What is your partner's occupation? _____

e) CHILDREN

i) Please give the following information regarding your children:

Sex	Age	Living at home or away	Achievement(s)/ problems

ii) Have you had any miscarriages? YES ☐ NO ☐   Dates: _____
Did you have any aftereffects (medical or psychological)? _____

f) OTHERS IN HOME

Are there any others who are regular members of the household? YES ☐ NO ☐
Details: _____

APPENDIX B: McGILL COMPREHENSIVE PAIN QUESTIONNAIRE INTERVIEWER GUIDE©

DATE OF INTERVIEW: _____

ADMINISTRATOR: _____

PATIENT'S NAME: _____

AGE: _____ DATE OF BIRTH:_____

ADDRESS: _____

PHONE NO.: Home: _____ Off: _____

POSTAL CODE: _____ SOCIAL INSURANCE NO.: _____

UNIT NO.: _____ MEDICARE NO.:_____

COMPENSATION INVOLVED:_____

COMPENSATION NO.:_____

FAMILY PHYSICIAN: _____

PHONE NO.: _____

REFERRING DOCTOR: _____

PHONE NO.: _____

REFERRING DIAGNOSIS: _____

COMMENTS: _____

PROBLEM LIST:

Problem(s)	Outcome measures	Date noted	Date resolved
ǂ	ǂ	ǂ	

PLAN:

Interventions	Responsible person	Date started	Date stopped
ǂ	ǂ	ǂ	

1. PAIN HISTORY

e) If answer to 1e, Patient Questionnaire page 1A, is NO, elaborate on any change in location, sensation, intensity, and time pattern frequency.

f) Have you had any X-rays done? YES ☐ NO ☐

Where	When	Body area(s)	Results
ǂ	ǂ	ǂ	

g) i) Have you had any length of time, since the pain began, when you have been pain free? YES ☐ NO ☐

If YES, date(s) of episode(s) _____

ii) Why do you feel that you had relief at this time (i.e. any physical, psychological or environmental changes)?

iii) Has this been a pattern? YES ☐ NO ☐

2. PAIN TREATMENTS

Have doctors ever suggested that your pain is imaginary? YES ☐ NO ☐   Have others suggested this? YES ☐ NO ☐   Comments:

10A

Have doctors ever acted as if you were faking the pain? YES ☐ NO ☐   Have others ever acted as if you were faking the pain? YES ☐ NO ☐   Comments:

3. PAST MEDICAL HISTORY

b) How do you usually react to illness? What kinds of thoughts? What kinds of emotions? Do you play it down? Do you talk to others about it? or have to depend on them?

c) Have any of your blood relatives or persons with whom you have been closely associated suffered from past or present health problems (pain conditions, chronic or major medical disorders, depression, alcoholism, suicide, hospitalizations for mental disorder(s), psychosis)?

Relative or friend	Disorder	Successful treatment (if any)
⨎	⨎	

d) Emotional Well-being

   i) Were there any episodes of sadness or anxiety lasting more than one or two weeks, prior to the start of your pain condition? YES ☐ NO ☐   If YES, obtain details of circumstances, symptoms, duration and treatment(s) if any.

   ii) Were there any episodes of feeling "high" lasting more than one or two weeks? YES ☐ NO ☐   If YES, obtain details.

   iii) Have there been any distressing, emotional experiences that you were concerned you could not cope with? YES ☐ NO ☐   If YES, obtain details.

5. MEDICATION

Regarding 5a and b, Patient Questionnaire pages 2A-3A, elaborate on any important drug adverse effects: _____

6. PAIN DESCRIPTION

Regarding 6a, Patient Questionnaire page 4A

a) Using the body map filled in by the patient (use additional body maps e.g., perineum, if necessary) add the following information:

   i) Mark the place where pain is with a (·). If a whole area hurts, shade in that area with light pencil strokes (/////).

   ii) If the pain radiates anywhere else use a dotted line and arrow to show how this usually occurs (- - - - →).

   iii) If the pain is internal (inside the body) put "I" beside the spot or area. If the pain is external (surface) put "E" beside the spot or area. If both put "EI."

   iv) If there are areas of increased or decreased sensation indicate this by putting " + S" or " − S" next to the area involved.

   v) Areas of peculiar sensations other than pain may be indicated by putting "PS" next to the area indicated.

   vi) Any areas where touching can begin, increase or decrease the pain (trigger zones) can be indicated by the letter "T."

b) Does the pain feel as if it is located in: check (√)   ☐ bone   ☐ joint
   ☐ muscle   ☐ nerve   ☐ skin   ☐ other _____

c) If pain is widespread are there any areas that are free of pain? _____

d) Choose *one* word group:
- ☐ continuous, steady, constant
- ☐ rhythmic, periodic, intermittent
- ☐ brief, momentary, transient

e) The following words represent pain of increasing intensity:
1. mild, 2. discomforting, 3. distressing, 4. horrible, 5. excruciating.
Choose the word which best describes:

Your pain right now _____

Your pain at its worse _____

Your pain at its least _____

The worst toothache you ever had _____

The worse headache you ever had _____

The worst stomachache you ever had _____

f) Tell me which words best describe your *present* pain. Leave out any word group that is not suitable. Use only a single word in each appropriate group—the one that applies *best*. Indicate answer with a check (√).

1
1. flickering ☐
2. quivering ☐
3. pulsing ☐
4. throbbing ☐
5. beating ☐
6. pounding ☐

2
1. jumping ☐
2. flashing ☐
3. shooting ☐

3
1. pricking ☐
2. boring ☐
3. drilling ☐
4. stabbing ☐
5. lancinating ☐

4
1. sharp ☐
2. cutting ☐
3. lacerating ☐

5
1. pinching ☐
2. pressing ☐
3. gnawing ☐
4. cramping ☐
5. crushing ☐

6
1. tugging ☐
2. pulling ☐
3. wrenching ☐

7
1. hot ☐
2. burning ☐
3. scalding ☐
4. searing ☐

8
1. tingling ☐
2. itchy ☐
3. smarting ☐
4. stinging ☐

9
1. dull ☐
2. sore ☐
3. hurting ☐
4. aching ☐
5. heavy ☐

10
1. tender ☐
2. taut ☐
3. rasping ☐
4. splitting ☐

11
1. tiring ☐
2. exhausting ☐

12
1. sickening ☐
2. suffocating ☐

13
1. fearful ☐
2. frightful ☐
3. terrifying ☐

14
1. punishing ☐
2. gruelling ☐
3. cruel ☐
4. vicious ☐
5. killing ☐

15
1. wretched ☐
2. blinding ☐

16
1. annoying ☐
2. troublesome ☐
3. miserable ☐
4. intense ☐
5. unbearable ☐

17
1. spreading ☐
2. radiating ☐
3. penetrating ☐
4. piercing ☐

18
1. tight ☐
2. numb ☐
3. drawing ☐
4. squeezing ☐
5. tearing ☐

19
1. cool ☐
2. cold ☐
3. freezing ☐

20
1. nagging ☐
2. nauseating ☐
3. agonizing ☐
4. dreadful ☐
5. torturing ☐

9. PAIN MODIFIERS

  a) From 9a on Patient Questionnaire page 5A, elaborate on any pain increasers or decreasers (noting situation(s), intensity, duration of pain change).

  g) From 9g on Patient Questionnaire page 6A, ask for details of pain behaviour (verbal, nonverbal).

10. EFFECTS OF PAIN

  b) i) What is your family income from all sources?
     iv) Clarify details of health insurance coverage.

  c) From 10c i) and ii) on Patient Questionnaire page 7A review and clarify nature of legal proceedings if necessary.

  f) From 10f ii) on Patient Questionnaire page 8A, if patient is overweight check diet history (i.e. type of diet, success, failure).

  g) From 10g v) on Patient Questionnaire page 8A review and clarify any alcohol-related problems.

  h) How often did you have sexual intercourse before your pain condition? Now? Does your pain interfere with sexual relations (e.g., change in sexual interest of patient or partner, or physical disability due to limited range of movement or anticipated pain, etc.)?

  i) MOOD: Consult Depression Inventory and elaborate responses, if necessary.

     i) Has your mood changed since the pain began? YES ☐ NO ☐ If YES, how?
     ii) What is your mood, on the whole, these days?
     iii) Do you feel unhappy most of the time?
     iv) Do you feel better in the A.M.? ☐ P.M.? ☐ same? ☐
     v) Do you have crying spells? YES ☐ NO ☐ How often?
     vi) Do you feel life is not worthwhile? YES ☐ NO ☐
     vii) Do you have any thoughts of harming yourself? YES ☐ NO ☐ If YES, elaborate on method, immediacy, etc.)
     viii) Do you feel irritable more often these days? YES ☐ NO ☐ If YES, for what situations?
     ix) Tell me how you express your anger (clarify whether the patient recognizes the emotion, how soon and how it is dealt with).

  j) ATTITUDE TOWARDS PAIN

     i) What do *YOU* feel is the cause of the pain?
     ii) How has your pain been explained to you?
     iii) How often in a day do you think about your pain? Could you describe those thoughts?
     iv) Are there any situations where you find that you are often thinking about pain?
     v) Are there people with whom you discuss your pain problems? YES ☐ NO ☐ With whom? How often? How do they respond?
     vi) Has this pain problem affected your feelings about yourself as a person? YES ☐ NO ☐ How?
     vii) Does religious faith help you to cope with the pain problem? YES ☐ NO ☐ If YES, in what way?
     viii) Are there thoughts, memories, or fantasies that you can think about which help you cope with your pain? YES ☐ NO ☐ Could you describe them?
     ix) What other methods do you use that help you cope with the pain problems?

k) FAMILY BURDEN

    i) What do members of your family no longer do because of your pain problem?

    ii) Would there be any changes if you no longer had the pain?
YES ☐ NO ☐   If YES, specify.

    iii) What do family members do when they realize you are in pain?

    iv) Do family members encourage you when you are trying to do something constructive about your life? YES ☐ NO ☐   Details:

11. PERSONAL HISTORY

  a) iv) Were either of your parents unavailable to you during your childhood (e.g., absence, illness—physical or emotional, etc.) YES ☐ NO ☐   If YES, specify age as a child, duration, reason.

  c) iv) While you were growing up was frustration frequently expressed verbally or physically in your family? YES ☐ NO ☐   Details:

    v) How did members of your family act when you were ill (e.g., sympathetic or not, angry, increased attention, ignored)?

    vi) What pleases you about yourself?

    vii) What displeases you about yourself?

d) MARRIAGE OR PERSON(S) LIVING WITH

    ii) Are there any areas of conflict with your partner regarding:

☐ finances	☐ legal	☐ physical illness
☐ children	☐ sex	☐ house
☐ parents-in-law	☐ personality	☐ religion
☐ work	other/elaboration of above	

    iii) Have you ever come to blows?

    iv) Have you ever separated?

    v) What pleases you about your partner?

12. PATIENT'S EXPECTATIONS

a) What are your life goals at this time? (Specify several, if possible.)

b) What do you expect from this consultation?

c) If complete relief of your pain is not possible at this time, would partial relief and/or learning how to cope with your pain be an acceptable goal? YES ☐ NO ☐ If YES, this will probably involve the Pain Center Staff teaching you new techniques for coping with pain during your usual activities as well as strategies for organizing your activities. Unlike many treatments, you will be expected to be an active participant. This means that you will be given assignments between sessions at the Center, and expected to keep records of activities related to pain. Would this be acceptable to you? Do you think you will try to get help elsewhere?

d) Any questions you would like to ask me? (Note questions)

13. PATIENT'S BEHAVIOR DURING THE INTERVIEW

a) Cooperative? Quality of rapport?

b) Ability to understand questions

c) Pain behavior during interview, e.g., grimaces, complaining, fidgeting, or favoring body area:

14. PATIENT'S MOOD DURING THE INTERVIEW

    ☐ sad   ☐ happy   ☐ angry   ☐ little emotion   ☐ anxious

15. EXAMINER'S IMPRESSIONS

SUBJECT INDEX

Subject Index

Activity
and pain behavior measurement, 156
underreporting of, 166–167,169
Activity Pattern Indicator, 149,150,151
compared with diary form, 150
Acupunctural analgesia, and sensory decision
theory, 21
Acute injury, pain behavior in, 155
Acute pain, 11
and affective distress, 122
and anxiety, 122
versus chronic pain, and pain chart,
223–225
and Finnish Pain Questionnaire, 90,91
laboratory pain as model for, 12
Adaptation level concept, 18,22,254,255
Affect
and acute pain, 122
and disabled patient, 192,193
pain language as measure of, 119–127
Affective quality of pain, 3–4,7
and depression, 100,101
dissociated from sensory qualities, 253
and emotional disturbance, 138
and Finnish Pain Questionnaire, 89,91
and McGill Pain Questionnaire, 42,43,44,
49; see also McGill Pain
Questionnaire
and Minnesota Multiphasic Personality
Inventory, 139–140
and pain intensity, 42,43
and tension versus migraine headaches, 99
Amnesia, for pain, 212
Analgesic(s), see also Narcotic analgesics;
specific name
in comparing clinical with laboratory pain,
9
and drug request point, 11,245
in laboratory studies, 9,11
mood-altering properties of, 20
requirements, postoperative, 90,112,114,
115,117
response to, and pain chart, 209–210
and sensory decision theory, 19–20,21
Anxiety
and acute pain, 122
and chronic pain, 123
and noxious stimuli, 10
and pain, 140–141

and pain threshold, 19
and sensory decision theory, 19
and tourniquet pain test, 30
Assessment, pain
goals of, 233
and McGill Comprehensive Pain
Questionnaire, 235
Attitudes
and pain threshold, 18–19
of scientists, 260,261
Attitudes Toward Disabled Persons (ATDP)
test, 191–192
Aversion threshold, versus pain threshold, 11
Avoidance behaviors, in chronic headache
pain, 157,159
laboratory techniques in assessment of,
160–161,162

Back pain, low
and detection using verbal pain
measurement, 79–84
and Finnish Pain Questionnaire, 89–90
Back Pain Classification Scale (BPCS),
80–84
administration of, 80–81
relationship of, to Minnesota Multiphasic
Personality Inventory scores, 81
reliability of, 83
scoring of, 80,81
validity of, 81–82
Beck Depression Inventory, and
postoperative pain, 112,113
Behavior modification, in chronic pain,
200–201
Behavioral change, in treatment of chronic
benign pain, 165
Behavioral time-sampling, 128
Benzodiazepines
and pain threshold, 20
and sensory decision theory, 20
side effects of, and self-report, 169
Biases, random, in verbal pain measurement,
71,74
Biofeedback, in tension headache, 98,101
Bodily harm, fear of, 140
Body image; see also Self-image
assessment of, in chronic pain, 227–231

Body Parts Problem Assessment (BPPA)
  scale, 227–231
  calibration of scale on, 230
  correlation of, with index of somatization,
    229
  correlation of, with McGill Pain
    Questionnaire, 229
  meaning of score on, 229
  as outcome measure, 229
  scoring of, 228
  as tool for focusing awareness, 230–231

Cancer patients, pain language, 123–124
Card sort method of pain assessment, 195
Central nervous system depressant
    medication, and self-report, 169
Checklist inventory, in assessment of chronic
    headache behavior, 157,159,162
Children, measurement of pain in, 176,
    183–189; *see also* Infants
  in concrete operational stage, 185–187
  lack of study of, 183
  in preoperational stage, 184–185
  problems in, 183,185,187
Chlorimipramine, and tourniquet pain test,
    28
Chronic benign pain
  and behavioral change, 165
  factors distorting self-report, 165–171
Chronic pain
  versus acute pain, and pain chart, 223–225
  and alcohol use, 169
  and anxiety, 122
  critical issues in, 145
  body image in, assessment of, 227–231
  and central nervous system depressant
    medication, 169
  definition of, 11
  and delineation of patient subgroups using
    Minnesota Multiphasic Personality
    Inventory and McGill Pain
    Questionnaire, 129–130,131–134
  and depression, 101,120,122,123,
    140–141,167
  and Finnish Pain Questionnaire, 89–90
  graded exposure to, 159
  meditation practices for self-regulation of,
    229,230–231
  and McGill Pain Questionnaire, 120–127,
    129,131–134
  and pain behavior, 155; *see also* Pain
    behavior assessment, in chronic pain
  pain language as a measure of, 119–127
  phobia's similarity to, 159
  and relationship between verbal pain,
    139–140
  and sensory decision theory, 22–23

  and Situational Pain Questionnaire, 22–23
Chronic pain patients, testing of, under
    laboratory conditions, 248,254–255
Chronic pain states
  behavioral modification in, 200–201
  classes of disability compensation patient,
    198,201,202
  and disabled persons, 200,201–202
  and impairment, 200
  treatment of, 201–202
Chronic pain syndrome, 11
Clinical pain, 1
  with assessment of laboratory pain, in ideal
    verbal pain measurement, 72,75
  compared with laboratory pain, 8–10,27,
    105–110
  and McGill Pain Questionnaire, 108–109
  and pain behavior measurement, 145–154
  relationship of, to laboratory pain, 8–11
  separation of, into acute and chronic, 11
Clinical research
  emphasis on motivational-emotional
    aspects, 246
  integrating with laboratory research,
    246–248
  and laboratory research, relationship
    between, 241,243–249
  measurements in, 244–245; *see also*
    specific name; type
Clinical trials
  and simple descriptive scales, 36
  and visual analogue scales, 34–35
Cluster analysis
  and chronic headache, and McGill Pain
    Questionnaire, 99,100–101
  and Minnesota Multiphasic Personality
    Inventory, 129–130
Coding systems, in nonverbal expression of
    pain, 178
Cognitive strategies, 255–256
Cold pressor test, 10,252–253
Color coding, of pain chart, 217,218
Color scales, in pain assessment in children,
    185
Compensation, *see also* Disability
    compensation patients
  of human subjects, 278
Complaints, pain, 156,157,159,206
Comprehensive pain questionnaire, 233–236,
    1A–14A
Concrete operational stage, pain
    measurement in, 185–187
Conversion, and low back pain, 81,83
Correlational methods, 8,9
Crying, as index of pain in children, 184
Culture
  and pain expression, 174
  and pain threshold, 19

Declaration of Helsinki, The, 262–263
Depression, 140–141,225
    and acute pain, 122,123
    and affective qualities of pain, 100,101
    and avoidance behaviors, 159
    and chronic pain, 101,120,122,123,
        140–141,167
    and distortion of self-reporting, 167
    postoperative, 115,116,117
    and sensory decision theory, 22
Descriptor Differential Scale, 74,75
Descriptors, pain; *see also* Language, pain;
        Verbal pain measurement
    classification of, 41–45
    and culture, 59
    ideal-type model of, 50–51
    structure of, 49–54
Diagnosis
    differential, role of laboratory pain in, 12
    and pain language diffusion, 124–125
Diary
    activity, 166–167
    Activity Pattern Indicator compared with,
        150
    headache, 97,159
    in pain behavior measurement, 147,
        149,150
Diazepam
    and pain threshold, 20
    and sensory decision theory, 20
    side effects of, and self-report, 169
Disabled persons
    and affective states, 192,193
    attitudes toward, 191–192
    and motivation for recovery, 193–194
    pain assessment in, 194–196
    and patient-spouse illness orientation, 192
    and self-image, 195–196
Disability(ies)
    attitudes toward, 191–192
    and chronic pain states, 200
    versus impairment, 199
Disability compensation patients
    and distortions in self-report, 168–169
    and Emory Pain Estimate model, 198–199
    and pathology behavior correlates, 198
    and patient-based behavior assessment,
        198
    and physician-based pathological
        assessment, 198
    and treatment, 201–202
    and vocational disability evaluation,
        199–200
Disability rating, in vocational disability
        evaluation, 200
Discriminability, 15,16–17
    and acupunctural analgesia, 21
    and analgesics, 19–20,21

and anxiety, 19
and anxiolytics, 20
and chronic pain patient, 22–23
in depression, 22
and Situational Pain Questionnaire, 23
and transcutaneous electrical nerve
    stimulation, 21
variables reputed to influence, 20–21
Distress score, in Finnish Pain
    Questionnaire, 90,92
Diurnal variation, and sensory decision
    theory, 21–22
Dolormetrics, 256
Drawings, in pain measurement
    of children, 186–187,195
    of disabled persons, 195
Drive mobilizer, pain as, 244
    in disabled persons, 192–193,194
Drug request point
    in bridging gap between laboratory and
        clinical pain, 245
    definition of, 11

Education, nursing, Finnish Pain
    Questionnaire in, 92
Emory Pain Estimate model, in disability
    compensation patients, 198–199,201
    reliability of, 198
Emotional disturbance
    and Back Pain Classification Scale, 79–84
    and pain description, 137–141
    and Minnesota Multiphasic Personality
        Inventory, 138–139
Endocrine effects, and sensory decision
    theory, 21–22
Endogenous opioids, and sensory decision
    theory, 22
Endurance, pain
    and pain sensitivity range, 11
    as pain-specific factor, 9
Ethics, 1,7,241–242,247,259–265
    and avoiding exploitation of human
        subjects, 261–263
    basic principle of, 263–264
    and children, 187
    and chronic pain models, 11–12
    and coercion of subjects, 260–261
    and compensation of subjects, 264
    and informed consent, 262,264
    and motivations in pain research, 259–261
    and scientists' attitudes, 260,261
    and subject's sense of obligation, 260–262
Evaluative descriptors
    in Finnish Pain Questionnaire, 89,91

Evaluative descriptors *(contd.)*
  in McGill Pain Questionnaire, 42,43,44,
    49; *see also* McGill Pain
    Questionnaire and Minnesota
    Multiphasic Personality Inventory,
    140
  and pain intensities, 42,43
Exercise, and discriminability, 22
Expressions of pain, nonverbal, *see*
    Nonverbal expressions of pain

Facial Action Coding System, 178
Facial expressions of pain, 173,174–175
  and display rules, 177
  and Factial Action Coding System, 178
  in infants, 175–176
Factor analysis
  definition of, 63
  of McGill Pain Questionnaire, 63–70,
    106–107,139,140
Fear
  of bodily harm, 140
  of pain, in children, 184
Finnish Pain Questionnaire, 59,85–93
  in acute pain, 90–91
  in chronic pain, 89–90
  classification of words in, 85,86–88
  in low backpain, 89–90
  and nurses' estimation of postoperative
    pain, 91–92
  in postoperative pain, 90–91
  with visual analogue scale, 85,90,93

Headaches, chronic; *see also* Migraine
    headaches; Tension headaches
  and affective scales, 99
  assessment of pain behavior in, *see* Pain
    behavior assessment, in chronic
    headache
  diagnostic division of, 97,98,101
  and McGill Pain Questionnaire, 98–101
  and sensory qualities, 97–100
  and treatment, 98,101
Health care utilization, and assessment of
    pain behavior, 149,151
Health professonals, and distortions in self-
    reporting, 167
Hester vocational evaluation system, 200
Human subjects; *see also* Ethics
  avoiding exploitation of, 261–263
  compensation of, 264
  and informed consent, 262,264
Human subjects research committees,
    263,264
Hypervigilance models, 255
Hypnoanalgesia, and pain threshold, 18

Hyposensitive patients, 207,208,211
Hysterical personality disorder, 225

Impairment(s)
  and chronic pain states, 200
  definition of, 199
  versus disability, 199
  rating of, in vocational disability
    evaluation, 199–200
Indirect psychophysical approach, 8–12
Infants
  and behavioral differences in pain
    response, 176
  facial expressions of pain in, 175–176
  indices of pain in, 184
  pain measurement in, 183–184
  pain perception in, question of, 183–184
Insensitivity, pain, 211
Intensity, pain, 1–2
  emphasis on, versus sensory qualities,
    97,98
  and McGill Pain Questionnaire, 42,43,
    45–46
  and measures of change, 45–46
  and temporal pain chart, 205,206–207
Ischemic methods, 10,252–253

Kinesthetic scales, in pain behavior
    measurement, 146

Labor pain, and McGill Pain Questionnaire,
    46
Laboratory methods of pain measurement,
    1,7–13,188; *see also specific method*
  historical aspects of, 7
  and stimulus, 7,8
  and threshold sensation, 7,8
Laboratory pain, 1
  and assessment of analgesic efficacy, 72
  with assessment of clinical pain, in ideal
    verbal pain measurement, 72,75
  compared with clinical pain, 8–10,27,
    105–110
  and differential diagnosis, 12
  and McGill Pain Questionnaire, 106–107,
    108–109
  as model for acute pain, 11,12
  relationship to clinical pain, 8–11
  value of, 72
Laboratory research
  on clinical pain patient, 248,254–255
  and clinical research, relationship between,
    241,243–249,251–265
  integrating with clinical research, 246–248
  sensory-discriminative aspects of, 246

and time frame, 247
Language, pain; *see also* Descriptors, pain
  and affect, 119–127
  in cancer patients, 121
  in cancer versus benign patients, 123–124
  in children, 184–185,186,194
  and ideal pain assessment, 71–77
  in medical versus psychiatric patients,
    121–122, 137–138
  in psychiatric patient, 120–122
Learned helplessness, 159
Low back pain, *see* Back pain, low
Low Back Pain Questionnaire, 234

McGill Comprehensive Pain Questionnaire,
    235–236
  Interviewer Guide of, 235,10A–13A
  Patient Questionnaire of, 235,1A–9A
  as teaching aid, 236
McGill Pain Assessment Questionnaire, 234
McGill Pain Questionnaire (MPQ), 4,
    41–47,145–146,234,245,254
  administration of, convenience of,
    107–108
  appraisal of, 55–61
  in assessment of sensory qualities of
    chronic headache, 98–101
  Body Parts Problem Assessment
    correlated with, 229
  and children, 186
  and chronic pain, 120–127,129
  and clinical pain, 108–109
  cluster analysis of, 99
  in comparison of laboratory and clinical
    pain, 108–109
  concurrent validity of, 57–58
  construct validity of, 57
  and culture, 59
  and delineation of patient subgroups,
    131–134
  and dental treatment pain, 108
  discriminant validity of, 58
  face validity of, 56
  factor analytic studies of, 63–70,
    106–107,139,140
  and Finnish Pain Questionnaire, 85,86–88
  and ideal pain measurement, 73,75
  internal structure of, 58–59
  and laboratory pain, 106–107
  in low back pain, 108
  in measure of affect, in chronic pain,
    120–127
  and measures of change, 45–46
  and memory loss or distortions, 100
  modification of, 59
  modification of, in laboratory pain, 106
  pain descriptors in, 41–45,49–54

and pain experience, direct measures of,
    45
paper-and-pencil administration of,
    107–108,109
and personality differences, 100
and postoperative pain, 111,112–117
relationship between Minnesota
    Multiphasic Personality Inventory
    and, 57,68–69,129–136
reliability of, 55–56,117,119,126
sensitivity of, 117,119,126
simplified version of, 139–140,141
usefulness of, 46,259
validity of, 56,57–58,117,126
versus visual analogue scale, 111–117
Magnitude estimations, 12,268
Marijuana, analgesic effects of, 20
Medical patients, *see* Language pain; in
    medical versus psychiatric patients
Medication rate, as index of pain behavior,
    156,157
Medications; *see also specific name; type*
  effect of, in self-reporting, 169
Meditation practices, for self-regulation of
    chronic pain, 229,230–231
Memory distortions, 212
  and checklist assessment of pain behavior,
    159
  and McGill Pain Questionnaire, 100
Migraine headaches; *see also* Headaches,
    chronic; Pain behavior assessment, in
    chronic headache
  versus tension headaches, 97–102
Mimicry techniques, 10
Minnesota Multiphasic Personality Inventory
    (MMPI)
  and chronic pain, 129
  and Conversion V (Hs-Hy), 81
  in delineation of patient subgroups,
    129–130,131–134
  depression scale of, 131,132,139
  disadvantages of, in medical settings,
    79,138
  and effective-evaluative versus sensory
    descriptors, 139–140
  and factor analysis, 68–69
  hypochondriasis scale of, 131,132,
    139,140
  hypomania scale of, 140
  hysteria scale of, 132,139,140
  low back scale of, 81
  multivariate analysis of, 129–130
  and pain descriptors and emotional
    disturbance, 138–139
  paranoia scale of, 140
  psychoasthenia scale of, 131,139
  psychopathic deviant scale of, 131,
    133,139

Minnesota Multiphasic Personality Inventory
   (contd.)
   relationship of, to Back Pain Classification
      Scale scores, 81
   relationship between McGill Pain
      Questionnaire and, 57,68–69,
      129–136
   schizophrenia scale of, 131, 133, 139
Mood, effect of analgesics on, 20
Motivation(s)
   in pain research, 259–261
   for recovery, of disabled persons, 193–194
Motivational-affective dimension of pain,
   3–4,245,246,247,248
Motor responses, as index of pain in infants,
   184
Multidisciplinary treatment programs, 233
Multiple Affect Adjective Checklist, 193
Myofascial pain dysfunction syndrome, 255

Narcotic analgesics
   pain tolerance as parameter in evaluation
      of, 11
   and self-report, 169
Neurophysiological model, 246
Neurotic triad scales, and chronic pain,
   131,133–134
Neuroticism, and tourniquet pain test, 30
Nonverbal expressions of pain, 173–179
   in children, 184
Nonverbal measures of pain, in children,
   185,186–187,194,195
Nonverbal measures of pain behavior,
   173–179
   brief history of, 174–175
   and discrete signs of pain, 175–176
   and global judgments, 175
   and individual differences in sensitivity to
      pain expressions, 176–177
   problems with, 178
   and voluntary control of nonverbal
      expressive behavior, 177–178
Noxious stimuli
   and manipulation of psychosocial
      variables, 10
   responses to, in sensory decision theory,
      17–22
Nurses
   education of, and Finnish Pain
      Questionnaire, 92
   and estimation of postoperative pain,
      91–92

Observation(s)
   of activity, and self-reporting, 166–167
   of pain, during experience of, 212

Orthopedic patients, and spatial pain chart,
   215–225

Pain; see also Acute pain; Chronic pain;
      Clinical pain; Laboratory pain
   anticipation of, and behavior, 156,
      161–162
   childrens' concepts of, 185–187,194
   as drive mobilizer, 192–193,194,258
   model for quantification and classification
      of, and disability patients, 198
   as multidimensional phenomenon,
      245–246
   as sensation, 2,3
   theories of, see specific theory
   unique qualities of each, 2,41
Pain behavior
   in acute injury, 155
   and avoidance, 157,159
   in children, 184
   and depression, 159
   in disability compensation patients,
      198,200
   in Emory Pain Estimate model, 198
   nonverbal measurement of, 173–179
   self-report of, see Self-report of pain
      behavior
Pain behavior assessment, in chronic
      headache, 155–163
   and activity levels, 156
   and avoidance behavior, 157,159,
      160–161,162
   checklist inventory in, 157,159,162
   and comparison of types of behavior and
      subjective experience, 158,159
   and complaint behavior, 156,157,159
   and diary, 159
   laboratory techniques in, 160–161,162
   and medication rate, 156,157
   and self-help or ameliorative behaviors,
      157
Pain behavior assessment, in chronic pain,
      145–154
   and activity Pattern Indicator, 149,
      150,151
   approaches to, 146
   and body position measures, 148
   and diary, 147,149,150
   and direct observation, 147,148
   and health care utilization, 149,151
   and recredentialling, 149–150
   and say-do distinctions, 146–147,148,
      149–152
   self-report in, factors distorting, 165–171;
      see also specific factor
Pain chart, and spatial properties of pain,
   215–225

and acute versus chronic pain, 223–225
and apportionment of symptoms, 218–219
composition of, 217
and deep and superficial pain, 223
definition of, 215–216
filling out, 223
grading systems of, 223
multipurpose format of, 218
and psychopathology, 225
purpose of, 217–223
structure of, 217
Pain chart, and temporal aspects of pain,
    205–213,215,217
and analgesic response, 209–210
calibration of, 206–207
clinical problems presented, 212–213
in clinical research, 210–211
in experimental research, 211–212
horizontal x-axis of, 208–210
hourly clinical, 208,209
long-term, 209–210
pain free, with noxious stimulation, 211
and serum lipid changes, 210–211
and variation in pressure-pain sensitivity,
    207–208
vertical y-axis of, 206
Pain induction methods, 252–253; *see also*
    specific method
classification of, 11
comparative perspective required in, 253
convergent validity of, 257
discriminant validity of, 252
and total pattern of pain response, 12
Pain measurement; *see also specific method*
absolute measures that increase the
    validity of pain comparisons between
    groups and within groups over time,
    72–73,75,76
comparative perspective required in, 253
concepts of, 1–5,253–254
laboratory methods of, *see* Laboratory
    methods of pain measurement
relative, problems with, 72–73
Pain Profile, 234
Pain recall, 100,120,159,212
Pain sensitivity range, 11
Pain-specific factors, 9
Perception, pain, in infants, 183–184
Performance accuracy, and verbal pain
    measurement, 71–72,75
Personality
and pain threshold, 19
and sensory decision theory, 19,23
and verbal measurement, 100
Phobia, chronic pain's similarity to, 159
Placebo, and sensory decision theory, 17–18
Poker Chip Tool, 185
Postoperative pain
and Finnish Pain Questionnaire, 90–91

and McGill Pain Questionnaire, 111,
    112–117
nurses' estimation of, 91–92
and pain measurement, mood, and narcotic
    requirements, 112–117
and visual analogue scale, 111,112
Preoperational children, measurement of pain
    in, 184–185
Pressure algometer, 207–208
Progressive relaxation, in tension headaches,
    98,101
Psychiatric patients, pain language of, versus
    medical patients, 121–122,137–138
Psychological component of pain, 15; *see*
    also Motivational-affective dimension
elements affecting, 15–16
emphasis in clinical studies, 7,8,246
Psychosocial Pain Inventory, 234
Psychosocial variables in laboratory-induced
    pain, 10–11

Qualities of pain, 7, *see specific quality*
Questionnaires, *see specific name*

Random biases, in verbal pain measure,
    71,74
Rating scales, pain intensity, in measurement
    of pain behavior, 146
Recredentialling, 149–150
Rehabilitation, pain as variable in, 192–194
Rehabilitation medicine, pain assessment in,
    191–196; *see also* Disabled persons
Report criterion, 15,17
and age, 18
and analgesics, 19–20
and anxiety, 19
and anxiolytics, 20
and chronic pain, 23
and culture, 19
in depression, 22
and sex, 18–19
and Situational Pain Questionnaire, 23
and suggestion, 18
and transcutaneous electrical nerve
    stimulation, 21

Say-do distinction, in pain behavior,
    146–147,149–152
Scientific inference process, 248
Scientists', attitudes of, 260,261
Self-image; *see also* Body image of disabled,
    195–196
Self-report of pain
advantages of, 173
limitations of, 173–174

Self-report of pain behavior
  and activity level, 166–167,169
  and chronicity, 167
  and depression, 167
  factors distorting, 165–171
  and financial compensation, 168–169
  and health professionals, 167
  and medication, 169
  and spouse, 167–168
  stimulus effects on, 167–168
Sensory decision theory, 2,15–25,254
  and acupunctural analgesia, 21
  and analgesics, 19–20
  and anxiolytics, 20
  and attitude and anxiety, 18–19
  and diurnal variation, 21–22
  and endocrine and neurotransmitter effects,
      21–22
  introduction to, 16–17
  in myofascial pain dysfunction, 255
  and Situational Pain Questionnaire, 22–23
  and suggestion, 17–18
  and transcutaneous electrical nerve
      stimulation, 21
Sensory-discriminative dimensions of pain,
      245,246,247,248
  separation from hedonic qualities, in verbal
      pain measurement, 72,74,75,76
Sensory modalities, assessment of, 73–74
Sensory quality of pain
  in chronic headache pain, 97–102
  dissociated from affective qualities, 254
  emphasis in laboratory studies, 7,8
  and Finnish Pain Questionnaire, 89,91
  and McGill Pain Questionnaire, 42,43,
      44,49; *see also* McGill Pain
      Questionnaire
  and Minnesota Multiphasic Personality
      Inventory, 139–140
  and pain intensities, 42,43
  and psychiatric patient, 121
  and tension versus migraine headache,
      98–100,101
Serum lipid changes, and pain chart,
      210–211
Signal detection theory, *see* Sensory decision
      theory
Situational Pain Questionnaire, 22–23
Somatization index, Body Parts Problem
      Assessment scale correlated with, 227
Spatial propeties of pain, and pain chart, *see*
      Pain chart, and spatial properties of pain
Specificity theory of pain, 2,3
Spouse
  and distortion in self-report of pain
      intensity, 167–168
  and illness orientation, 192

State-Trait Anxiety Inventory State form, in
      postoperative pain, 112
Stimulus effects, on self-reporting of pain
      behavior, 167–168
Stress Neuromyelopathic Syndrome,
      221–223
Structural model of pain descriptors, 49–54
Suggestion
  and pain threshold, 17–18
  and sensory decision theory, 17–18

Tactile analogue scales, in pain behavior
      measurement, 146
Team research, 247
Temporal aspects of pain, and pain chart, *see*
      Pain chart, and temporal aspects of pain
Tension headaches, *see also* Headaches,
      chronic; Pain behavior assessment, in
      chronic headache
  biofeedback for, 98,101
  versus migraine headaches, and sensory
      qualities, 97–102
  progressive relaxation for, 98,101
Threshold, pain
  and acupunctural analgesia, 21
  and age, 18
  versus aversion threshold, 11
  and cold pressor test, 252–253
  and culture, 19
  definition of, 2,8,11
  and diazepam, 20
  and hypnoanalgesia, 18
  and ovulatory cycle, 21
  and pressure, 252–253
  and sex, 18–19
  and shock, 252–253
  and suggestion, 17–18
Tolerance, pain
  and cold pressor test, 252–253
  definition of, 2,8,11
  as parameter in evaluation of narcotic
      analgesics, 11
  as parameter in evaluation of pain relief,
      11
  and pressure, 252–253
  and shock, 252–253
Tooth pulp stimulation method, 10
Tourniquet pain test, 10,27–31,245
  development of, 27–28
  sensitivity of, 28–29
  standardization of, 29,30
Transcutaneous electrical nerve stimulation
      (TENS)
  and sensory decision theory, 21
  and tourniquet pain test, 28

Up-time, self-report of, 166–167
Up-time clock, 166

Valper vocational evaluation system, 200
Verbal pain measurement, 41–93,111,146;
   see also specific method
  and detecting psychological disturbances
    with low back pain, 79–84
  in Finnish, *see* Finnish Pain Questionnaire
  ideal, properties of, 71–73,74,75,76
  and ideal pain measurement, 71–77
Visual analogue scale, 33–37
  and acute pain, 90,91
  and changes, immediate, 90,93
  with children, 194–195
  and chronic pain, 90
  compared with other methods, 36,254

concept and behavior of, 33,34,36
  definition of, 33
  design of, 34
  with Finnish Pain Questionnaire, 85,90,93
  versus McGill Pain Questionnaire,
    111–117
  in pain behavior measurement, 146
  and postoperative pain, 111,112
  reliability of, 117
  sensitivity of, 33,35
  sources of error in, 35–36
  uses of, 34–35,146
  validity of, 117
Vocational disability evaluation, 199–200

Wakefield Depression Scale, 123